# EMERGING

# INFECTIONS

2

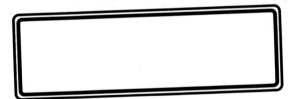

# EMERGING INFECTIONS

# 2

*Edited by*

## W. Michael Scheld
Division of Infectious Diseases
University of Virginia Health Sciences Center
Charlottesville, Virginia

## William A. Craig
William S. Middleton Memorial Veterans Hospital
Madison, Wisconsin

## James M. Hughes
National Center for Infectious Diseases
Centers for Disease Control and Prevention
Atlanta, Georgia

ASM PRESS    *Washington, D.C.*

**Cover photo:** Leptospirosis associated with pulmonary hemorrhage. A single leptospire in alveolar space is seen by immunostaining in a lung sample from a patient who died of a pulmonary hemorrhage. Naphthol-fast red with hematoxylin counterstain was used. Original magnification, ×250. (Courtesy of Sherif R. Zaki, Division of Viral and Rickettsial Diseases, National Center for Infectious Diseases, Centers for Disease Control and Prevention.)

To our spouses:

Suss Scheld,
Judy Craig,
and
Pam Hughes

# CONTENTS

# CONTRIBUTORS

**Sean F. Altekruse** • Foodborne and Diarrheal Diseases Branch, Division of Bacterial and Mycotic Diseases, National Center for Infectious Diseases, Centers for Disease Control and Prevention, Atlanta, Georgia 30333

**Timothy J. Barrett** • Division of Bacterial and Mycotic Diseases, National Center for Infectious Diseases, Centers for Disease Control and Prevention, 1600 Clifton Road NE, Atlanta, Georgia 30333

**Charles B. Beard** • Division of Parasitic Diseases, National Center for Infectious Diseases, Centers for Disease Control and Prevention, Atlanta, Georgia 30333

**Mary Chamberland** • Division of Viral and Rickettsial Diseases, National Center for Infectious Diseases, Centers for Disease Control and Prevention, Atlanta, Georgia 30333

**David T. Dennis** • Bacterial Zoonoses Branch, Division of Vector-Borne Infectious Diseases, National Center for Infectious Diseases, Centers for Disease Control and Prevention, P.O. Box 2087, Fort Collins, Colorado 80522

**Michael Dunne** • Department of Clinical Research, Pfizer Central Research, Eastern Point Road, Groton, Connecticut 06340

**Clare A. Dykewicz** • Division of AIDS, STD, and TB Laboratory Research, National Center for Infectious Diseases, Centers for Disease Control and Prevention, Atlanta, Georgia 30333

**Scott B. Halstead** • Medical Science and Technology Division, Office of Naval Research, 800 N. Quincy Street, Arlington, Virginia 22217-5660

**Debra L. Hanson** • Division of HIV/AIDS Prevention, National Center for HIV, STD, and TB Prevention, Centers for Disease Control and Prevention, Atlanta, Georgia 30333

**Erik L. Hewlett** • Departments of Medicine and Pharmacology, University of Virginia School of Medicine, Box 419, Health Sciences Center, Charlottesville, Virginia 22908

**James M. Hughes** • National Center for Infectious Diseases, Centers for Disease Control and Prevention, Atlanta, Georgia 30333

**Harold W. Jaffe** • Division of AIDS, STD, and TB Laboratory Research, National Center for Infectious Diseases, Centers for Disease Control and Prevention, Mail Stop A25, 1600 Clifton Road NE, Atlanta, Georgia 30333

**Jeffrey L. Jones** • Division of HIV/AIDS Prevention, National Center for HIV, STD, and TB Prevention, Centers for Disease Control and Prevention, Atlanta, Georgia 30333

**Dennis D. Juranek** • Division of Parasitic Diseases, National Center for Infectious Diseases, Centers for Disease Control and Prevention, Atlanta, Georgia 30333

**Jonathan E. Kaplan**    •    Division of HIV/AIDS Prevention, National Center for HIV, STD, and TB Prevention, Centers for Disease Control and Prevention, Atlanta, Georgia 30333

**Rima F. Khabbaz**    •    Division of Viral and Rickettsial Diseases, National Center for Infectious Diseases, Centers for Disease Control and Prevention, Atlanta, Georgia 30333

**Donald J. Krogstad**    •    Department of Tropical Medicine, Tulane School of Public Health and Tropical Medicine, New Orleans, Louisiana 70112

**James W. LeDuc**    •    National Center for Infectious Diseases, Centers for Disease Control and Prevention, Atlanta, Georgia 30333

**J. Dick MacLean**    •    McGill University Centre for Tropical Disease, Montreal General Hospital, 1650 Cedar Avenue, Room D7-153, Montreal, Quebec, Canada H3G 1A4

**Bradley A. Perkins**    •    Division of Bacterial and Mycotic Diseases, National Center for Infectious Diseases, Centers for Disease Control and Prevention, 1600 Clifton Road NE, Atlanta, Georgia 30333

**C. J. Peters**    •    Division of Viral and Rickettsial Diseases, National Center for Infectious Diseases, Centers for Disease Control and Prevention, Mail Stop A26, 1600 Clifton Road NE, Atlanta, Georgia 30333

**David A. Relman**    •    Veterans Affairs Palo Alto Health Care System, 154T, 3801 Miranda Avenue, Palo Alto, California 94304

**Peter M. Schantz**    •    Division of Parasitic Diseases, National Center for Infectious Diseases, Centers for Disease Control and Prevention, Mail Stop F22, 4770 Buford Highway, Atlanta, Georgia 30341

**Lawrence B. Schonberger**    •    Division of Viral and Rickettsial Diseases, National Center for Infectious Diseases, Centers for Disease Control and Prevention, Mail Stop A39, 1600 Clifton Road NE, Atlanta, Georgia 30333

**Thomas J. Spira**    •    Division of AIDS, STD, and TB Laboratory Research, National Center for Infectious Diseases, Center for Disease Control and Prevention, Mail Stop A25, 1600 Clifton Road NE, Atlanta, Georgia 30333

**David L. Swerdlow**    •    Foodborne and Diarrheal Diseases Branch, Division of Bacterial and Mycotic Diseases, National Center for Infectious Diseases, Centers for Disease Control and Prevention, Atlanta, Georgia 30333

**Robert V. Tauxe**    •    Division of Bacterial and Mycotic Diseases, National Center for Infectious Diseases, Centers for Disease Control and Prevention, 1600 Clifton Road NE, Atlanta, Georgia 30333

**Yao-Lung Tsai**    •    Department of Tropical Medicine, Tulane School of Public Health and Tropical Medicine, New Orleans, Louisiana 70112

**Victor C. W. Tsang**    •    Division of Parasitic Diseases, National Center for Infectious Diseases, Centers for Disease Control and Prevention, Mail Stop F22, 4770 Buford Highway, Atlanta, Georgia 30341

**Patricia P. Wilkins**    •    Division of Parasitic Diseases, National Center for Infectious Diseases, Centers for Disease Control and Prevention, Mail Stop F22, 4770 Buford Highway, Atlanta, Georgia 30341

# FOREWORD

Emerging infectious diseases are a continuing threat to the health of U.S. citizens and of people around the world. They cause suffering and death and impose an enormous financial burden on society. The recent outbreak of a new and virulent strain of influenza virus in Hong Kong raised the specter of a pandemic and illustrated the potential danger posed by these diseases to all countries. This incident also illustrated, yet again, the need for the United States to work closely with other countries and the World Health Organization (WHO) to ensure that there is adequate global capacity to detect and address such outbreaks.

Today we see a global resurgence of infectious diseases, including the identification of new infectious agents, the reemergence of old infectious agents such as *Mycobacterium tuberculosis*, and the rapid spread of antimicrobial resistance. The factors that contribute to the resurgence of these diseases, including increasing global travel, the globalization of the food supply, population growth and urbanization in conjunction with changes and challenges in human behavior and demographics, ecological and climatic changes, and the evolution of drug-resistant microbes, show no signs of abatement. We also face the threat of bioterrorism and must be prepared to respond to it.

In 1995, I had the opportunity to chair a workgroup on emerging diseases for a committee of the National Science and Technology Council (NSTC) which was charged with conducting a government-wide review of our ability to protect our citizens from emerging infectious diseases. The NSTC committee—the Committee on International Science, Engineering, and Technology—issued a report that concluded that existing mechanisms for surveillance of, response to, and prevention of outbreaks of new and reemerging infectious diseases were inadequate, both at home and abroad. The report made specific recommendations that became the basis of a 1996 Presidential Decision Directive that established a new national policy. The Directive called for a coordinated U.S. government response to address the growing health and national security threats posed by infectious diseases. The new policy acknowledged that domestic health and international health are intimately linked, that microbes do not respect borders, and that the United States cannot protect the health of its citizens without playing a leadership role in international health.

We know that the challenge ahead outstrips the means available to any one agency, organization, or country. However, if we pool our talents and resources, a great deal may be accomplished. This is well illustrated by the great success of smallpox eradication and the ongoing polio and guinea worm eradication programs.

These principles of collaboration and coordination are being applied both at home, where U.S. agencies have coordinated the effort to address emerging infectious diseases among themselves as well as with partners at the state and local levels, and overseas, where agencies are working with the WHO and other international partners to improve global health communications, set standards for global surveillance of antimicrobial resistance, and share experience and training on disease prevention and control on a regional basis.

The challenges ahead will demand our continued attention. Our goal is to ensure that we are able to protect outselves and the global community from emerging pathogens whenever and wherever they may arise.

**David Satcher**
**Surgeon General of the United States**
**Assistant Secretary for Health**

# PREFACE

As a result of improvements in sanitation and overall living conditions during the early part of the 20th century and the subsequent introduction of many vaccines and antibiotics, tremendous progress has been made in the prevention and control of infectious diseases. Globally, smallpox has been eradicated and target dates have been established for the eradication of poliomyelitis and dracunculiasis. In the United States, the annual incidence of several vaccine-preventable diseases is at an all time low.

In spite of these successes, infectious diseases remain the leading cause of death worldwide and the third leading cause of death in the United States. The World Health Organization (WHO) estimated that approximately 17 million (33%) of the 52 million deaths that occurred worldwide in 1997 were caused by microbial agents. Infectious diseases are the third leading cause of death in the United States. Human immunodeficiency virus (HIV) infection is among the leading causes of death in the United States among persons between the ages of 25 and 44 years.

The Institute of Medicine (IOM) published a report entitled "Emerging Infections: Microbial Threats to Health in the United States" in the fall of 1992. This report, developed under the leadership of Joshua Lederberg and Robert Shope, identified the important factors that contribute to disease emergence and reemergence. These factors include changes in human demographics and behaviors, advances in technology and industry, economic development and changes in land use, increases in travel and commerce, microbial adaptation and change, and deterioration in the public health system at the local, state, national, and global levels.

Recognizing the intense interest and scientific and public health importance of new and emerging infectious diseases, the program committee of the Interscience Conference on Antimicrobial Agents and Chemotherapy (ICAAC) and the officers of the Infectious Diseases Society of America (IDSA) organized joint sessions during ICAAC and the IDSA annual meeting beginning in 1995. These joint sessions on new and emerging pathogens were immensely popular, attracting audiences in excess of 4,000, and were planned carefully to span the gamut among new and emerging bacteria, viruses, fungi, and parasites with appropriate discussions on national and international strategies for control.

The chapters in *Emerging Infections 2* were derived primarily from presentations given at the sessions on new and emerging infections at the 1997 ICAAC and are updated and fully referenced for this volume, the second in a series. These chapters focus on a variety of diseases that pose major clinical and public health challenges today; some have been recognized for a century or more, while others have been identified during the past 25 years. Some affect healthy persons, while others primarily affect immunosuppressed persons. Some are important problems in the

United States, while others cause disease primarily in other parts of the world. Approximately half of these diseases are zoonotic or vector borne, reflecting the current importance of these modes of transmission. The epidemiology of each has been influenced by one or more of the factors identified in the IOM report. Because of the nature of the "global village" in which we live, we cannot afford to be ignorant or complacent about any of them.

Experiences with these diseases dramatically remind physicians, microbiologists, researchers, public health officials, policy makers, and the public of the critical importance of ensuring the availability of the capacity to detect, respond to, and control these infections. The ability to address these emerging and reemerging microbial threats requires adequate surveillance and response capacity, ongoing research and training programs, strengthened prevention and control programs, and repair of the public health system at the local, state, national, and international levels. Some of the United States' contributions to strategies to address these threats at the global level are outlined in the last chapter. The challenges that these diseases will continue to pose demand a multidisciplinary approach and a supply of trained clinicians, microbiologists, pathologists, biomedical researchers, rodent and vector biologists, ecologists, behavioral scientists, and public health officials. The challenges also require funds to support the people and facilities needed to meet them. This is especially true in the developing world because poverty and malnutrition make populations especially susceptible to emerging and reemerging infections.

Future challenges are difficult to predict but certainly include more problems with antimicrobial-resistant infections, the threat of another influenza pandemic, and the increasingly complex challenges of food-borne disease resulting from the globalization of the food supply. The global HIV epidemic will put large numbers of people at risk for currently recognized and new opportunistic infections. The roles of hepatitis B and C viruses in chronic liver disease and hepatocellular carcinoma, human papillomavirus in cervical cancer, and *Helicobacter pylori* infection in peptic ulcer disease and gastric cancer are now well established. Additional chronic diseases will certainly be found to have an infectious etiology, providing important new opportunities for disease prevention in the future. Food and blood safety will continue to be priorities and to pose challenges.

Based on the continued importance of new and emerging infectious diseases as defined by the 1992 IOM report, symposia on these topics are planned for future ICAACs. We plan production of an annual volume on new and emerging infections based on the presentations at each year's ICAAC. This volume, the second in the series, should serve as a valuable source of current information for persons responsible for coping with infectious diseases in the new millennium.

**W. Michael Scheld**
**William A. Craig**
**James M. Hughes**

# ACKNOWLEDGMENTS

We thank everyone who has helped us in the preparation of this volume. Most importantly, we thank all of the authors for their outstanding contributions. As editors, we are particularly grateful to those members of the Interscience Conference on Antimicrobial Agents and Chemotherapy (ICAAC) Program Committee who assisted us in coordinating topic and speaker selection for and/or moderating the joint symposia on emerging infections during the 1997 ICAAC: Tom Bergan, John Conly, and Barbara Murray. Numerous other colleagues provided helpful discussion, advice, and criticism. We are also grateful to our secretaries, Susan Shaker, Susan Waisner, and Darlene Shannon. We thank Ken April of ASM Press for coordinating production of the book. And, finally, we thank our families for their understanding and support during this undertaking.

*Emerging Infections 2*
Edited by W. M. Scheld, W. A. Craig, and J. M. Hughes
© 1998 ASM Press, Washington, D.C.

*Chapter 1*

# New-Variant Creutzfeldt-Jakob Disease and Bovine Spongiform Encephalopathy: the Strengthening Etiologic Link between Two Emerging Diseases

*Lawrence B. Schonberger*

This chapter updates an article written in June 1997 and is based on the accumulating data available in late November 1997 (32). There is increasing evidence for an etiologic link between the bovine spongiform encephalopathy (BSE) epizootic in the United Kingdom and the emergence of a new variant form of Creutzfeldt-Jakob disease (nvCJD). This tightening link and the many scientific uncertainties about BSE and nvCJD underscore the importance for increased surveillance for these emerging diseases in many countries, including the United States. They also indicate that full compliance in this country with a 1997 U.S. Food and Drug Administration regulation prohibiting the use of most mammalian protein in the manufacture of ruminant feed remains prudent for protecting the health of both animals and the public (16).

Both CJD in humans and BSE in cattle are invariably fatal, subacute, degenerative diseases of the brain that are classified as transmissible spongiform encephalopathies (TSEs) (18, 29). They are regarded as the same type of disease process. The leading etiologic hypothesis for these diseases is that they result from the accumulation in affected brains of the transmissible agent, which consists of an abnormal form of a host-encoded glycoprotein. In 1982, this transmissible agent was named a "prion" because of its novel, proteinaceous, infectious properties that distinguished it from viruses, plasmids, and viroids (30).

Since 1968, when CJD in humans was first reported to be transmissible to chimpanzees, there has been continued speculation about the possibility of natural transmission of this disease to account for the over 85% of CJD cases that appear to occur sporadically with no known source of infection (20). However, no natural

---

*Lawrence B. Schonberger* • Division of Viral and Rickettsial Diseases, National Center for Infectious Diseases, Centers for Disease Control and Prevention, Mail Stop A39, 1600 Clifton Road NE, Atlanta, GA 30333.

route for transmission of CJD has been convincingly demonstrated. To explain both the similar incidence of CJD (about one case per million population per year) found in many different geographic areas of the world and the absence of apparent environmental risk factors, prominent investigators have hypothesized that the vast majority of CJD cases (i.e., those classified as sporadic with no known environmental source of infection) result from de novo spontaneous generation of the self-replicating prion protein. Further, this process may be facilitated by an occasional somatic mutation that increases the usually rare stochastic fluctuations in the structure of the normal cellular form of the prion protein (18, 29).

## THE BSE EPIZOOTIC IN THE UNITED KINGDOM

BSE was first diagnosed as part of an epizootic in the United Kingdom in November 1986 (37). The epizootic curve of confirmed BSE cases in Great Britain (England, Scotland, and Wales), by quarter of the year, through September 1997, illustrates both the rapid rise in the number of new cases until the peak consecutive two quarters beginning October 1992 and then a subsequent decline (Fig. 1). For the first 6 months of 1997, the total of just over 2,100 reported cases was 10.6% of the number during the peak consecutive two quarters (33, 36).

The BSE epizootic began earlier than is indicated in Fig. 1, probably as early as April 1985, when suspected cases were retrospectively recognized, or possibly

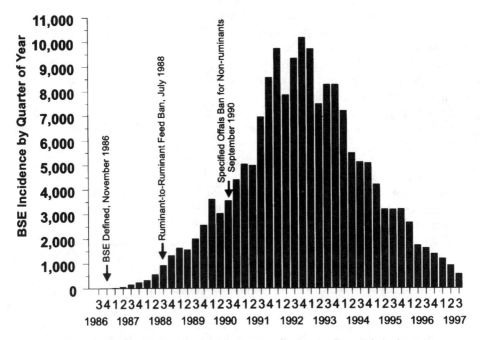

**Figure 1.** Confirmed BSE, by quarter of year of onset, in Great Britain from 1 September 1986 to 30 September 1997 (reported through 28 November 1997). Adapted from references by Wilesmith et al. (35, 36) and Smith (33).

as early as 1983 (12, 37). In addition, the epizootic was probably slightly less explosive than depicted because of underreporting before the new disease became officially notifiable in June 1988, and possibly for 1 or 2 years after this time (2). In August 1988, government compensation for cattle slaughtered on account of BSE was begun at a level of 50% of the value for confirmed cases, and this new compensation program also may have led to improved reporting.

By November 28, 1997, about 170,000 head of cattle in over 34,000 herds had been diagnosed with BSE in Great Britain (33, 36). Provisional data as of September 10, 1997, indicated over 2,900 additional cattle diagnosed with BSE in Guernsey, Jersey, the Isle of Man, and Northern Ireland (36).

The source of the BSE epizootic is uncertain. The leading hypothesis is that it resulted from feeding cattle rendered protein, such as meat-and-bone meal, produced from the carcasses of scrapie-infected sheep in the early 1980s, after most rendering plants abandoned the use of organic solvents in the preparation of this feed (26). This hypothesis best explains the occurrence of the epizootic predominantly in the United Kingdom, where the ratio of the numbers of sheep to cattle and the rate of endemic scrapie are both high. An alternative hypothesis is that the epizootic resulted from feeding cattle rendered protein produced from the carcasses of possible rare endemic cases of BSE. Although the existence of such endemic cases has not been documented, a prominent expert in BSE has argued that the hypothesized de novo spontaneous generation of the self-replicating protein in humans may also occur in cattle and account for rare sporadic cases of BSE (19). Indirect support for this latter hypothesis comes from several observations: (i) an experimental challenge study of cattle parenterally injected with U.S. scrapie-infected material produced a cattle disease clinically and pathologically different from the BSE occurring in the United Kingdom (9), (ii) there is an absence of reported experimental transmission or molecular studies linking British strains of the scrapie agent with BSE (9, 11), and (iii) transmission of BSE by oral challenge of cattle was documented with ≤1 gram of BSE-infected bovine brain (9). In addition, Bruce and coworkers have reported that mouse-strain-typing studies (based on both incubation periods and pathologic features) have uncovered the "BSE signature" only in transmissions from animals suspected or known to have been infected with BSE and specifically not in 35 sheep and 2 goats with naturally occurring scrapie (5). Variation in strains among the sheep sources also was reported. It has been suggested in support of the hypothesis that scrapie rather than endemic BSE was the source of the BSE epizootic that the rendering process may have altered a scrapie agent or selected for a possible preexisting BSE-like scrapie strain (4). Regardless of the validity of these hypotheses about the original source of the BSE epizootic in the United Kingdom, there is convincing evidence and general agreement among investigators that feeding rendered bovine meat-and-bone meal to young calves amplified the spread of the disease (5, 26, 37).

The key measures to control the BSE epizootic in the United Kingdom included a ban on using ruminant protein for ruminant feed (introduced on July 18, 1988) and a ban on using brain, spinal cord, and other specified bovine offals in feed for nonruminant animals and poultry (introduced in September 1990) (Fig. 1) (25). This latter ban differs from another specified bovine offals ban, instituted in November 1989, that forbade use of certain bovine tissues for food for human consumption (26). The beneficial effects of the 1988 feed ban on the BSE epizootic provided epidemiologic confirmation of the hypothesis that the use of bovine meat-and-bone meal was amplifying the spread of disease. For example, the approximate annual number of cases of BSE, by year of birth, rose from 10,000 to 51,000 between 1984 and 1987 but declined from 28,000 to 4,000 between 1988 and 1990. Because experimental studies have confirmed that the incubation period after oral exposure to infectious feed is 2 to 8 years, some increase in this latter number may be expected as cases continue to occur in the 1990 birth cohort through 1998 (26).

## THE nvCJD EPIDEMIC IN THE UNITED KINGDOM

On March 20, 1996, an expert advisory committee to the United Kingdom government, the Spongiform Encephalopathy Advisory Committee, announced its "great concern" that the agent responsible for the ongoing BSE epizootic might have spread to humans. This was based on recognition of 10 persons with onset of an apparently new variant form of CJD during February 1994 through October 1995 (34). The advisory committee's concern raised the possibility that the 10 cases could represent the beginning of a delayed, BSE-related epidemic of nvCJD in humans that might parallel the course of the epizootic of BSE in cattle. As the basis for diagnosing nvCJD, the initially published proposal for its existence described an apparently newly recognized brain pathologic profile found by histologic examination of brain tissue (39). This profile included, in both the cerebellum and cerebrum, numerous kuru-type amyloid plaques surrounded by vacuoles (Fig. 2) and prion protein accumulation at high concentration, indicated by immunocytochemical analysis. Because all 10 initial cases of nvCJD also showed the classic spongiform pathologic features of CJD, there was little question that the illnesses were appropriately classified as CJD.

In addition to the newly recognized pathologic profile, the unusually young age of the patients and several atypical clinical features supported the proposal that a new variant of CJD had emerged. These reported clinical features included prominent behavioral changes at the time of clinical presentation with subsequent onset of neurologic abnormalities, including ataxia within weeks or months, dementia and myoclonus late in the illness, a duration of illness of at least 6 months, and nondiagnostic electroencephalographic changes (39).

The initially recognized 10 patients with nvCJD were reported to reside in widely scattered areas of the United Kingdom. Review of these patients' medical histories, genetic analyses, and consideration of other possible causes did not provide an adequate explanation for these cases. Nevertheless, there was also no clear epidemiologic link to BSE reported, such as an increased prevalence of eating cattle brain or other foods derived from cattle or of an occupational or other exposure to cattle or to their tissues (26, 39).

Since the initial announcement of possible nvCJD in the United Kingdom, additional case-reports have accumulated, validating the publicized concerns in 1996 about the presence of an ongoing epidemic. On November 3, 1997, the Department of Health in England reported a total of 22 cases of nvCJD identified among res-

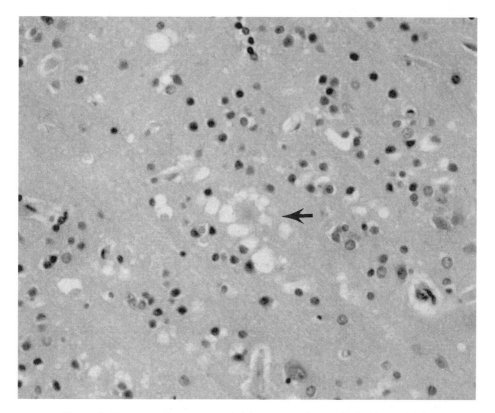

**Figure 2.** Kuru-type plaque surrounded by a zone of spongiform change in the frontal lobe of a patient with nvCJD (arrow). The sample was stained with hematoxylin and eosin. Photomicrograph courtesy of J. W. Ironside.

idents of the United Kingdom through September 1997 (14). Eleven of the 12 additional cases reported since March 20, 1996, were confirmed on the basis of the previously described characteristic brain pathologic profile. For the 12th case, brain tissue was unavailable for study, but the patient was a teenager who had a compatible clinical course. She was classified as a probable case of nvCJD with the caveat that criteria for such cases could not yet be fully validated (14).

This total of 22 reported British patients with nvCJD included 13 females and 9 males. Their median age at onset was 28 years (range, 16 to 48 years). The median age at death was 29 years (range, 19 to 50 years). This latter median and range were determined without excluding the one patient among the 22 who was still alive as of September 30, 1997; she was over age 30 but unlikely to live beyond age 50. Remarkably, 13 of these 22 patients died at younger than 30 years of age. These 13 unusually young patients with CJD included 5 patients who had onset at less than 20 years of age. Four of the 13 died as teenagers (12, 14, 38).

Whereas more than half the patients with CJD in the United States die within 6 months of onset of illness, the median duration of illness for the 22 British patients with nvCJD was 14 months (range, 8 to 38 months) (12, 38, 41).

Because the median duration of illness with nvCJD was 14 months and brain tissue to confirm the diagnosis was usually obtained after death, the illustrated pattern of occurrence of the 22 case patients, by year of onset, is likely to change and should be interpreted accordingly (Fig. 3); subsequently identified cases will likely have onset of disease in the more recent years, 1995 to 1997.

The lower number of confirmed cases of nvCJD with onset in 1996 compared with either 1994 or 1995 and the absence of confirmed cases in 1997 through September do not necessarily mean that the outbreak is waning. Analyses based on models of epidemic curves indicate that the observed annual numbers of cases by onset and by death may also be consistent with a true, rapidly rising incidence of disease, if reporting delays of confirmed cases are about equal to the duration of illness. The existence of such reporting delays of confirmed cases is supported by a report that only 4 of the 14 initial nvCJD cases were confirmed before death and that for 2 of these 4 cases, the confirmation occurred less than 3 months before death (12).

These reporting delays can affect the appropriate interpretation of the epidemic curve of nvCJD in the United Kingdom. If, for example, a 15-month delay (onset of illness to the confirmation of nvCJD) is likely for each case-patient whose illness lasts 15 months, then such a case would need to have an onset before July 1996 for probable confirmation by September 1997. The reason for this is that if such a case-patient's onset of illness were in the last half of 1996, the patient would still be alive in September 1997 and unlikely to have a neuropathologically confirmed diagnosis. Through September 1997, the number of reported nvCJD cases with onset in the first half of 1996 that had a 15-month or less duration of illness was

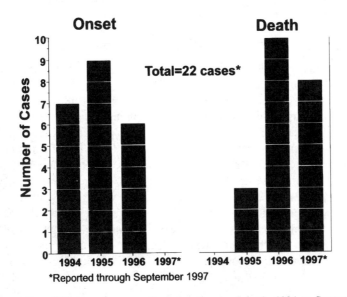

**Figure 3.** nvCJD cases, by year of onset and year of death, 1994 to September 1997. Data are from the Department of Health of the United Kingdom (14), Cousens et al. (12), and Will (38). One patient was still alive.

4, or 0.67 cases per month during this 6-month period in 1996, compared with 8 such cases with onset during the 24-month period beginning January 1994, or 0.33 cases per month. Thus, the rate of such cases was higher during the 1996 period than in the previous 2 years, but the numbers are too small to convincingly demonstrate that an increase in incidence has, in fact, been occurring. Additional evidence which supports a conclusion that the number of cases with onset in 1996 may be greater than depicted in Fig. 3 is that 5 of the 16 cases with onset in 1994 and 1995 had illnesses lasting 21 months or longer. Such long-duration illnesses would probably not be confirmed by September 30, 1997, even if their onset was in the first month of 1996.

With regard to the absence of reported confirmed cases with onset in 1997, it is important to consider that the shortest duration of illness for a nvCJD case with onset in 1994 or 1995 was 9 months (one case). For any patient with a 9-month illness to die and for the illness to be confirmed by the end of September 1997, the onset would likely need to be before January 1997. Thus, for reports through September 30, 1997, the absence of any nvCJD cases with onset in 1997 does not provide reassurance that the incidence of the disease is declining.

None of the 22 patients with nvCJD in the United Kingdom died in 1994, compared with 3 in 1995, 10 in 1996, and 8 in 1997 through September (Fig. 3). Although the absolute number of cases in 1997 is smaller than in 1996, the 1996 data are less complete and hence also do not provide evidence that the outbreak is waning. Rather, these data suggest a slightly rising or stable rate of new deaths in 1997 compared with 1996 after a sharp rise in such deaths in 1996 compared with 1995. A slightly rising rate of new deaths, however, remains consistent with a sharply rising rate of newly ill cases if there are delays in the reporting of such new cases.

In February and also in September of 1997, the government of the United Kingdom reported that 10 patients had died of nvCJD in 1996. This unchanging number of reported nvCJD cases since early February 1997 suggests that delays in confirming and reporting cases after a patient with nvCJD dies remains only a potential, not an actual, additional problem for properly interpreting the epidemic curve. If such delays after death in confirming and reporting cases remain short and if the long duration of illnesses were, in fact, currently obscuring an increasing incidence of disease in the epidemic curve, then based on the duration of illnesses observed for cases with onset in 1994, one can expect that such an increase in the incidence of nvCJD would likely become apparent during 1998. For example, if the incidence were rising exponentially according to one possible model of the epidemic, then by the end of 1998, the expected number of reported confirmed cases with onset in 1996 should be closer to 13 cases than to 6 cases, the number presently shown in Fig. 3 for 1996. With the data presently available, it remains too early to draw firm conclusions about the number of nvCJD cases that will occur in the United Kingdom.

## nvCJD OUTSIDE THE UNITED KINGDOM

In early April and again in May of 1996, consultants meeting at the World Health Organization in Geneva called for establishment of ongoing surveillance programs worldwide to better determine the geographic distribution of both BSE and nvCJD, thereby better clarifying the possible relationship of these two diseases (7).

Through November 1997, the only reported non-British person with definite nvCJD was a 26-year-old French man with onset of CJD in 1994. His 23-month-long illness resembled the illness in the British cases and was confirmed neuropathologically as nvCJD in 1996. He had traveled outside France only once, and that was to Spain in 1990. He was described as a mechanic who had no particular contact with cattle (8).

This case was originally reported as raising a question about the possible causal relationship between BSE and nvCJD because at the time only 16 cases of BSE had been reported from France. As other evidence favoring an etiologic relationship between BSE and nvCJD has increased, this case has begun to suggest that continental Europe is not free of the risk for an occasional case of nvCJD from BSE despite its relatively low number of reported BSE cases. As of September 1997, there were fewer than 400 reported BSE cases in continental Europe, including 27 reported cases in France (36). The probable existence of such a risk for an occasional case of nvCJD increases the importance of surveillance for both BSE and nvCJD throughout continental Europe and of the institution of control measures to reduce the probability of BSE infectivity in human food. In light of the potential for long illness to temporarily alter the shape of the developing epidemic curve in the United Kingdom, the case in France also supports concerns that just under 2-year delays from onset to the confirmation and reporting of nvCJD may not be rare.

## CJD SURVEILLANCE IN THE UNITED STATES

In the United States, where the U.S. Department of Agriculture has reported no evidence of BSE in any U.S. cattle (13), the Centers for Disease Control and Prevention (CDC), with the help of many others, has been seeking evidence for either the presence or absence of nvCJD through several CJD surveillance mechanisms (22). These mechanisms have included active CJD surveillance in April and May 1996 conducted by surveillance teams that were in place as part of the Emerging Infections Programs in Connecticut, Minnesota, Oregon, and the San Francisco Bay area of California and as part of a food safety program in metropolitan Atlanta, Georgia; the overall 1993 population for these five sites was 16.3 million (6). (Emerging Infections Programs were established in 1994 through cooperative agreements between CDC and state health departments to conduct special surveillance and laboratory/epidemiologic projects and to pilot and evaluate prevention programs.) CJD surveillance in the United States also has consisted of analyses of the multiple cause-of-death data obtained from CDC's National Center for Health Statistics and follow-up reviews since April 1996 of available clinical and neuropathologic information on patients younger than 55 years of age who died after 1993 (22, 32). In late September 1996, CDC in collaboration with the American Association of Neuropathologists augmented CJD surveillance by alerting the U.S. neuropathologist members of the association about the importance of their reporting any suspected cases of the nvCJD, regardless of the patient's age or the initial clinical diagnosis (32). Finally, widespread publicity and concern about nvCJD have led to spontaneous calls about suspected cases of nvCJD to CDC from the public, physicians, and newspaper reporters. Despite the increased surveillance and attention concerning this new disease entity, as of the end of November 1997 no evidence has been found for the occurrence of nvCJD in the United States.

The U.S. CJD mortality data underscore the uniqueness of the cluster of nvCJD cases in the United Kingdom with a median age at death of 29 years. In addition to illustrating the extreme rarity of CJD deaths in patients under 30 years of age, the age distribution and death rates for the total of 3,904 CJD deaths reported in the United States (1979 to 1995) show a dramatic rise in the CJD death rates beginning at about age 50, a decrease in such rates for those 80 years old and older, and a peak number of CJD deaths in the 65- to 69-year-old age group (median age, 68 years) (Fig. 4). In the United States over the 17-year period from 1979 to 1995, the annual CJD death rate for persons younger than 30 years of age was less than five cases per billion, and no CJD death occurred in a teenager. For the 6-year period 1990 to 1995, these data included only one CJD death in a patient less than 30 years old, a patient who died in 1993 and who had been previously identified as part of an ongoing surveillance for CJD among recipients of pituitary-derived human growth hormone. Another recipient of pituitary-derived human growth hormone who died at under 30 years of age was identified among the partial

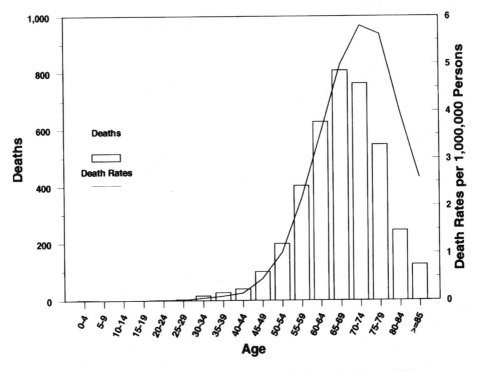

**Figure 4.** CJD deaths and death rates by age group in the United States, 1979 to 1995.

(about 85% complete) national mortality data for 1996 available in November 1997. No one else was younger than 30 years of age among the 218 reported CJD deaths in these 1996 data. One patient less than 30 years of age who died of CJD in 1997 was recently reported spontaneously to CDC; neuropathologic follow-up of this patient, however, ruled out nvCJD.

## EVIDENCE FOR AN nvCJD RELATED TO BSE

The currently available pathological, clinical, and epidemiologic information on the newly described variant of CJD provides convincing evidence that it is, in fact, a novel variant. This conclusion is supported by the following observations: (i) an increasing concurrence among neuropathologists and CJD experts that they have not previously seen the pathologic profile of the nvCJD described by Will and Ironside (3, 17, 39); (ii) the relatively consistent and distinct clinical features of nvCJD in comparison with sporadic CJD, such as the unusually long duration of illness, the prominent early psychiatric symptoms with delayed evolution of neu-rologic signs, and the absence of the diagnostic electroencephalogram pattern of CJD (40, 41); (iii) the extraordinary young age of the patients with nvCJD, partic-ularly the occurrence of five cases among teenagers in the United Kingdom within a 3-year period; and (iv) the absence of documented cases outside of France and the United Kingdom through November 1997 or anywhere in the world with onset before 1994, especially given both the worldwide publicity about nvCJD and the results to date of CJD surveillance in the United States.

Recently, the evidence that this apparently novel variant of CJD is causally linked to the ongoing BSE epizootic in the United Kingdom has also become convincing but with an important caveat. This caveat is that the final results of two ongoing studies of this link will not give a different picture than the investigators' recently published initial results, a possibility that has been reported to be unlikely (1, 5, 21).

Overall, the epidemiologic evidence remains consistent with causation and grows more supportive as cases of nvCJD continue to occur confined primarily to the United Kingdom, as would be predicted if such cases were, in fact, related to the BSE epizootic. The absence of any confirmed cases of nvCJD in geographic areas free of BSE is similarly consistent with causation. Further, the interval between the most likely period for the initial extended exposure of the population to potentially BSE-contaminated food (1984 to 1986) and onset of initial cases (1994 to 1996) is consistent with known incubation periods for CJD (3, 10). Although the young age of slaughter of most BSE-infected animals would help to reduce any possible infectivity of food derived from their tissues (26), Anderson and colleagues (2) estimated that approximately 446,000 infected animals entered the human food chain in the United Kingdom before the specified bovine offal ban of late 1989. Approximately 283,000 more entered before the end of 1995.

Among the stronger evidence supporting a causal link between BSE and nvCJD are transmission studies of BSE to macaques. These studies showed that the disease which developed after a 3-year incubation period in three rhesus macaques that had been inoculated with a single pool of BSE-infected cattle brain homogenate was strikingly similar, both clinically and neuropathologically, to nvCJD. The neuropathologic similarities included the distribution of spongiform changes and the morphologic features of plaques (23).

In October 1996, Collinge and colleagues (11), using the approach of Parchi and colleagues (28), described a new molecular marker for tracing the passage of individual prion protein strains within and between species. Their marker consisted of the pattern of bands on a Western blot test of the prion protein from proteinase K-treated brain extracts. They reported that the prions of 10 nvCJD cases had strain characteristics distinct from prions of any of 26 sporadic CJD cases or 7 iatrogenic CJD cases. These strain characteristics, they reported, resembled those of known BSE-infected animals, including cattle, mice, domestic cat, and a macaque (11). Deslys and coworkers (15) and then Parchi and colleagues (27) subsequently confirmed that Western blot analyses of the prion protein distinguished the one reported French nvCJD patient from those with sporadic or iatrogenic CJD. Parchi and colleagues reported, however, that this finding was based solely on an unusual glycoform pattern, rather than on differences in the mobility of the bands.

In October 1997, Bruce and coworkers (5) substantially strengthened the evidence for a link between BSE and nvCJD by reporting interim results of their prion strain-typing studies of six cases of sporadic CJD, including two cases in dairy farmers (aged 61 and 64 years) who had owned cattle with BSE, and three cases of nvCJD in mice. These strain-typing studies are based on the incubation times and brain lesion profiles in three inbred lines and one cross strain of mice. The reported results from the study of the line of mice associated with the shortest incubation period showed differences between the cases of nvCJD and all six cases of sporadic CJD. These results also confirmed the striking similarity of incubation times and brain lesion profiles associated with each of the cases of nvCJD and the previously studied cases of BSE. The remaining lines of mice that had been inoculated in this study were still under observation. Consistent with previous studies of the BSE agent, some of a second line of mice inoculated with the agent of nvCJD were reported as developing signs of disease.

Bruce and coworkers summarized results of their previous transmissions of the BSE agent from eight unrelated cattle with BSE and from three domestic cats and two exotic ruminants with TSEs attributed to the BSE agent. These transmissions were reported as showing remarkably similar incubation times and lesion profiles. This "BSE signature" was also seen in studies of mice injected with brain from two sheep, a goat, and a pig that had been experimentally infected with BSE but not in similar studies of 40 animals with naturally occurring TSEs that were not BSE, including 35 sheep and two goats with scrapie (5).

Also in October 1997, Hill and coworkers (21) provided further corroborating evidence that nvCJD was distinct from sporadic CJD and iatrogenic CJD and related to BSE. Their evidence was derived from studies of a large number of prion transmissions, using both transgenic mice expressing the human prion protein gene (*PRNP*) and their nontransgenic counterparts. The authors reported, for example, that 33 (77%) of 43 wild-type mice developed prion disease after inoculation with the agent of nvCJD compared with none of 60 wild-type mice after inoculation with the agent of sporadic CJD, although both groups of patients had methionine at codon 129 of their *PRNP* gene (codon 129 genotype is thought to influence susceptibility to CJD). In addition, Western blot analyses of the prion proteins in the wild-type mice inoculated with nvCJD were indistinguishable from those observed in the wild-type mice inoculated with BSE and similar to those previously described in several other species inoculated with BSE (21).

Some reported evidence for the link between nvCJD and BSE by Hill and coworkers provided a mixed message about the link because it indicated a substantial species barrier against BSE infections of humans. Such a barrier had been indicated previously by an apparently low molecular compatibility between the BSE prion protein and the normal, nonpathogenic form of the human prion protein as determined by cell-free conversion reactions (31). The evidence reported by Hill and coworkers for a substantial species barrier included the long mean incubation period of 602 days in 10 of 26 transgenic mice inoculated with BSE, compared with 228 days in 25 of 56 transgenic mice inoculated with the agent of nvCJD. Despite this difference in incubation period, the study appeared to demonstrate the susceptibility of humans to BSE infection. The authors indicated that the two groups of ill mice shared unusual clinical features, including long duration of illness and backwards walking as well as the otherwise typical clinical features of mouse scrapie. The investigators were unable to confirm, however, the prion disease diagnoses in the BSE-inoculated mice by a highly sensitive Western blot test of brain tissue; the test did not demonstrate the presence of pathogenic prion protein in the mice. This result complicates the interpretation of the study. As acknowledged by Hill and coworkers, second-passage studies to confirm the reported transmission of BSE to the transgenic mice will be important (21).

Similar to the French patient with nvCJD, all 14 tested cases of nvCJD described by Zeidler and colleagues were homozygous for methionine at codon 129 of their *PRNP* gene, despite a valine-methionine polymorphism of the *PRNP* gene at codon 129 among the general population (11, 15, 41). Cattle genes do not carry this polymorphism at the equivalent site to codon 129; they code only for methionine (41). This difference may be responsible for some of the BSE-to-human species barrier observed in the transgenic mice experiments; the transgene in the mice experimentally injected with BSE prions carried valine (21). It has been suggested that the ability to transmit a prion disease between species is in part determined by the homology of the structures of the interacting proteins coded by their prion protein genes (with the region containing codon 129 of particular importance) (24, 31, 41). Methionine homozygosity at codon 129 is a risk factor for nvCJD because it presumably confers increased susceptibility. It has been suggested that transgenic mice with methionine homozygosity at codon 129 could be more susceptible to prion disease from BSE inoculations, but these studies have not been reported (21).

## CONCLUSIONS

The accumulating experimental and epidemiologic data provide increasingly strong support for a causal link between BSE and nvCJD, but the likely causal link is not definitely established at the time of this writing. The continuing assessment of this link will be assisted by completion of the standard strain-typing studies of the agent of nvCJD in mice and the confirmation of the apparent transmission of BSE to transgenic mice expressing the human *PRNP* gene with valine at codon 129. In addition, this evidence for a causal link will be strengthened by the demonstration of the greater susceptibility of similar transgenic mice with methionine at codon 129. In 1998, surveillance of nvCJD in the United Kingdom may indicate whether the early epidemic of nvCJD is increasing exponentially, similar to the early epizootic of BSE. If it is, this tragic observation would provide additional compelling evidence for an etiologic link between these two emerging diseases. Ongoing surveillance of both CJD and BSE in many countries of the world, including the United States and especially in the United Kingdom, remains critical for continuing the assessment of this link and for determining to what extent the agent of BSE may be causing disease in humans.

In the meantime, the continued application of the series of measures in the United Kingdom and the United States designed to minimize the risk for disease transmission is justified (3) because of the strong evidence and general acceptance that feeding ruminant animal proteins to cattle played an important role in amplifying the BSE epizootic in the United Kingdom (9, 26, 37) and because of the existing evidence for a probable risk of transmission of BSE to humans. In the United States, the Food and Drug Administration issued a final regulation in June 1997 that prohibits the use of most mammalian protein in the manufacture of ruminant feed. Full compliance with this ban remains prudent to protect the health of both animals and the public (16).

**Acknowledgments.** I thank R. G. Will, CJD Surveillance Unit, Edinburgh, Scotland, for providing data on patients with nvCJD and Ermias Belay, National Center for Infectious Diseases (NCID), Centers for Disease Control and Prevention (CDC), and the staff of state and local health departments who were responsible for collecting data in this report on young patients with CJD in the United States. The author also acknowledges the essential support of the following staff of the NCID, CDC: Robert Holman for analyses of the U.S. mortality data, James Dobbins for assistance in assessing the possibility of an exponential rise in nvCJD cases in the United Kingdom, John O'Connor for editorial assistance, and Karoyle Colbert and Voughn Trader for technical support.

## REFERENCES

1. **Almond, J., and J. Pattison.** 1997. Human BSE. *Nature* **389:**437–438.
2. **Anderson, R. M., C. A. Donnelly, N. M. Ferguson, M. E. J. Woolhouse, C. J. Watt, H. J. Udy, S. MaWhinney, S. P. Dunstan, T. R. E. Southwood, J. W. Wilesmith, J. B. M. Ryans, L. J. Hoinville, J. E. Hillerton, A. R. Austin, and G. A. H. Wells.** 1996. Transmission dynamics and epidemiology of BSE in British cattle. *Nature* **382:**779–788.
3. **Brown, P.** 1997. The risk of bovine spongiform encephalopathy ('mad cow disease') to human health. *JAMA* **278:**1008–1011.
4. **Bruce, M., A. Chree, I. McConnell, J. Foster, G. Pearson, and H. Fraser.** 1994. Transmission of bovine spongiform encephalopathy and scrapie to mice: strain variation and the species barrier. *Philos. Trans. R. Soc. Lond. Biol. Sci.* **343:**405–411.
5. **Bruce, M. E., R. G. Will, J. W. Ironside, I. McConnell, D. Drummond, A. Suttie, L. McCardle, A. Chree, J. Hope, C. Birkett, S. Cousens, H. Fraser, and C. J. Bostock.** 1997. Transmissions to mice indicate that 'new variant' CJD is caused by the BSE agent. *Nature* **389:**498–501.
6. **Centers for Disease Control and Prevention.** 1996. Surveillance for Creutzfeldt-Jakob disease—United States. *Morbid. Mortal. Weekly Rep.* **45:**665–668.

7. **Centers for Disease Control and Prevention.** 1996. World Health Organization consultation on public health issues related to bovine spongiform encephalopathy and the emergence of a new variant of Creutzfeldt-Jakob disease. *Morbid. Mortal. Weekly Rep.* **45:**295–296, 303.

8. **Chazot, G., E. Broussolle, C. I. Lapras, T. Blattler, A. Aguzzi, and N. Kopp.** 1996. New variant of Creutzfeldt-Jakob disease in a 26-year-old French man. *Lancet* **347:**1181. (Letter).

9. **Collee, J. G., and R. Bradley.** 1997. BSE: a decade on—part 1. *Lancet* **349:**636–641.

10. **Collee, J. G., and R. Bradley.** 1997. BSE: a decade on—part 2. *Lancet* **349:**715–721.

11. **Collinge, J., K. C. L. Sidle, J. Meads, J. Ironside, and A. F. Hill.** 1996. Molecular analysis of prion strain variation and the aetiology of 'new variant' CJD. *Nature* **383:**685–690.

12. **Cousens, S. N., E. Vynnycky, M. Zeidler, R. G. Will, and P. G. Smith.** 1997. Predicting the CJD epidemic in humans. *Nature* **185:**197–200.

13. **Davis, A.** 1997. U.S. surveillance for bovine spongiform encephalopathy (BSE). *DxMonitor Animal Health Report* (Fall 1997), p. 11.

14. **Department of Health, United Kingdom.** 1997. Monthly Creutzfeldt-Jakob figures: November 3, 1997. Department of Health, London, United Kingdom.

15. **Deslys, J.-P., C. I. Lasmezas, N. Streichenberger, A. Hill, J. Collinge, D. Dormont, and N. Kopp.** New variant Creutzfeldt-Jakob disease in France. *Lancet* **346:**30–31.

16. **Food and Drug Administration.** 1997. Substances prohibited from use in animal food or feed; animal proteins prohibited in ruminant feed; final rule. *Fed. Regist.* **62**(108):30936–30978.

17. **Gambetti, P., and B. Ghetti.** June 1997. Personal communication.

18. **Gajdusek, D. C.** 1996. Infectious amyloids: subacute spongiform encephalopathies as transmissible cerebral amyloidoses, p. 2851–2900. *In* B. N. Fields, D. M. Knipe, P. M. Howley, R. M. Chanock, J. L. Melneck, T. P. Monath, B. Roizman, and S. E. Straus (ed.), *Virology,* 3rd ed. Lippincott-Raven, Philadelphia, Pa.

19. **Gibbs, J. C.** 1996. Debate: is BSE endemic? Presented at the International Symposium on Spongiform Encephalopathies: Generating Rational Policy in the Face of Public Fears, Washington, D.C., 13 December 1996.

20. **Harries-Jones, R., R. Knight, R. G. Will, S. Cousens, P. G. Smith, and W. B. Matthews.** 1988. Creutzfeldt-Jakob disease in England and Wales, 1980–1984: a case-control study of potential risk factors. *J. Neurol. Neurosurg. Psych.* 51:1113–1119.

21. **Hill, A. F., M. Desbruslais, S. Joiner, K. C. L. Sidle, I. Gowland, J. Collinge, L. J. Doey, and P. Lantos.** 1997. The same prion strain causes vCJD and BSE. *Nature* **389:**448–450.

22. **Holman, R. C., A. S. Khan, E. D. Belay, and L. B. Schonberger.** 1996. Creutzfeldt-Jakob disease in the United States, 1979–1994: using national mortality data to assess the possible occurrence of variant cases. *Emerg. Infect. Dis.* **2:**333–337.

23. **Lasmezas, C. I., J.-P. Deslys, R. Demalmay, K. T. Adjou, F. Lamoury, D. Dormont, O. Robain, J. Ironside, and J.-J. Hauw.** 1996. BSE transmission to macaques. *Nature* **381:**743–744. (Letter.)

24. **Masters, C. L., and K. Beyreuther.** 1997. Tracking turncoat prion proteins. *Nature* **388:**228–229.

25. **Ministry of Agriculture, Food, and Fisheries.** 1996. A progress report on bovine spongiform encephalopathy in Great Britain, p. 1–51. *In Bovine Spongiform Encephalopathy in Great Britain. A Progress Report,* May 1996. Ministry of Agriculture, Food, and Fisheries. Weybridge, England.

26. **Nathanson, N., J. Wilesmith, and C. Griot.** 1997. Bovine spongiform encephalopathy (BSE): causes and consequences of a common source epidemic. *Am. J. Epidemiol.* **145:**959–969.

27. **Parchi, P., S. Capellari, S. G. Chen, R. B. Petersen, P. Gambetti, N. Kopp, P. Brown, T. Kitamoto, J. Tateishi, A. Giese, and H. Kretzschmar.** 1997. Scientific correspondence: typing prion isoforms. *Nature* **386:**232–233.

28. **Parchi, P., R. Castellani, S. Capellari, B. Ghetti, K. Young, S. G. Chen, M. Farlow, D. W. Dickson, A. A. F. Sima, J. Q. Trojanowski, R. B. Petersen, and P. Gambetti.** 1996. Molecular basis of phenotypic variability in sporadic Creutzfeldt-Jakob disease. *Ann. Neurol.* **39:**767–778.

29. **Prusiner, S. B.** 1996. Prions, p. 2901–2950. *In* B. N. Fields, D. M. Knipe, P. M. Howley, R. M. Chanock, J. L. Melnick, T. P. Monath, B. Roizman, and S. E. Straus (ed.), *Virology,* 3rd ed. Lippincott-Raven, Philadelphia, Pa.

30. **Prusiner, S. B.** 1982. Novel proteinaceous infectious particles cause scrapie. *Science* **216:**136–144.

31. **Raymond, G. J., J. Hope, D. A. Kocisko, S. A. Priola, L. D. Raymond, A. Bossers, J. Ironside, R. G. Will, S. G. Chen, R. B. Petersen, P. Gambetti, R. Rubenstein, M. A. Smits, P. T. Lansbury,**

**Jr., and B. Caughey.** 1997. Molecular assessment of the potential transmissibilities of BSE and scrapie to humans. *Nature* **388:**285–288.

32. **Schonberger, L. B.** 1998. New variant Creutzfeldt-Jakob disease and bovine spongiform encephalopathy. *Infect. Dis. Clin. North Am.* **12:**111–122.

33. **Smith, M.** 1997. Unpublished data.

34. **Statement by the U.K. Spongiform Encephalopathy Advisory Committee.** March 20, 1996. House of Commons. Her Majesty's Stationery Office, London, United Kingdom.

35. **Wilesmith, J., T. Chillaud, and G. O. Denny.** 1996. Bovine spongiform encephalopathy update. *DxMonitor Animal Health Report* (**Summer 1996**):3–4.

36. **Wilesmith, J., T. Chillaud, and G. O. Denny.** 1997. International bovine spongiform encephalopathy update–United Kingdom update and other BSE affected countries. *DxMonitor Animal Health Report* (**Fall 1997**):4–5.

37. **Wilesmith, J. W., G. A. H. Wells, M. P. Cranwell, and J. B. M. Ryan.** 1988. Bovine spongiform encephalopathy: epidemiological studies. *Vet. Rec.* **123:**638–644.

38. **Will, R. G.** 1997. Unpublished data.

39. **Will, R. G., J. W. Ironside, M. Zeidler, S. N. Cousens, K. Estibeiro, A. Alperovitch, S. Poser, M. Pocchiari, A. Hofman, and P. G. Smith.** 1996. A new variant of Creutzfeldt-Jakob disease in the U.K. *Lancet* **347:**921–925.

40. **Zeidler, M., E. C. Johnstone, R. W. K. Bamber, C. M. Dickens, C. J. Fisher, A. F. Francis, R. Goldbeck, R. Higgo, E. C. Johnson-Sabine, G. J. Lodge, P. McGarry, S. Mitchell, L. Tarlo, M. Turner, P. Ryley, and R. G. Will.** 1997. New variant Creutzfeldt-Jakob disease: psychiatric features. *Lancet* **350:**908–910.

41. **Zeidler, M., G. E. Stewart, C. R. Barraclough, D. E. Bateman, D. Bates, D. J. Burn, A. C. Colchester, W. Durward, N. A. Fletcher, S. A. Hawkins, J. M. Mackenzie, and R. G. Will.** 1997. New variant Creutzfeldt-Jakob disease: neurological features and diagnostic tests. *Lancet* **350:**903–907.

*Emerging Infections 2*
Edited by W. M. Scheld, W. A. Craig, and J. M. Hughes
© 1998 ASM Press, Washington, D.C.

*Chapter 2*

# Hantavirus Pulmonary Syndrome in the Americas

## C. J. Peters

Hantaviruses have a worldwide distribution and result in severe public health problems by causing hemorrhagic fever with renal syndrome (HFRS) in many areas of Asia and Europe. More recently the hantaviruses of the Americas (Table 1; Fig. 1) are being recognized as a numerous and growing group of rodent-borne viruses that cause a disease called hantavirus pulmonary syndrome (HPS). The American viruses all belong to the genus *Hantavirus* of the family *Bunyaviridae*. They result in chronic inapparent infections in their specific rodent reservoir and have both genetic and antigenic similarities. There are differences in epidemiology, which seem to be related mainly to the habits and geographic distributions of the hosts and in the clinical syndrome, although the diseases have all been identifiable as HPS. There are recent general reviews of hantaviruses (32, 92, 122, 141, 142) and their molecular genetics (129), but this chapter emphasizes some of the recent findings in the Americas.

## DISCOVERY OF HPS AND SIN NOMBRE VIRUS

Hantaviruses belong to four phylogenetic and antigenic groups corresponding to the phylogeny of their reservoirs (30, 140, 148, 176). These include viruses from three subfamilies of the rodent family Muridae (Fig. 2): Arvicolinae (voles), Murinae (Old World rats and mice), and Sigmodontinae (New World rats and mice). The fourth group is represented by a single virus, Thottopalayam virus, thought to be a shrew or insectivore virus rather than a rodent virus. Progress in discovery of new hantaviruses was slow because of the difficulty in isolation of these agents. Only two hantaviruses were known in the Americas before 1993: Prospect Hill virus from the meadow vole *Microtus pennsylvanicus* and Seoul virus from the Old World rodent *Rattus norvegicus* (180). Neither Prospect Hill virus nor other related

---

*C. J. Peters* • Division of Viral and Rickettsial Diseases, National Center for Infectious Diseases, Centers for Disease Control and Prevention, Mail Stop A26, 1600 Clifton Road, Atlanta, GA 30333.

**Table 1.** Hantaviruses of sigmodontine rodents in the Americas

| Rodent reservoir | Name of virus[d] | Disease | Disease distribution (references) |
|---|---|---|---|
| Akodon azarae | Pergamino | Not known | 94, 95, 97 |
| Bolomys obscurus | Maciel | Not known | 94, 95, 97 |
| Calomys laucha | Laguna Negra | HPS | Paraguay, Bolivia (46, 80, 174) |
| Oligoryzomys chacoensis | Bermejo[b] | Not known | 94, 95, 97 |
| Oligoryzomys flavescens | Lechiguanas | HPS | Central Argentina (94, 95, 96, 97, 119, 120) |
| Oligoryzomys longicaudatus (southwestern Argentina[a]) | Andes | HPS | Argentina, Chile (18, 43, 89, 100, 101, 171, 156) |
| Oligoryzomys longicaudatus (northwestern Argentina[a]) | Oran | HPS | Northwestern Argentina (34, 97) |
| Oligoryzomys microtis | Rio Mamore | Not known | 7, 69 |
| Oryzomys palustris | Bayou | HPS | Southeastern United States (17, 85, 87, 110, 157, 158) |
| Peromyscus leucopus (Atlantic coast[a]) | New York | HPS | Eastern United States (13, 66, 67, 146) |
| Peromyscus leucopus (central plains[a]) | Blue River | Not known | 109 |
| Peromyscus maniculatus ("grassland" form[a]) | Sin Nombre | HPS | United States and western Canada (26, 39, 41, 112, 114, 187) |
| Peromyscus maniculatus ("forest" form[a]) | Monongahela | HPS | Eastern United States (147) |
| Reithrodontomys megalotis | El Moro Canyon | Not known | 63 |
| Reithrodontomys mexicanus | Rio Segundo | Not known | 62 |
| Sigmodon alstoni | Caño Delgadito | Not known | 51 |
| Sigmodon hispidus (eastern form[a]) | Black Creek Canal | HPS | Southeastern United States (16, 56, 130, 134) |
| Sigmodon hispidus (western form[a]) | Muleshoe[c] | Not known | 132 |
| Unknown | HU39694 | HPS | Argentina (95, 97) |
| Unknown | Juquitiba | HPS | Brazil (36, 76, 164) |

[a]Different geographic forms or races of several rodent species in the table may actually represent phylogenetically distinct subspecies or even species. Taxonomy is under revision.
[b]Bermejo hantavirus lineage is closely related to Lechiguanas virus.
[c]Muleshoe hantavirus lineage is closely related to Black Creek Canal virus.
[d]Some of these agents are closely related and may not be considered separate species in the future.

vole hantaviruses (142) have been associated with human disease in the Americas, although Puumala virus from the bank vole causes HFRS in Europe. Seoul virus infection from contaminated laboratory rats or from wild rats in Asia is common and is associated with HFRS. Although Seoul virus is widely distributed in rats in the Americas (32, 91, 122, 162, 168, 169), the disease has been infrequently recognized (57, 61).

In 1993 an epidemic of unexplained adult respiratory distress syndrome in the southwestern U.S. was serologically linked to hantaviruses (88). This finding led to the use of reverse transcription and PCR (RT-PCR) to detect and analyze viral

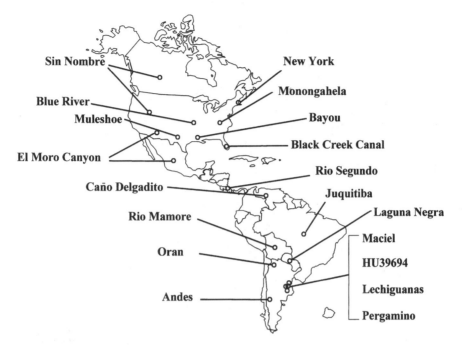

**Figure 1.** Recognized hantaviruses associated with sigmodontine rodents. These are provisional viral species and may be revised in the future. The dot indicates site of identification, but the potential range of the viruses will depend on the distribution of the rodent host (compare SNV in Fig. 4). (Courtesy of Jim Mills.)

RNA directly in clinical specimens and rodent material, circumventing the need for laborious cultivation in the description of the agent (112). The disease was found to be a new clinical entity (39, 108), HPS, caused by a previously undiscovered virus, Sin Nombre virus (SNV) (41) with the deer mouse (*Peromyscus maniculatus*) as its reservoir (26). SNV is the prototype of a group of viruses associated with sigmodontine rodents, and this viral phylogenetic group is uniquely linked to HPS (10, 112, 113) (Fig. 1 and 2).

## HOW DO WE IDENTIFY AND CLASSIFY HANTAVIRUSES?

Subsequently, many hantaviruses have been found using this same approach with modification of the original PCR primers (Table 1; Fig. 1). Positive indirect fluorescent antibody (IFA) tests had been reported from several North American rodent species for more than a decade, and additional testing has provided even more candidates for RT-PCR testing (180). Once the presence of a novel virus is inferred by finding phylogenetically distinct genetic sequences, the agent is customarily named for a geographic feature of the site where it was initially identified. Unfortunately, many of these viruses are known only from a limited amount of genetic sequence information, perhaps only a few hundred of their 12,000 to 13,000 nucleotides. Nevertheless, limited genetic fragments have usually yielded the same

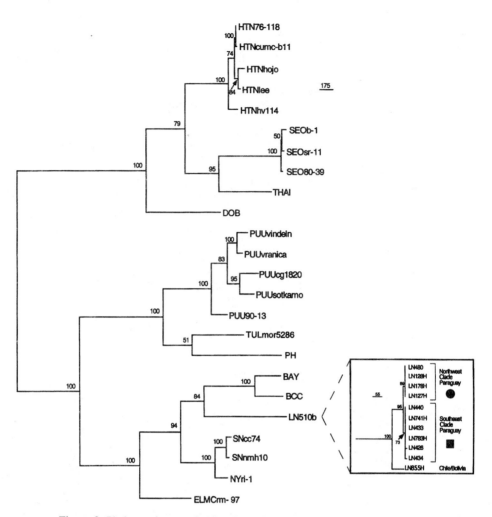

**Figure 2.** Phylogenetic tree of rodent-borne hantaviruses derived from maximum parsimony analysis of the open reading frame on the M RNA segment that codes for the glycoprotein precursor, GPC. The viruses are all associated with rodents in the family Muridae. The upper branch shows Hantaan (HTN), Seoul (SEO), Thailand (THAI), and Dobrava (DOB) viruses from rodents of the subfamily Murinae; these are known only from Europe and Asia with the exception of Seoul virus which has a worldwide distribution with the spread of its reservoir, *R. norvegicus*, from its origins in Asia (91). The middle branch has Puumala (PUU), Tula (TUL), and Prospect Hill (PH) viruses from rodents of the subfamily Arvicolinae or voles; these are present in Europe, Asia, and the Americas. The lower branch contains Bayou (BAY), Black Creek Canal (BCC), Laguna Negra (LN), Sin Nombre (SN), NY (New York), and El Moro Canyon (ELMC) viruses from American rodents of the subfamily Sigmodontinae. The inset shows a magnified analysis of Laguna Negra isolates based on a smaller RNA fragment amplified from tissues of humans and rodents. Note the distinctly different LN855H strain from a Chilean patient thought to be have been infected in Bolivia. The LN855H virus differs from the Paraguayan viruses by 16% of the 521 nucleotides examined, but has a 100% identical predicted amino acid sequence. The sigmodontine hantaviruses often show a pattern of much greater variation of nucleotides than amino acids, both within and among virus species. (From reference 80.)

classification of the viruses when compared to the complete gene segment (80, 110, 113, 130, 140, 148) or to serology (29, 30). Each of the three RNA segments comprising the virus genome also give the same phylogenetic relationships (80, 98, 130, 148). There is evidence for reassortment of RNA segments among the same viral species in the field (60, 98, 135, 138) and in the laboratory (133) but it appears that stable interspecific reassortment is restricted among the viruses examined to date, and recombination has not been incriminated as a source of genetic variability.

The use of phylogenetic analysis alone has limitations even though it is an exceedingly powerful technique to infer the evolutionary history of the viruses. There are no established limits of variation that define a viral species, and some of the viruses that are named in Table 1 may eventually not be considered as independent species. For example, amino acid sequences of the M segments of Sin Nombre and New York viruses differ by only 4.3% (see "Vaccines" below) (67, 109, 147). If one compares the available sequence of 381 amino acids from the M segment of Monongahela virus to that of other SNV variants, one also sees how close these viruses are: there is a 2.9 to 3.4% difference from New York virus and a 4.7 to 5.5% difference from Blue River virus. Strains of each of these viruses clearly define different lineages, but are they different viral species? Similarly, the viruses from *Oligoryzomys* species in South America are closely related (97). Lechiguanas virus (*Oligoryzomys flavescens*) differs from the proposed Bermejo virus (*O. chacoensis*) by only 1.6% in the amino acid sequence coded by the fragment of the M segment analyzed and from Andes virus (*O. longicaudatus*) by 4.6%. Interestingly, Andes virus in southern Argentina and Oran virus in northern Argentina share *O. longicaudatus* as their putative reservoir species; the two rodent populations are disjunct and may represent different subspecies as has usually been the case when one rodent apparently is associated with two hantaviruses.

The usual approach to zoonotic viruses such as arthropod- or rodent-borne viruses is to isolate viral strains from patients and from nature and then to compare the resulting virus isolates by serology (the neutralization test usually provides the most specific results) (155). In addition, viruses are tested by inoculating candidate vectors and reservoirs in the laboratory to demonstrate that they are competent to maintain and transmit the virus in nature (124). This approach has led to a useful paradigm that has generality: neutralization tests, repeated isolation from a given reservoir/vector, and the behavior of the virus when inoculated in the natural hosts are congruent and unequivocally identify different virus species.

The Old World hantaviruses have shown the correlation of serology with host association, and in addition their genetic sequences have agreed (30, 140, 142, 176). Only a handful of New World hantaviruses have been isolated from rodents of the Sigmodontinae subfamily: SNV (41, 138) and Black Creek Canal (134), Bayou (87), Caño Delgadito (51), New York 1 (146), and Laguna Negra (80) viruses. Limited examination by neutralization tests has correlated with the phylogeny and the usual reservoir (29). The hantaviruses are not only difficult to isolate but also, for reasons not well understood, infectious virus content is not readily quantified in human or rodent tissues and secretions (27). This has limited the studies on virus excretion by natural reservoirs (52, 93, 179), and only a single study has been performed on sigmodontine-derived hantaviruses (75); the findings of chronic infection and virus excretion in the implicated natural reservoirs have provided confirmation of the biologic plausibility of the virus-host pairings which had been suggested by virus isolation and identification of viral sequences in rodent tissues.

In most instances the individual viruses identified by genetic sequences have each had a single defined rodent host, although when transmission rates are high there has been spillover into other species (24, 26, 107, 135).

## HOST RELATIONSHIPS OF HANTAVIRUSES

The regular geographical patterns of genetic variation of a given virus and the correspondence of virus and rodent phylogeny are strong evidence for coevolution of these parasites with their hosts over millions of years (109, 112, 113). This general relationship predicts that cross-species transfers should be uncommon and generally epidemiologically ineffective. These are very old viruses, and their emergence reflects recognition on the part of the biomedical community.

A few viruses are under intensive study to define their ability to adopt alternate hosts in shorter term situations. For example, Monongahela virus has been found in several *P. maniculatus* captured in areas where *P. leucopus* does not occur. It has also been found in *P. leucopus* in zones where the ranges of the two rodents overlap, suggesting the possibility that the virus may be able to use a closely related host. Similar suggestive data exist for Dobrava virus, an Old World hantavirus that is thought to be primarily associated with *Apodemus flavicollis* but which may also utilize the primary Hantaan virus host *Apodemus agrarius* in or near areas of rodent reservoir overlap (6, 166).

The taxonomy of rodents presents many problems, just as does the taxonomy of viruses. The mitochondrial DNA of *Peromyscus* rodent species was analyzed with an immediate need to correct the significant misidentification of *P. maniculatus* and *P. leucopus* that occurs even by museum-trained crews collecting specimens for hantavirus genotyping. Of course, it was also a goal to identify subspecies of rodents and correlate those with virus genotypes; this was achieved and the data for *P. leucopus* have provided remarkable insights (109). These data confirm the biological specificity of viruses for their host species and subspecies (Table 2), but they also suggest that host switching between closely related species may occur rarely. This event was inferred by finding that a virus associated with *P. leucopus*, the New York virus (66, 67, 146), was phylogenetically more closely related to *P. maniculatus* viruses such as the Monongahela virus from *P. maniculatus nubiterrae* (147) or even SNV itself (109). The divergence may well have begun 10,000 years ago, at the end of the last ice age in New England.

This should not be interpreted to mean that viruses readily move back and forth between rodent hosts; the stable and characteristic genetic constitution of viruses repeatedly found in the same host are inconsistent with this view (Fig. 2). A vivid example is provided by SNV and Prospect Hill virus. They are phylogenetically quite distinct (Fig. 2), as are their respective sigmodontine and arvicoline hosts (113, 129, 176). The home ranges of both these rodent species have overlapped for centuries without virus crossover. In fact, Prospect Hill virus is more closely

**Table 2.** HPS recognition in South America

| Location | Virus | Year of cases | Year linked to HPS | Transmission | Circumstances |
|---|---|---|---|---|---|
| Brazil (Juquitiba) | Juquitiba | 1993 | 1993 | Family cluster | Clinicians plus capacitated national laboratories and reference laboratories (35, 76, 113, 164) |
| Argentina (Salta Province, northwestern area [Salta and Jujuy provinces]) | Oran | 1984–1993 | 1994 | Endemic | Local clinicians recognize new pulmonary syndrome before definition of HPS; later, capacitated national laboratory confirms (34, 96, 97) |
| Argentina, central area (Buenos Aires and Santa Fe Provinces) | Lechiguanas | 1988–1992 | 1994 | Sporadic | Aggressive hemorrhagic fever surveillance; capacitated national laboratory (95, 96, 119, 120) |
| Paraguay (western) | Laguna Negra | 1995 | 1995 | Epidemic | Recognized by local clinicians; reference laboratory (80, 174) |
| Argentina and Chile | Andes | 1993–1995 | 1995 | Sporadic | Clinicians plus capacitated national laboratories and reference laboratory (89, 100, 101) |
| Argentina, (southern area [Rio Negro, Nequen, and Chubut Provinces]) | Andes | 1996 | 1996 | Epidemic | Clinicians plus capacitated national laboratories (43, 95, 116, 117) |
| Chile (southern zone) | Andes | 1997 | 1997 | Epidemic | Clinicians and referral of samples to capacitated regional and reference laboratories (18, 33, 156) |
| Uruguay | Unknown | 1997 | 1997 | Small number of reports | Clinicians and referral of samples to capacitated regional laboratories (117a) |

related to viruses such as Puumala and Tula viruses, which are associated with Eurasian arvicolines.

Infection of the rodent is thought to have no important effects on fitness of the host to reproduce and survive in nature. Overt illness has not been described, although there is one report of minor histologic changes. Five wild-caught, sero-positive *Peromyscus leucopus* mice were found to have lymphohistiocytic infiltrates in the portal zones of the liver, reminiscent of those seen in human HPS. They were also said to have edema of the alveolar septae of the lung as well as hyper-chromasia of the nuclei of the alveolar lining cells or type I pneumocytes (103). Nevertheless, seropositive *Peromyscus maniculatus* mice were found to be capable of the same maximum exercise limits as seronegative animals (115). Furthermore, in field studies using capture-mark-release techniques, seropositive deer mice sur-vive as well as their seronegative counterparts (1, 136) and no effects of Seoul virus were found on survival, growth, or fertility of urban rats (23).

Although the tissue sites of virus replication have been defined for Hantaan and Black Creek Canal viruses in their natural reservoirs (75, 93), the immunologic means by which viruses persist in their rodent hosts are unknown. Hantaviruses produce lifelong infection in their reservoirs, but they do not result in prolonged or persistent virus circulation in the blood as do many members of the arenavirus family (44). There is a humoral immune response with neutralizing antibodies produced, and concurrently virus disappears from the circulation. It is possible that virus avoids serum neutralizing antibodies as it is shed on mucosal surfaces by directional maturation across epithelium as has been demonstrated in some in vitro cell culture systems (131); similarly, the mechanisms by which an effective im-munoglobulin A (IgA) response is evaded and infected cells escape cytotoxic T cell lysis are not understood (5, 42).

The application of new methods of virus detection and the incorporation of viral genetic information into the classical virus species paradigm (140, 155) has led to a situation in which knowledge of new viruses, disease potential, reservoir host(s), and classification of the American hantaviruses has advanced enormously in the last 5 years but in which there remain a substantial number of unanswered questions.

## SEROLOGICAL CROSS-REACTIVITY AND DIAGNOSIS OF AMERICAN HANTAVIRUSES

The most commonly used serological tests are the IFA test and more recently the enzyme-linked immunosorbent assay (ELISA). Both tests are moderately cross-reactive and thus are useful in screening for previously unidentified viruses as well as for diagnosis of a spectrum of known viruses. For example, the discovery of the sigmodontine rodent viruses was based on cross-reactive serological tests using antigens prepared from both the Arvicolinae and Murinae rodent associated hanta-viruses (88). The cross-reactivity between arvicoline viruses (such as Prospect Hill virus) and viruses from rodents of the subfamily Sigmodontinae (such as SNV) is high, whereas the viruses from rodents of the subfamily Murinae cross-react with SNV less well, as might be expected from their more distant phylogenetic relationship (Table 2). The IgM ELISA must be run in the IgM capture format to avoid the problems associated with other IgM tests.

The IFA test may be unreliable at lower titers and require confirmation, particularly in serosurveys of asymptomatic rodents or humans (162). It has largely been supplanted by the ELISA, which is more objective and more readily standardized and has fewer false-positives as well as greater sensitivity. All of the known American sigmodontine rodent hantaviruses elicit antibodies that react in both IgM capture and IgG ELISAs using SNV antigens (47, 88). There are minor differences in reactivity in the IgG or IgM ELISA tests and the signal strength is slightly higher with sera from some North American and South American viruses when tested on homologous as compared to SNV antigens.

The virus neutralization test is relatively specific but does have some cross reactivity among phylogenetically related viruses (29, 30, 90, 140, 176), and diagnostic results on early sera can be misleading (102). It is too time consuming and difficult to perform for routine diagnostic use.

Western blot tests with recombinant antigens have been developed to provide rapid and specific diagnostics (65, 79). Other serological tests which have been applied to the diagnosis of hantavirus infections include focus reduction, inhibition of the naturally occurring viral hemagglutinin, passive hemagglutination, inhibition of antigen accumulation in microtiter wells, high-density particle agglutination, and several ELISA formats (30, 88, 102, 140, 142, 160). Particularly notable are focus reduction, which eliminates the need for plaques when performing neutralization tests with these difficult agents, and hemagglutination inhibition, which has not been used with American hantaviruses but which is an inexpensive and rapid technique (102, 160).

Virus isolation is not practical for diagnosis, and indeed there are no human isolates of any of the New World hantaviruses. RT-PCR usually detects viral RNA in sera or blood clots for the first 7 to 10 days of illness (68). Although sensitive primers for RT-PCR amplification of sigmodontine hantavirus genetic sequences from rodent or human tissues have been designed (80), optimum sequences are often different among the viruses, particularly in clinical specimens in which RNA concentrations are generally lower. Immunohistochemistry has been particularly valuable in confirming the etiological relationship of SNV to HPS (112), in establishing the pathogenesis of HPS (187), and in retrospective diagnosis of cases (185); it seems to be broadly cross-reactive if appropriate monoclonal and polyclonal antisera are used judiciously (142).

In the experience of the Centers for Disease Control and Prevention (CDC), the best approach to HPS diagnostics is to employ an IgM capture ELISA, which is virtually always positive on the first sample available from a patient and has an exceedingly low rate of false positives (88). We also test for IgG antibodies using a recombinant SNV antigen (47). There is no need to use the local strain of virus. The different sigmodontine-derived viruses are quite closely related at the amino acid level. The dominant antigen in diagnostic ELISAs is the nucleocapsid protein, and the nucleocapsid proteins of these viruses share at least 81% amino acid identity. When individual virus nucleocapsid proteins are compared at the amino acid level, SNV is quite close to the New York virus (93.5%) and also to Bayou (86.9%),

Andes (86.0%), and Laguna Negra (85.4%) viruses. South American viruses are even more closely related to one another; for instance, Laguna Negra and Andes virus nucleocapsid proteins are quite closely related, with 90.5% amino acid identity (111a). All sera from HPS patients infected with a heterologous virus have been positive with SNV antigens, but some of the South American viruses may give slightly higher optical density with an antigen such as Laguna Negra virus (86a). RT-PCR is useful for genotyping viruses but is expensive and cumbersome for routine diagnosis, and cross-contamination must be guarded against.

In the case of rodents, we use serology exclusively to monitor infection. Occasional rodents will be RT-PCR positive and antibody negative (8, 112) but this does not affect interpretation of rodent infection prevalence importantly. Indeed, antibody screening is useful to select the rodents one wishes to investigate further for analysis of the species of viral RNA present. Once the rodent-virus relationships are established, identification of the rodent species and seropositivity are enough. If epidemiologic linkage is sought, then sequencing of RT-PCR products from many rodents and patients may be needed in a particular investigation (8, 70, 116, 117). In addition, we always sequence PCR products to exclude the possibility of contamination.

## HOW WERE ADDITIONAL AMERICAN HANTAVIRUSES DISCOVERED?

In the United States the publicity surrounding the 1993 outbreak in the Southwest resulted in intense interest by the medical system. Availability of a special hotline over 6 months resulted in 21,443 calls and submission of 280 samples from patients suspected to have HPS from outside the initially involved states; 21 confirmed cases were found and they included the samples yielding Bayou (17), Black Creek Canal (16), and New York viruses (13, 154). Additional cases continue to be added to a nationwide registry of HPS cases maintained by CDC (Fig. 3).

Hantavirus infection had been suspected in Argentina and Brazil by IFA-based serosurveys of rats (104, 127) and humans (127, 169, 170) in the 1980s, and the presence of Seoul virus in several cities of South America was established by antibody studies supplemented with isolation of the virus from a rat captured in Brazil (90). Indeed, studies of laboratory rats (168) and animal caretakers (169) in Argentina found high-titered neutralizing antibodies that strongly suggested infection of the laboratory rats with transmission to humans. Tests of field rodents, mainly using Hantaan antigen in the IFA test, gave inconclusive data suggesting the possibility of infection (168), but studies of hemorrhagic fever suspects using ELISA and IFA produced evidence of acute human hantavirus cases with renal involvement (119).

After the association of SNV with the newly described HPS (39, 112), an intensive education campaign was undertaken in the U.S. to disseminate information on recognition and prevention of the syndrome (12, 181). The presence of a rodent-borne disease with high mortality in the United States required prevention guidelines for ordinary citizens (12), virus laboratory workers (14), and rodent workers (15, 106). Presentations at major meetings such as the Interscience Conference on

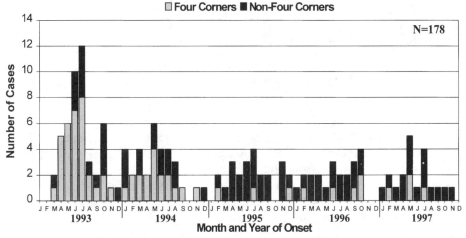

**Figure 3.** HPS in the United States showing secular trend. The epidemic was recognized in the Four Corners states in 1993, and there was increased transmission there in 1994 as well. More recently a greater proportion of cases have occurred in other states. There is a tendency for greater transmission in summer months, but cases are seen all year. (Courtesy of Joni Carson.)

Antimicrobial Agents and Chemotherapy and outreach by providing diagnostic reagents to selected laboratories reached physicians and virologists working in many areas of South America and led to recognition and laboratory confirmation of cases of HPS in several countries (10, 120, 174). Because of the limited infrastructure for low-temperature preservation of samples, formalin-fixed material for immunohistochemistry (IHC) was often an important element in the diagnosis.

Laboratories with an interest in rodent-borne hemorrhagic fevers (119, 120), thoughtful clinicians (34, 89), targeted searches for hantaviruses (90, 94, 95, 170), and local epidemics (11, 43, 174) were among the routes to recognition (Table 2). On balance, the key element is usually the clinician (Table 2). Two of the sites recognized an unusual clinical syndrome before the 1993 HPS outbreak in the U.S.; one was a mixed etiology outbreak including leptospirosis (34) and the other eventually provided the first recognition of Andes virus (89, 100).

These historical facts provide an empirical basis for planning future surveillance in other areas of South America. When well-trained, alerted clinicians in a given area begin to suspect HPS as a diagnosis in their patients and submit samples for testing, those samples can efficiently be examined in regional or international reference laboratories. If positive results are obtained, this demonstrates both a potential public health problem and an embryonic surveillance system. Provided that there is sufficient infrastructure, the situation becomes ready for transfer of ELISA diagnostic technology and reagents. The addition of RT-PCR to the laboratory armamentarium is optional, provided the local infrastructure will fully support that technology. RT-PCR is not needed to diagnose HPS but is desirable in selected situations to ascertain which virus(es) is causing human disease and to answer selected research questions. RT-PCR is useful only when coupled with DNA sequencing of the products because of the need for genetic information to interpret the resulting product and exclude contamination.

## EPIDEMIOLOGY OF AMERICAN HANTAVIRUSES, PARTICULARLY SIN NOMBRE VIRUS

The epidemiology of all hantavirus infections is basically that of rodent infection, rodent virus shedding, and rodent-human contact. This apparently simple equation is in fact quite complicated and poorly understood. Large rodent population surges may lead to hantavirus epidemics, and there are several examples of this relationship (11, 32, 111, 121); however, systematic studies correlating rodent population size, rodent infection prevalence, and human disease are lacking.

In general, rodents carrying a given hantavirus will be infected wherever they are found (32, 122, 141). For example, in North America the deer mouse (*P. maniculatus*) is found to be infected over most of its range (105, 107) whenever a sufficient number of rodents is sampled to yield a good estimate of seroprevalence. Infection prevalence will, of course, vary with age, sex, season, population density, intraspecific and interspecific competition, and climate. However, there are remarkable differences in prevalence of infection that are not readily explained. For example, positive animals have not yet been obtained from Alaska. In the Channel Islands off the coast of California, seroprevalence as high as 58 to 71% was found on some islands, but others had no positive rodents among the 37 to 91 animals tested from each island (78).

In the southwestern U.S., the number of deer mice trapped and their seroprevalence varies with ecologic zone, and pinyon juniper forest at an average altitude of 1,980 m was a prolific zone (107). This is important since many humans reside in rural sites in this zone and many of the 1993 and 1994 cases came from that area (Figs. 3 and 4). It may be possible to map risk of infection at an even finer resolution within that biome by applying remote sensing with high-resolution Landsat thematic mapper images (21).

Of course, in any given location there are many variables that may be important in human risk. The average deer mouse seroprevalence in a number of large studies is around 10%, but the findings in the southwestern United States during the 1993 epidemic were around 30% (26, 107). This was attributed to the crowding of the rodent populations. This intuitive proposition may be true when the number of animals is very high, but formal studies have failed to demonstrate a relation at usual rodent densities (1, 36, 40, 78, 107). In preliminary analyses of short-term data, these studies regularly find asynchronous changes in deer mouse and other rodent populations at sites that are geographically near to one another. In these same studies, it was difficult to predict changes in seroprevalence based on population density. Infection prevalence may decrease as newly weaned animals join the general population. The antibody prevalence may rise as rodent numbers fall because of adverse conditions: newly weaned, seronegative animals are not forthcoming as breeding decreases and older, seropositive animals retreat to preferred habitats (1, 56) and persist without adverse effects of their infection. Important new

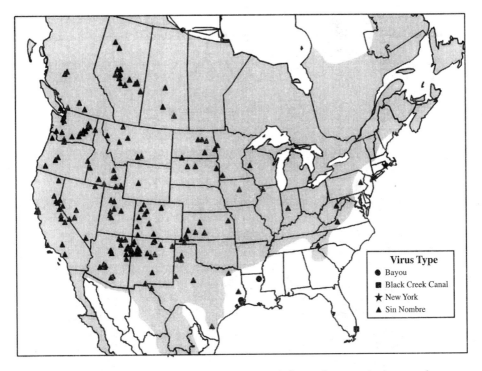

**Figure 4.** HPS in North America. Shaded area indicates the recognized range of the deer mouse, *Peromyscus maniculatus*, and triangles identify cases known or thought to be from SNV. Infections acquired outside the range of the deer mouse are caused by other viruses. (Courtesy of Joni Carson; rodent distribution is from reference 9a.)

information is expected to arise as rodent populations are increasing in the Four Corners area (the area where Colorado, Utah, New Mexico, and Arizona meet) because of the excessive rains and unusually warm winters following the El Niño conditions in 1997 (183).

New infections can be traced in these field studies of free-living rodents repeatedly captured and released; some animals first become RT-PCR positive in blood samples, then are simultaneously RT-PCR and antibody positive, and finally have only antibodies in their blood samples (8); correlates of infectivity for humans and other rodents are lacking in these field studies, but laboratory studies (52, 75, 93, 179) suggest that the period soon after infection is the most dangerous in terms of shedding virus in urine and throat swabs, as well as for transmission when caged with susceptible rodents.

One important epidemiological aspect of rodent behavior is their relation to humans. The significance of rodent behavior for human disease is well documented for the rodent-borne arenaviruses (44), but these interactions are equally important for hantaviruses. The propensity for deer mice to enter houses was an important rodent behavior in determining the risk of HPS; in the southwestern United States in 1993, more deer mice than house mice were trapped inside buildings (26). Systematic studies of rodent behavior and interactions with human dwellings are usually eschewed in favor of ecological research in undisturbed environments, leading to a knowledge gap that needs to be corrected (55). For example when radiotelemetry is combined with other techniques, deer mice can be shown to adopt buildings that furnish food and repeatedly enter them although trap capture rates do not reflect this (37).

Of course, many infections will occur outdoors, particularly in more rural lifestyles and with other rodents that may not enter houses as readily as the deer mouse. For example, in the SNV epidemic in the United States in 1993, 17 of 32 (53%) cases were female, but the overall figures for 1994 to the present are only 37/99 (37%) female. The figures for Andes virus in Chile also show a male preponderance with 75% male patients (156), as do those for Argentina (120). Interestingly, 9 of 16 (56%) patients in the Andes epidemic involving person-to-person transmission were women (171).

Infection among rodents is mainly from combative encounters often associated with bite wounds (24, 26, 54, 56, 107), but transmission to humans is probably largely from small-particle aerosols (122, 161, 180). There may be a risk equation in which recently infected rodents (often younger and male) are the major danger to humans because of their greater virus excretion, and infections of longer duration with lower-titered virus in secretions are important in the more intimate and direct setting of bite wounds of competing rodents. This differential could also explain the apparent paradox of finding many infected rodents but relatively few human cases (122). The hantaviruses are the only group of the hemorrhagic fever viruses that do not have a recognized mechanism for tightly coupled vertical transmission (124). It has been suggested that mites could be involved in hantavirus ecology (159), but no credible laboratory evidence has been presented to support this idea (93).

The best-studied American example of HPS epidemiology is that of SNV infection. In the case of SNV, entry of the reservoir, deer mice, into human habitation and sparsely used outbuildings is thought to be important (3, 26). Infected rodents are often trapped in case households, and comparison of genetic sequences may strongly suggest that the rodents are the source of the human virus infection (26, 27, 70, 80, 112, 174). A case control study in 1993 showed that the major risk factor for disease was the number of rodents trapped in and immediately around the household using a standardized protocol (189). There was no evidence of focality of rodent infection, and indeed infected rodents were often found in or very near control houses. Presence of rodent harborage around homes had no statistically significant relation to the risk of human infection (25). The other significant findings mainly related to a rural life style and included peridomestic cleaning activities and agricultural pursuits. There was an excess of Native Americans among the early U.S. HPS patients, probably due mainly to their rural lifestyle in biogeographic zones favorable to the deer mouse reservoir, although genetic susceptibility and other factors have not been closely examined. Subsequent experience is consonant with these findings: the people who are infected are usually exposed to infected rodents during their home activities in rodent-infested houses and outbuildings, as a consequence of their occupation, or during recreational activities (83).

The capricious nature of infection of the individual (in contrast to the overall risk to a population) is exemplified by a study of mammalogists (3). Less than 1% of professional biologists who handled thousands of known hantavirus reservoirs had antibodies reactive with SNV antigens, and only a single person had an illness history consistent with HPS. Only one person knew of a fatal case of HPS in another rodent worker, and that case had already been retrospectively diagnosed at CDC. Yet, the CDC HPS case registry contains several field biologists, reflecting the low but definite risk of infection and the high case fatality of HPS. A study in the southwestern United States among those thought to have some occupational risk for hantavirus infection found no hantavirus antibodies among 494 persons sampled (190). This emphasizes the difficulty inherent in preparing guidelines for occupational and other potential exposures to hantaviruses.

## PERSON-TO-PERSON TRANSMISSION OF HANTAVIRUSES

Strong evidence has established that hantaviruses in Europe and Asia are not transmissible from human to human, and the same pattern has emerged in the United States. During the 1993 epidemic of HPS, no case of disease or of sero-conversion was observed among hospital workers, including those performing re-suscitation on patients (167). Nevertheless, chains of apparent interhuman spread were observed in 16 of 20 patients in an Andes virus outbreak in southern Argentina in 1996–1997 (43, 116, 117, 171, 177, 178). Epidemiological observations established that the spread was plausible; a case-control study identified contact with another case rather than with rodents as a major risk factor; ecological studies showed the absence of substantial numbers of reservoir rodents or of rodent sign within houses; and molecular genetic studies demonstrated a close similarity of the viral genome among patients tested. There is little room for doubt that person-to-person transmission occurred, particularly to a physician infected by a patient who had traveled to the capital city many miles from the area of endemicity. The mechanism of spread was not established, but close contact was present in all cases, and the most common period of contact seemed to be before or shortly after hospitalization. No evidence of hantavirus infection was found when 126 health care workers from one of the two towns involved or 13 clinically normal household contacts of patients were tested for antibodies (172). In a 1997 Chilean outbreak, no compelling evidence implicating interhuman transmission of Andes virus was found in spite of a lack of precautions by health care workers (18, 19).

These findings prompted a review of the U.S. case registry at CDC (173). Among 160 confirmed HPS patients in North America, 5 clusters comprising 12 persons with illness occurring within 8 weeks of one another were identified. In three instances rodent trapping showed infected *P. maniculatus* to be present, and the other two had been sleeping and working in a rural environment in which rodent infestation was noted. Contacts of 40 HPS patients have been tested for antibodies; only six of 320 had evidence of recent infection, and these were among the clusters identified from the registry. Four had IgG antibodies and one (also included in the clusters) had a retrospective diagnosis of HPS. Although five health care workers were among the patients in the 1996 Andes virus epidemic (171), only one patient in the U.S. registry had a medically related occupation, and this nurse had evidence of rodent droppings in her home; retrospective chart review found no indication that she had cared for a patient with adult respiratory distress syndrome or HPS. Interhuman transmission of most hantaviruses must be exceedingly rare if it occurs at all.

The problem of interhuman transmission of Andes virus will not be easily resolved by future research. An integrated medical, epidemiological, ecological, pathogenetic, and genetic approach is needed. Some comments on each part of the approach follow.

1. Field epidemiology is absolutely essential to the process. Only a firsthand, carefully collected description of a large number of Andes virus index cases and their contacts will provide the basic information needed for interpretation of events.

2. Study of the rodents present and their proximity to humans will be needed, but infected rodents may be present and not highly infectious (75), confounding the situation. Rodent sampling will always be delayed by the incubation period of the index case (typically 1 to 4 weeks). Unless a prospective plan is in place, it will be further delayed until the putative secondary cases are recognized and often delayed even longer by communication and logistic restraints. Furthermore, the presence of large populations of infected rodents will make interpretation of the epidemiological data difficult. For example, in the case of Bolivian hemorrhagic fever, interhuman transmission was not suspected during early town-based epidemics because of the presence of so many rodents and such frequent rodent transmission of the causative arenavirus. Only when rodent-transmitted disease was minimized by control of the reservoir within towns was it possible to see the relatively frequent interhuman transmission of the disease (44).

3. Molecular biology will be helpful but will not entirely resolve the routes of infection because of the inherent genetic properties of hantaviruses. There is a high natural error rate in all RNA polymerases so that movement of a hantavirus to another selective milieu such as a different host can readily select for small differences in genotypes. Furthermore, the selective pressures on rodent viruses within a small geographic area will tend to stabilize a relatively narrow genotypic spectrum. This will make it difficult to reliably genetically differentiate between transmission from a small genetic pool of viruses in the resident rodents from spread from rodent to an index case and then to a secondary case. These difficulties are compounded by the need to have a large number of virus genotypes from

the region to assess the diversity of the virus and by the possibilities for rodents to enter or leave the suspected areas of transmission between the infection events and the necessarily delayed sampling of the reservoir fauna.

4. One approach would be to study the virology of the patient and attempt to quantitate virus excretion in different situations. Although this approach has been used to assess risk from several hemorrhagic fevers (123), it is even more limited when applied to hantaviruses. Hantaviruses are usually difficult to isolate and more so to quantitate from primary material. Thus, secondary measures such as quantitative RT-PCR will be needed as surrogate markers for infectious virus excretion. Although there has been some correlation between these values in experimental systems, particularly where virion-sense RNA was measured, there are disparities, and more work is needed (75). In particular, SNV RNA has been detected in bronchoalveolar lavage and in blood, but there is no evidence to suggest contagiousness (68, 173). The current situation is similar to the use of hepatitis B antigen as a surrogate for hepatitis B virus infectivity.

5. Careful pathological examination, including ultrastructure and immunohistochemistry of well-preserved materials, may yield clues to the pathogenesis of Andes and other hantaviruses that would be helpful in understanding why interhuman transmission may have occurred in a particular episode.

A major question facing clinicians is what to do about personal protection and patient isolation. Until systematic observations resolve the uncertainties as to transmissibility, the reasoned answer to those likely to be faced with HPS cases caused by the "new" viruses is to employ the recommended universal precautions. The occurrence of other diseases such as pneumonic plague should prompt respiratory precautions until a definitive diagnosis is made. In South America, a private room is advisable if available, and additional respiratory precautions may be desirable (118). It seems likely that some time will be needed to ascertain whether the 1996 epidemic of Andes virus in Patagonia represents a unique event or a pattern for Andes virus; either of these outcomes is consistent with the findings with another group of rodent-borne viruses, the arenaviruses (44). It is important to know whether to anticipate frequent interhuman transmission of such a lethal disease because the administration of intravenous ribavirin to contacts at the first sign of fever would be a therapeutic modality worth investigation. Although ribavirin did not have marked effects when given to HPS patients with SNV infection (20), its use with the earliest observable clinical signs could well have greater benefit.

## CLINICAL PICTURE OF SIN NOMBRE VIRUS INFECTION

SNV is the commonest cause of HPS in North America, and more than 150 cases have been recognized. The few cases of New York or Monongahela virus infection recognized are indistinguishable from SNV infection. The clinical presentation of HPS following SNV infection is highly characteristic and differs from that of other overwhelming respiratory diseases (39, 86, 108). The early recognition of cases is, however, difficult. A prodrome of fever, myalgia, and malaise lasting 4 to 6 days (as short as 1 day or over a week in some cases) precedes the onset of pulmonary edema. Nausea, vomiting, and/or abdominal pain are often present and may mimic a surgical abdomen. Dizziness is surprisingly common in HPS as compared to other diseases (108) and has even been a dominant clinical feature in occasional SNV or Juquitiba virus infection (35, 76, 84, 113, 164). This may have an experimental counterpart in the invasion of the labyrinth of experimentally inoculated rats and guinea pigs by Seoul virus (151). Findings that have not been associated with SNV infection are coryza, prominent cough at the onset of illness, facial flushing, and conjunctival suffusion.

The cardiorespiratory phase is ushered in by progressive leakage of high protein fluid into the pulmonary interstitium and alveoli with accompanying hypoxemia, tachypnea, and tachycardia. Patients may have presented for medical consultation earlier because of the severity of their constitutional symptoms and been sent home with a lack of objective findings. At this stage of illness, there is usually some combination of tachycardia, tachypnea (remembering that this measurement is often not taken or assumed to be normal and so noted), fever, and mild hypotension. Reports of auscultation of the chest have often indicated only a few rales or other unimpressive findings.

Radiography of the chest is typical and very helpful in the differential diagnosis, with a progression from subtle interstitial findings such as peribronchial haze and Kerley B lines through frank bilateral alveolar edema; normal findings or asymmetrical involvement occasionally occur briefly during the early stages (81, 108). Pleural effusions are usually present. Thrombocytopenia is almost universal and provides an important clue to look more carefully for HPS, whether screening patients with only fever and myalgia (143), working with patients in the emergency room with a differential diagnosis of influenza or pneumonia (108), or dealing with adult respiratory distress syndrome (108) cases, or even comparing suspected HPS to confirmed HPS (38). Unfortunately, the thrombocytopenia may not be found on initial presentation. A recent review of admission clinical laboratory values of adult respiratory distress syndrome (ARDS) patients suspected of HPS found that thrombocytopenia and hemoconcentration were independent statistical predictors of HPS even though both values might be normal in any given HPS patient (38). Every patient with a platelet count less than 150,000/mm$^3$ and a high-normal or elevated hematocrit (>49) had HPS, although 47% of HPS patients did not meet this criterion. A left shift (with normal or elevated leukocyte count) and atypical lymphocytes are usual but similarly may not occur until the disease is well established and the patient is in mortal danger. The triad of thrombocytopenia, left shift (with circulating myelocytes), and circulating immunoblasts is very suggestive of HPS (86). Other common findings are hemoconcentration, hypoalbuminemia, metabolic acidosis, slightly elevated aspartate aminotransferase, elevated lactate dehydrogenase, and in severe cases lactic acidosis.

The kidney is usually not involved in a major way. There is often some proteinuria and abnormal urinary sediment, but azotemia is generally not inordinate considering the circulatory compromise. There is laboratory evidence of a coagulopathy with thrombocytopenia accompanied by abnormal partial thromboplastin time and sometimes a prolonged prothrombin time. Overt bleeding or evidence of disseminated intravascular coagulation is seen in a minority of cases (126, 187).

The differential diagnosis should include leptospirosis, rickettsial diseases, viral hemorrhagic fevers, and adult respiratory distress syndrome from any number of causes including mycoplasmas, pneumonic plague, and influenza A (38, 125). Inhalation anthrax may pursue a rapidly downhill course but should be relatively easy to exclude because it is usually a mediastinitis rather than a pneumonic process. Because of the possibility of several treatable diseases, antibiotic therapy which might include doxycycline should be undertaken until definitive diagnosis is established.

The disease progresses rapidly once the lungs begin to flood with high-protein, high-permeability edema fluid and death commonly ensues within 24 to 48 hours of hospital admission or even sooner. The immediate cause of death is hypoxia and/or circulatory compromise (59). Hypotension and shock represent an independent clinical problem because they occur even in patients whose hypoxemia is controlled by medical therapy. The cause of the circulatory collapse is not known, but the commonly seen pattern of low cardiac output, high systemic vascular resistance, and hypotension differs markedly from the findings in septic shock.

Treatment is supportive. Major elements are management of hypoxia, fluid balance, and shock. Respiratory difficulties may progress rapidly and demand hour-by-hour attention to blood oxygenation and regulation of inspired oxygen concentration; about two thirds of patients will require intubation and mechanical ventilation. Patients have major hemoconcentration from fluid loss into the lungs and pleural cavity, yet infused fluids will exacerbate the pulmonary edema. The amount of fluid resuscitation should be calibrated to maintain filling pressure to support the circulation; because of the capillary leak, monitoring often will require a pulmonary artery catheter to establish pulmonary wedge pressure. Shock is managed by correcting hypoxemia, maintaining cardiac filling pressure, and administration of inotropic agents (59). Fluids should be administered with particular caution and careful monitoring, and cardiostimulatory drugs may be indicated earlier in the course of disease than in conditions such as sepsis.

During the Korean War, steroids were felt to have a favorable effect on the outcome of HFRS, and a randomized trial supported this opinion to some degree (137). Later, a Chinese study showed little effect (129a). It is difficult to accept the utility of steroids in a different hantavirus disease, given the several clinical trials that have shown no benefits in septic shock and adult respiratory distress syndrome as well as the deleterious effects in cerebral malaria; a controlled trial would be needed in HPS (72). The antiviral drug ribavirin has had a positive effect in HFRS (74), and both Sin Nombre and Black Creek Canal viruses are sensitive in vitro (136a). Nevertheless, the clinical course of HPS proceeds more rapidly than that of HFRS and intravenous ribavirin did not have a marked effect on the course of HPS in open-label trials (20); the drug is under more careful evaluation in a randomized, double-blind trial sponsored by the National Institute of Allergy and Infectious Diseases in selected clinical research centers in the United States. Both extracorporeal membrane oxygenation and inhaled NO have been used in therapy, but there are insufficient data to evaluate their efficacy (86).

A search for mild disease during the 1993 epidemic (143) and among the household contacts of HPS cases (173, 189) indicates that most SNV infections result in HPS. Seroprevalence is also low among these groups and other normal persons (overall ~0.3%). The case fatality ratio has apparently been decreasing among reported cases after the discovery of the disease. More than half of those discovered in 1993 died, with a decline to about 40% in 1994 to 1996; of the 20 patients with confirmed cases in 1997, only 20% died.

Children are notably spared by SNV, an unexplained observation that has been made in other hantavirus diseases (9, 84). A 4-year-old child is the youngest known person to have an SNV infection, and he had very mild illness that would not meet the criteria for HPS (2). The national HPS case registry contains nine cases of patients under 18 years of age (ages 11 to 16 years, 6% of the total); clinical findings were similar to those in adults.

There is little experience with HPS in pregnancy; only two of five women delivered normal, uninfected infants, and both mothers had mild disease. The other three mothers were intubated, and one died; two suffered fetal death in utero, and the third bore a live premature infant who died at 6 months of age. One of the fetuses was negative for hantaviral antigens, and the premature infant had no serological evidence of active infection (53, 73).

## STATUS OF HPS IN DIFFERENT REGIONS AND COUNTRIES IN THE AMERICAS

Although most HPS cases in North America have occurred in the western United States and Canada, sporadic cases have been confirmed in several eastern states, including New York, Pennsylvania, Virginia, West Virginia, North Carolina, Florida, and Louisiana. Most cases are associated with SNV; the deer mouse (*P. maniculatus*) reservoir is most common in the western United States and Canada (Fig. 4). All investigated cases within the known range of the deer mouse have been caused by SNV or a closely related hantavirus such as Monongahela virus (Table 1). New York virus, also closely related to SNV, is associated with the white-footed mouse (*P. leucopus*), found mainly in the eastern and central United States. Bayou and Black Creek Canal viruses have been implicated as causes of HPS in the southern United States (Fig. 4).

No HPS has been recognized in Mexico, Central America, or the Caribbean. The deer mouse range extends into Mexico, and SNV has been identified in stored organs from deer mice captured in Baja California (182a). *Sigmodon hispidus* and other sigmodontine rodents believed to be potential hosts for hantaviruses are widely distributed south of the Rio Grande, but the only other definite evidence of hantaviruses in Mexico or Central America is the presence of viral genetic sequences amplified from a harvest mouse, *Reithrodontomys mexicanus*, from Costa Rica (Table 1) (62). The Caribbean habitats are so extensively disturbed and their normal rodent fauna has been extensively replaced by Old World rodents such as *Rattus* and *Mus musculus* that the sigmodontine species carrying the viruses likely to cause HPS may not be present.

Elsewhere in South America, HPS is being identified with increasing frequency, both in endemic and epidemic form (Table 3). I will discuss its epidemiology in different countries and then discuss some of the distinct properties of the individual viruses.

## Argentina

This country has yielded the greatest number of HPS cases and the largest array of hantavirus genotypes of any country in the Americas, perhaps reflecting established capability in zoonotic diseases and an active molecular biology capability. Serological studies using an ELISA with SNV antigen clearly identified human disease (96) and several rodent species with hantavirus infection (94), and later RT-PCR detected the genetic signatures of seven viral genotypes (95, 97, 100). Andes virus from *Oligoryzomys longicaudatus* is a common cause of HPS (95, 100), and other hantaviruses including the human pathogens Lechiguanas, Oran, and HU39694 as well as the less well characterized Pergamino, Maciel, and Bermejo viruses have been identified (95, 97) (Table 1). The four *Oligoryzomys*-borne viruses are closely related phylogenetically and come from related reservoirs; eventually they all may not be regarded as independent species.

Retrospective studies conducted with sera obtained from patients in the course of viral hemorrhagic fever surveillance in central Argentina detected 13 acute hantavirus infections, including four with classic HPS and nine initially referred to as HFRS but largely representing mild disease (120); some of these patients have been found to be infected with Lechiguanas virus (42a, 97). Later several HPS cases in the same temperate zone in the Pampas and nearby Parana River yielded viral sequences designated as Lechiguanas virus (96, 97). A total of 32 cases have now been recorded from Buenos Aires and Santa Fe provinces including retrospective cases dating from 1991 to the present (Ministerio de Salúd y Acción Social de

**Table 3.** Estimates of HPS cases identified in the Americas as of March, 1998, by country of infection[a]

| Country | No. of cases |
| --- | --- |
| Canada | 25 |
| United States | 179 |
| Total North America | 204 |
| Argentina | 142 |
| Bolivia | 1 |
| Brazil | 6 |
| Chile | 44 |
| Paraguay | 34 |
| Uruguay | 2 |
| Total South America | 229 |

[a]Adapted from reference 118.

Argentina, April 1998). Many or most are presumed to be Lechiguanas virus infections.

Further to the south in the cooler, high Andean forested zone, Andes virus has caused sporadic cases of HPS and an unusual outbreak with interhuman spread in 1996 (89, 100, 116, 117, 171). A total of 44 HPS cases are reported from the geographic area, including Neuquen, Rio Negro, and Chubut provinces (Ministerio de Salúd y Acción Social de Argentina, April 1998).

Oran virus is suspected to be the main causative agent of HPS in the northern subtropical region around Oran in Salta and Jujuy provinces near Bolivia (34, 96, 97). That region has reported 74 HPS cases from 1991 to the present (Ministerio de Salúd y Acción Social de Argentina, April 1998).

Additional information on the clinical features of infection with Andes, Oran, and Lechiguanas viruses is awaited. Five pediatric cases collected from southern, northern, and central areas of Argentina HPS activity have been reported in detail (128) and official figures include 12 cases younger than 14 years of age and 18 younger than 17 years (8% and 12% of the total, respectively) (Ministerio de Salúd y Acción Social de Argentina, April 1998). Most normal human populations sampled have had a low (<1%) seroprevalence against SNV antigen by ELISA (120, 172).

## Bolivia

Recently, a suspected HPS patient presented in Chile with epidemiological antecedents suggesting infection after travel in one of several regions of Bolivia (46). After detection of IgM antibodies with SNV antigen, genetic sequences implicating Laguna Negra virus were amplified from his serum by RT-PCR, and he had a typical course of HPS. RT-PCR has also obtained sequences from *Oligoryzomys microtis* trapped in Bolivia in 1985 and 1992, and the name "Rio Mamore virus" has been proposed for the virus inferred to be present (7, 69) (Table 1). Hantavirus antibodies have been detected in human survey sera (169).

## Brazil

Serological evidence of acute Seoul virus infection in suspected leptospirosis patients has been reported from Brazil (61), and IFA serological surveys have found human antibodies reactive with hantaviruses (77, 90, 127, 165). In 1993, active surveillance for hantavirus disease found a cluster of three cases, brothers in a single family residing near Juquitiba, São Paulo state (35, 76, 164). RT-PCR analysis of frozen and immunohistochemistry testing of fixed lung tissue confirmed that one of the infected brothers did indeed have HPS and a newly recognized virus (Juquitiba virus) was present (113, 184b). Since then, two fatal cases of HPS have been identified from other areas of São Paulo state and one from Mato Grosso state (35a). Nothing is known about the reservoirs. Extensive serosurveys with an ELISA using SNV recombinant antigen have shown a relatively low prevalence of antibodies in several areas of Brazil (35a).

## Chile

HPS was first recognized in Chile in 1995, and since that time a total of 44 cases have been reported, mainly in the southern region of the country (33, 118). A number of these, including an epidemic of 23 HPS cases occurring in southern Chile between August and December 1997, have been identified as Andes virus infections by RT-PCR and sequencing of tissues or blood samples (18, 101, 156). The epidemic corresponded to a surge in rodent populations, possibly a consequence of synchronous flowering of bamboo plants and the increased food supply for *O. longicaudatus* and other rodents (111). There has been no reported nosocomial transmission (19) or definitive evidence of interhuman spread (18, 156), but several interesting clinical differences from SNV infection were noted (153, 156) (see "Andes virus" below). IgG ELISA antibodies reactive with SNV were found in 2 to 13% of local residents (163).

## Paraguay

In 1995, an outbreak of 17 confirmed cases of HPS occurred in the Paraguayan Chaco, and an additional six patients were also identified (174). The outbreak was thought to be related to unusually heavy rainfall leading to increased rodent populations. The most common rodent remaining at the time of the postoutbreak investigation, *Calomys laucha*, also had the highest hantavirus antibody prevalence and was later implicated as the reservoir of the agent causing the epidemic, Laguna Negra virus (80).

Antibodies reactive with SNV antigens were frequently found in asymptomatic persons. Among a convenience sample of area residents 21% of 127 Indians, 7% of 94 Paraguayans, and 10% of 89 Mennonite settlers were seropositive. The high prevalence of antibodies to hantaviruses has been confirmed in Indians living in the Gran Chaco region of Paraguay; using an immunoblot assay 40% of 193 were positive and in nearby Salta Province of Argentina 18% of 212 reacted (48). It is difficult to interpret such antibody results in asymptomatic people. Certainly they imply the existence of a hantavirus with low pathogenicity for humans. This raises the possibility that Laguna Negra virus could have a milder course in many infected persons, perhaps influenced by the genetic constitution of the exposed host. However, another equally likely interpretation is that other hantaviruses of low pathogenicity are present and infecting humans.

The problem in interpreting the results of these serosurveys can be understood from the nature of the tests. The IgG ELISA using SNV antigen detects antibodies in sera following infection with all known sigmodontine derived hantaviruses and also many sera from arvicoline-derived virus infections and even some sera from murine rodent hantavirus infections. Additional specificity could be obtained by testing against all local virus serotypes, but we do not know how many there are nor are the agents available for test antigens. The unavailability of a battery of local virus isolates would also frustrate the application of the neutralization test. Similar considerations would apply to other approaches with recombinant subunit antigens. None of the available tests have been validated with multiple serial human sera tested against an ensemble of relevant hantaviruses, nor does such a collection of sera exist.

## Peru

The varied ecological zones of Peru undoubtedly harbor many different sigmodontine rodents with their hantaviruses. No disease has yet been identified, although antibodies are found in several rodent species and in humans (154a). A virus, as yet unidentified, has been isolated from rodents collected in Iquitos (50a).

## Uruguay

Two HPS cases have been diagnosed; genetic sequences suggest that the virus is closest to Lechiguanas virus (115a). Hantavirus antibodies have also been reported in asymptomatic humans (169).

## Venezuela

Surveys undertaken with rodent sera obtained for arenavirus surveillance have indicated widespread hantavirus infection of the rodent *Sigmodon alstoni*, the reservoir of the Guanarito arenavirus. The Caño Delgadito hantavirus has been isolated from these rodents but not yet been associated with human disease (51). *Sigmodon alstoni* is widely distributed over the llanos and is common in the tall grass around human habitation and agricultural areas, making it a potentially dangerous virus carrier.

## CLINICAL AND EPIDEMIOLOGICAL FINDINGS IN HPS CAUSED BY OTHER VIRUSES

Less information is available on the clinical manifestations of human infections with other American hantaviruses derived from sigmodontine rodents (Tables 1 and 2; Fig. 1), but several basic elements of HPS as found in SNV infection recur with every virus studied and provide the basic definition of HPS:

1. Pulmonary edema. It begins as an interstitial process and develops into frank alveolar involvement with pleural effusions, usually accompanied by early manifestations of tachypnea, shortness of breath, and hypoxemia. Hemoconcentration is present secondary to the vascular leak.
2. Cardiovascular depression. In milder cases there is mild hypotension and tachycardia which might be attributed to hypovolemia and/or hypoxia, but in more advanced or more severe cases there is shock which is out of proportion to other abnormalities and persists even if hypoxemia and filling pressure are normalized. When studied, there has usually been myocardial depression and elevated systemic vascular resistance.

3. Thrombocytopenia is universal. Bleeding is not usually seen. There is often a prolonged PTT, but prothrombin time abnormalities or evidence of disseminated intravascular coagulation are not common.
4. Immune activation is evidenced by atypical lymphocytes in the blood and the presence of activated germinal centers in lymphoid tissues of fatal cases.
5. Leukocytosis or at least a left shift in the polymorphonuclear neutrophil series is present and often accompanied by such immature cells as myelocytes on the peripheral smear.

However, some notable differences from SNV infection have been found with several viruses (Table 4). Possible areas of differences include the degree of renal involvement, the extent of vascular instability manifest as cutaneous flushing and conjunctival injection, muscle involvement as assessed by serum creatine kinase levels, occurrence of childhood disease, and spectrum of disease severity. There is no reason, based on our knowledge of other hantaviruses, to think that there would be major variations in pathogenesis within a single virus species found in different areas of the Americas, but that supposition (or any assertion to the contrary) requires documentation. Some of the reported manifestations may reflect differences in observation or in host response as well as actual variations in pathogenic potential of the hantavirus. Furthermore, surveillance is different in each area. For example, based on findings during the 1993–1994 epidemic, sporadic cases in the U.S. are routinely tested for acute hantavirus infection only if they meet the surveillance case definition for HPS (11) which detects the vast majority of SNV infections (2, 143). During different hantavirus outbreaks, asymptomatic patient contacts and febrile patients with a variety of manifestations may be tested with positive (18, 153, 156) or largely negative results (143). In central Argentina, where Lechiguanas virus is active, patients were initially sought using a surveillance definition appropriate to Argentine hemorrhagic fever so that fever, thrombocytopenia, and hemorrhagic phenomena were emphasized (120).

## Bayou Virus

Soon after the recognition of SNV and the new clinical syndrome of HPS, samples from a suspicious case in Louisiana indicated hantavirus infection (17). RT-PCR of postmortem tissues was used to analyze the genome and establish that the causative agent was a newly recognized hantavirus related to but clearly distinct from SNV (110). Because the infection occurred outside the range of the deer mouse (Figure 4) and clinical features were atypical, an on-site investigation was performed with the state health department and local physicians. The patient was a bridge inspector with several potential sites of exposure to rodents.

His clinical course was complicated and occurred on a background of preexisting disease (85, 149). He was admitted initially for evaluation of fever, vomiting, weakness, and dizziness of 2 to 3 days' duration with normal white cell count, platelets, blood urea nitrogen, creatinine, arterial blood gases, urinalysis, and chest X ray as

**Table 4.** Clinical features of hantavirus infections[a]

| Virus | Location and yr | Clinical findings |
|---|---|---|
| Andes | Argentina, 1996 | Case fatality ratio, 10/20 (50%) |
| | | Flush of head and neck, 32%; conjunctival injection, 42% (43, 171) |
| Andes | Chile, 1997 epidemic; sporadic | Case fatality ratio, 18/33 (54%) |
| | | Additional four mild or asymptomatic infections found in investigation of 23 cases of HPS |
| | | Six HPS patients <17 yr of age (26% of epidemic and 18% total) |
| | | Petechiae and hematuria more common than in SNV cases (18, 45, 153, 156) |
| Bayou | Louisiana, Texas, 1993–1996 | Case fatality ratio, 1/3 |
| | | Renal failure; no hemodialysis |
| | | Mild increase in serum creatine kinase (17, 64, 85, 110, 149, 157) |
| Black Creek Canal | Florida, 1993 | Case fatality ratio, 0/1 |
| | | Renal failure; no hemodialysis |
| | | Modest elevation serum creatine kinase (16, 82, 130) |
| Juquitiba | Brazil, 1993 | Case fatality ratio, 2/3 |
| | | Two classic HPS cases |
| | | One case with extensive vertigo (35, 76, 113, 164) |
| Laguna Negra | Paraguay, 1995 | Case fatality ratio, 2/23 (8.7%) for confirmed cases |
| | | Case fatality ratio, 10/34 (29.4%) for confirmed and presumptive cases (80, 174) |
| Lechiguanas | Argentina, 1988–1998 | Some cases classic HPS; others milder, less typical; minor bleeding common |
| | | Many cases detected by Argentine hemorrhagic fever surveillance, others during HPS surveillance (97, 120) |
| Oran | Argentina (Salta Province), 1984–1998 | Endemic |
| | | Clinical data under review |
| | | Leptospirosis also present (34, 97) |
| HU39694 | Argentina | Single fatal case; site of infection unknown (97) |

[a]Most reported cases were typical of SNV infection, but variations were found in some cases.

well as mild hypertension. However, by the second hospital day he developed leucocytosis, thrombocytopenia, and rising blood urea nitrogen. The third day found him in shock, oliguric, hyperamylasemic, and with full-blown ARDS and disseminated intravascular coagulation. He died on the fourth hospital day with a serum creatinine level of 7.4 mg/dl. It appears that this patient was in the late prodrome of HPS when admitted to the hospital and demonstrates the rapid progression that is possible with the disease. The cause of the renal failure is unclear, but probably is part of the infective process; on the third hospital day the patient was reported to be passing scanty, concentrated urine in spite of intravenous hydration, even before an intravenous contrast computed tomography study was undertaken to evaluate his obtundation. Postmortem examination revealed the expected changes with only tubular necrosis found in the kidneys.

Two other Bayou virus-associated cases of HPS have occurred in Texas with seropositivity and diagnostic RT-PCR genetic typing (64, 157). Both resided in and worked outdoors in areas with drainage ditches and swampy habitats. Their clinical courses were typical of SNV infection except for mild renal failure. The second patient had clear-cut renal involvement with a creatinine rising from 1.9 to 3.6 mg/dl before returning to normal and a urinalysis showing 2+ protein and microscopic hematuria. The third patient had a transient creatinine increase from 0.6 to 1.9 mg/dl and 300 mg of urine protein per dl. Both had mildly elevated serum creatine kinase levels of 1,171 and 917 U/liter, respectively, but neither had muscle edema, discolored urine, pronounced muscle tenderness, or other signs that would suggest clinically significant rhabdomyolysis, particularly that could have led to the renal failure. The abnormal skeletal muscle enzymes may reflect direct viral involvement or cytokine effects on muscle.

While Bayou virus' clinical picture does appear to differ from that of SNV it is worth bearing in mind that about one fifth of non-Bayou, non-Black Creek Canal HPS cases in a preliminary examination of the case registry had a creatine kinase above 1000 U/ml or a maximal serum creatinine that exceeded 2.0.

Bayou virus is associated with the rice rat (*Oryzomys palustris*) (15, 87, 157, 158), which is restricted to the southeastern United States and is a nocturnally active resident of moist or swampy grassland habitats (175).

## Black Creek Canal Virus

This virus was recognized as the cause of an acute HPS case in southern Florida as part of U.S. national surveillance (16). Only one human infection has been identified. At the time of admission following a 4-day prodrome the illness was typical of SNV infection, except that elevated serum creatine kinase levels (maximum of 5,427 U/ml on day 9 of illness), proteinuria, microscopic hematuria, and azotemia were already present (82). The patient's course was uneventful, with extubation after 12 days and discharge 5 days later. He did not have oliguria, red urine, or any clinical evidence of a bleeding diathesis at any time during his illness; his admission serum creatinine level of 4.6 mg/dl reached a maximum of 4.7 mg/dl by the next day and on day 7 was normal.

The patient customarily spent late afternoons on the edge of a local grassland with scattered brush, a common habitat for the cotton rat (*Sigmodon hispidus*), the rodent that yielded an isolate of Black Creek Canal virus (134). This was a unique hantavirus by phylogenetic and antigenic criteria. Black Creek Canal virus RNA was detected in all 13 seropositive cotton rats captured near the site of the index case's infection, and the fragments of the genomes sequenced were closely related (130).

One interesting feature of the HPS patient's immune response was the failure to develop IgM antibodies against SNV, although high-titered IgG ELISA antibodies were present on admission (82). A convincing pattern of IgM and IgG antibodies to the homologous virus was demonstrated after its isolation. Black Creek Canal virus and SNV cross-react immunologically at the level of all three major structural virus proteins (nucleocapsid, N; glycoprotein 1, G1; glycoprotein 2, G2) although quantitative differences with SNV G1 and G2 were easily demonstrable when naturally infected rodent or human sera were tested (130). There are eightfold or greater differences in the cross-neutralization titers of the single Florida Black Creek Canal virus-infected human and SNV patients (29).

The cotton rat is a common inhabitant of grasslands of the southeast and south-central United States, Central America, and northern South America. However, hantavirus antibodies have been found almost exclusively in Dade County, Fla. (56, 105). In Dade County, the overall seroprevalence in *Sigmodon hispidus* is 11%, but the distribution of infected cotton rats was focal, perhaps reflecting congregation of older infected males in more favorable habitats (56). The closely related Muleshoe virus (132) was identified in cotton rats from the western part of their range, and these rodents may well represent a different taxon.

## Juquitiba Virus

Identification of a cluster of three cases in Juquitiba, São Paulo State, Brazil, in 1993 was the first confirmation of a suspicion that sigmodontine rodents in South America would be reservoirs of hantaviruses causing HPS (35, 76, 113, 164, 184a). The first patient identified, who suffered a mild illness with brief hospitalization, was unusual: he presented with fever and true vertigo without prominent systemic manifestations noted in the record.

The other two cases were very similar to one another and were classic examples of severe HPS. They reached a primary care facility with complaints of fever, malaise, myalgia, and shortness of breath. The second patient, 3 days after the index case, was found to have extensive bilateral infiltrates on chest X ray, somewhat surprising the attending physician. This led to his admission to a rural hospital and the administration of multiple antibiotics and intravenous fluids to correct the dehydration inferred from the gastrointestinal upset and the elevated hematocrit. By the next day he was dead from fulminant HPS. The third patient entered with similar complaints 13 days after the index case with X-ray findings and laboratory data resembling those of his brother, resulting in his referral to a tertiary care hospital. A similar sequence of events ensued with a fatal outcome.

The latter two patients exemplify the pitfalls and dilemmas of treating HPS. Neither appeared to be mortally ill on presentation, but chest X rays were indicative of a severe bilateral process. Both had findings such as fever and hemoconcentration that would lead the clinician to suspect the need for aggressive fluid therapy which combines with the fluid load often associated with administration of broad spectrum antibiotics to aggravate the pulmonary edema, perhaps inevitably so. The second patient was cared for in a rural health care center without radiologists, pulmonary specialists, critical care specialists, or intensive care units, which is the typical setting in which HPS presents.

Three of 49 contacts of the initial case cluster were found to have hantavirus antibodies (188). The reservoir of Juquitiba virus is as yet unknown. Preliminary studies have not identified antibody-positive rodents in the area where the cases occurred.

## Andes Virus

Andes virus has been associated with sporadic cases of HPS as well as clusters of disease. The first clinical recognition was in 1993 in Argentina with typical cases of HPS (89) leading to serological diagnosis and detection of the virus by RT-PCR and sequencing of tissue and blood samples (50, 96, 100, 101).

Interestingly, two of the six original cases were in a single family, and 2 of 25 family contacts were seropositive. One of these seropositive contacts was a 9-year-old girl with mild febrile disease and high IgM titers, probably representing an acute Andes virus infection without HPS (89, 128). A different member of the same family was in the first trimester of pregnancy when she had mild HPS but later delivered a normal-term infant with no serological evidence of hantavirus infection. Another woman who died of presumed Andes virus infection with a clinical diagnosis of HPS nursed her 7-month-old baby who was found to be hantavirus antibody positive at 15 and 33 months of age, raising the question of breast milk transmission.

From September to December 1996 an epidemic of Andes virus infection took place in southern Argentina (43) with 16 of the 20 identified HPS cases having an epidemiological link (171, 177) and representing person-to-person transmission of the virus (see "Person-to-Person Transmission of Hantaviruses," above) (116, 117). The clinical picture of the disease resembled SNV except that conjunctival injection and cutaneous suffusion of the head and neck were prominently commented on by attending physicians. Azotemia was not common or marked, nor was bleeding. The case fatality ratio was 50% (171). In the epidemic area of southern Argentina in 1996, only 3 persons were found to have hantavirus antibodies in a randomly selected serosurvey of 294 residents of El Bolson, and no additional seropositives were encountered among the total of 517 persons examined (172).

In Chile an epidemic of HPS caused by Andes virus occurred in July to December 1997 and provided another opportunity to study the consequences of human Andes virus infection. Six of the 23 cases (26%) in the epidemic were children less than 17 years of age, and three of them had petechiae, including one with a frank bleeding diathesis. One pregnant woman suffered disseminated intravascular coagulation, and both she and her fetus died.

When additional sporadic HPS cases of presumed Andes virus infection from Chile were compared to the epidemic cases, the only notable difference was the absence of children in the sporadic sample. Renal failure, flushing, conjunctival injection, and clinically evident bleeding (beyond the three children noted above and three adults with microscopic hematuria) were not features (45, 152, 153, 156). The mortality rate among the combined 33 cases was 54%.

Among 13 patients admitted to a single hospital, more intensive observations were possible, and the similarities to SNV infection were evident with the exceptions of the presence of children with HPS, frequent finding of cutaneous petechiae, uniform presence of petechiae on organ serosa at postmortem examination, and frequent pharyngeal congestion. All patients had platelet counts below $52,000/mm^3$ (153). Interestingly, nadir platelet counts less than 50,000 were found in only about half of U.S. HPS registry patients and half of the patients from Argentina with Andes virus infection. Early admission and treatment with large doses of steroids were thought to be associated with improved survival (153), but this suggestion is not supported by controlled data or statistics and requires testing by a randomized trial before acceptance (72).

During the epidemic investigation, blood samples were taken from 53 contacts of 14 patients. Two had evidence of recent or ongoing infection as evidenced by IgM antibodies; one was asymptomatic, and the other was suffering from mild febrile disease (no pulmonary symptoms and normal chest X ray) and clearly did not meet the case definition for HPS. Another asymptomatic contact had only IgG antibodies as evidence of infection in the distant past (156). In other surveys of sick persons, two IgM positive patients were found without evidence of HPS and with normal chest X rays.

Three family clusters were observed in the epidemic (156). In one group, all four members became ill within 5 days of one another and represent a commonly described phenomenon in hantavirus diseases, probably caused by a common source exposure to unusually infectious rodent(s).

In another rural cluster, the index patient became ill on 15 July 1997; his family departed to a small town 7 km away and never returned to the original home site after 27 July. His wife became ill on 2 August, 2-year-old son 7 days later, and 12-year-old son 16 days after his mother. The brother-in-law resided intermittently at the original home site and became ill on 4 September. All genetic sequences of a RT-PCR fragment of the M RNA segment were identical among members of the cluster tested and differed from several other clusters or cases tested. Although interpersonal transmission can be suspected, the cluster fails to convince for three reasons. (i) The epidemiology is consistent with all being infected from rodents at the original home site. (ii) A rodent irruption was taking place at the time. For example, trap success in the area was around 50% (the number of traps catching rodents divided by the number of traps set). Typical trapping forays in temperate climates during summer months have widely varying figures but most often are around 10%; during the 1993 epidemic in the southwestern U.S., figures of 20 to 30% were typical. For comparison, trap success in and near the towns in southern

Argentina in 1996, when interpersonal spread occurred, was 1 to 2%, and the highest success was at a distant park with 15%. Thus, there was ample opportunity for infection from rodents. (iii) Molecular biology will eventually add more information as more sequence data are obtained from cases and possibly from rodents. But without knowing more about the genetic variability in the rodents to which the family was exposed, it is impossible to conclude definitively that the same virus was spreading among family members. Trapping at the original home site was done more than 2 months after the index case's illness and yielded eight *O. longicaudatus*, of which one was seropositive. The new home site had been extensively treated with poison baits. (iv) No samples from the index case were studied for virus excretion. (v) No human tissues were collected in suitable condition for an ultrastructural search for virus particles.

Cases in one husband-wife pair were very suggestive of interhuman transmission. The man apparently became infected in a rural area and returned home already ill. Sixteen days later, his spouse was sick. She had not left the center of a city of 60,000 during the previous year and had not sighted any rodents, and the *O. longicaudatus* reservoir of Andes virus enters cities only exceptionally. When sequence banks for the virus strains in the area are constructed, it may be possible to make a better inference in this pair, but meanwhile one must ask if the wife might not have been exposed unknowingly to a reservoir brought into the city, perhaps in the market.

Among 319 health care workers, 3.7% had IgG ELISA hantavirus antibodies, and there was no difference among those caring for HPS patients or in the precautions taken (19). In urban residents of a town in the epidemic area, 2% of 144 normal persons had reactions in the IgG ELISA using cross-reactive SNV antigen, whereas samples of about 100 persons from each of three rural communities had a seroprevalence of 5.6 to 13.1% (163). The caveats for interpreting the seroprevalence as subclinical Andes virus infection are the same as those which apply to the interpretation of the Paraguayan data noted above (pages 39 and 40).

## Laguna Negra Virus

Most of our information about this virus comes from a single outbreak in Paraguay in 1995 (174). The clinical picture was typical of SNV infection, as was that of a single case infected in Bolivia and cared for in Chile (46). In the outbreak investigation 34 probable cases were identified, but samples were available for only 24; 23 of the 24 were confirmed. Among the 10 not available for testing, there were eight fatal cases without tissue for immunohistochemical antigen detection. The case-fatality ratio was only 8.7% for confirmed cases, but because of the unavailability of blood or tissues for postmortem confirmation of fatal cases, one might include all those patients meeting the case definition, which would give an overall figure of 29.4%. Thus, it is unclear whether the actual case fatality for this virus is lower than for SNV or, more likely, not very different.

Four of 27 (15%) household contacts of HPS patients were seropositive, and all were contacts of patient 1. In addition, 12.8% of 345 community residents were seropositive. (See "Paraguay" [pages 39 and 40] for pitfalls in interpretation.)

Rainfall had achieved a 10-year record high in May 1995 before precipitation returned to its usual low levels in June through September; the epidemic occurred from July 1995 through January 1996. No objective measurements were made of rodent populations, but local residents reported increases in rodent sightings during the epidemic. The dynamics may have been a consequence of increased rodent numbers resulting from the rainfall (water being a likely limiting factor in rodent populations in the plains of the chaco, either directly or through their food supply) followed by the dryer harvest season which would bring humans into greater contact with rodents and speculatively might lead to increased movement of rodents into proximity to humans. In any case, at the time of the investigation of the epidemic, evidence of rodent traffic was found in most of the homes examined, and the home of case one yielded four antibody-positive *Calomys laucha* mice. *C. laucha* was the commonest rodent trapped (22 of 78 total) and constituted five of the six antibody-positive rodents taken. Later, Laguna Negra virus was isolated from and identified in tissues of several *C. laucha* mice as well as human tissues from the outbreak (80).

*C. laucha* is a common savanna rodent with a northward extension from southern Brazil and Bolivia extending south throughout much of Paraguay and Uruguay and reaching Rio Negro province in southern Argentina. Interestingly, *C. laucha* and Laguna Negra virus furnish one of the few examples of a rodent host apparently not uniformly infected over its range. Frozen sera from almost 2,000 *C. laucha* mice collected during Argentine hemorrhagic fever studies yielded only three hantavirus seropositives, suggesting that Laguna Negra virus does not occur in populations of *C. laucha* from central Argentina (97a).

## Lechiguanas Virus

This virus has been identified with 11 cases of HPS in central Argentina (97). The spectrum of disease has not yet been defined, although it includes mild cases detected only as part of Argentine hemorrhagic fever surveillance. Some patients presented only fever, constitutional symptoms, thrombocytopenia, and proteinuria. The reservoir *Oligoryzomys flavescens* is a common rodent in central Argentina and also occurs on the island of Lechiguanas in the Parana river where a number of cases have occurred among nutria hunters and trappers.

## PATHOLOGY AND PATHOGENESIS OF AMERICAN HANTAVIRUSES

Hantavirus diseases leave relatively little histopathological evidence of cellular damage except in the kidneys, anterior pituitary, and right atrium of HFRS patients (186). In the case of HPS caused by SNV, the most important morphological findings are in the lungs, which are typically heavy with edema fluid and surrounded by pleural effusions. Microscopically they show marked edema, modest hyaline membranes, and an interstitial lymphocytic infiltrate with activated macrophages present (114, 187). Hemorrhage occurs but is not common, and diffuse alveolar damage is only seen in the minority of patients who die more than 2 weeks after onset (187). There are infiltrates in the portal triads, and lymphoid tissues are activated.

The pathogenetic features of hantavirus infections that lead to HFRS or HPS are thought to be mainly a consequence of the immune response to the viruses (88, 126). The viruses are not destructive to cells they infect in vitro, and indeed endothelial infection with SNV does not lead to increased permeability (150). Serious disease occurs at or shortly after initiation of the immune response. HPS patients suffer the sudden onset of massive high permeability pulmonary edema usually without hemoptysis; if they survive 24 to 48 hours, most will recover and leave the hospital within 10 to 14 days (39, 59). This clinical and pathological picture suggests a functional derangement in pulmonary microvascular permeability rather than a necrotizing process. In the case of HPS, the lung microvascular endothelial cells stain extensively for hantaviral antigens; definite but minimal staining for viral antigens is present in endothelial and other cells elsewhere in the body (187). Antigen is also extensively present in the germinal centers of the lymphoid system.

The lungs are notable for their content of T lymphocytes; $CD8^+$ cells are particularly prominent. These cells presumably reflect those circulating in peripheral blood of the patient early in the course of the disease and often identified as atypical lymphocytes (86, 114); they can be cultivated and cloned to yield $CD8^+$ lymphocytes suitable for analysis (42). A likely simplified scenario for pathogenesis of the disease is production of cytokines by activated, antigen-specific T lymphocytes which act directly on endothelial cells or in turn activate macrophages for cytokine elaboration. Human SNV-specific T-cell clones produce large amounts of gamma interferon when stimulated in vitro, and that cytokine as well as others are found in the serum of HPS patients (144, 145). Presumably as the acute immune activation decays, endothelial cells regain their integrity, and the patient improves.

Relatively little is known about the pathology and pathogenesis of infections with sigmodontine-derived hantaviruses other than SNV and the material that has been studied is insufficient to yield definitive conclusions. Preliminary histopathological and immunohistochemical examination of material from Bayou, Juquitiba, and Andes virus cases suggests a very similar pathogenesis as SNV but with a need for more specimens to allow proper analysis of the variations found (85, 174, 184c). For example, several Andes virus cases have shown much more extensive alveolar macrophage antigen presence than is seen in SNV infections (156, 184c).

## PREVENTION OF HPS

The control of the rodent reservoirs of these viruses in nature is simply not practical. An important measure of protection can be obtained by excluding rodent hosts (such as the deer mouse) that readily enter houses (12). Rodent-proofing of rural cabins can be achieved for approximately $400 and results in 85% or more reduction of rodent entry in field testing (55, 71). In addition, strategies can be devised to avoid known risk factors for HPS such as opening seasonally unoccupied cabins (3) or cleaning rodent-contaminated areas (12). It is likely that known risk factors for HFRS such as sleeping on floors, sleeping outdoors, threshing, and cleaning vacation homes are also risk factors for HPS and should be avoided (32, 125).

Because HPS occurs every year and in every part of North America, health education plays an important role in providing each citizen with the tools to protect against infection in different settings and activities (181). The educational efforts must be directed to the cultural and educational groups in the greatest risk areas. Once the epidemiology of HPS is better understood in South America, there may be important target populations for educational efforts.

Once a case occurs, there are a series of public health actions that follow and the opportunity to work through these state-by-state in the United States has been helpful in knowing how to begin in South America where most of the same considerations have come up. There is a need to support the family, particularly given the attendant publicity and the possibility of stigmatization of the survivors. There is specific, sensitive advice to be given concerning trapping and cleaning the residence or suspected site of infection. If Andes virus is suspected, there is a need to monitor close contacts and counsel them to immediately seek medical evaluation if fever develops. Finally, it is necessary to work proactively with the press to be sure the community receives an accurate and helpful message: the disease is uncommon even in epidemics and rodent avoidance measures can lessen the chances of infection even further. The national press is also useful in preventing untoward effects on tourism and exports from the affected region.

It is possible that we will be able to identify additional particularly risky human activities or dangerous rodent infection situations through continuing human epidemiological studies or ecological work with rodent populations. One such predictive factor could be the weather. The 1993 epidemic in the southwestern United States came after two consecutive El Niño events (121), and the current El Niño condition has been associated with increasing rodent populations in regularly monitored sites in the same geographic area (40). An effort is being made to reinforce multicultural health education efforts in the southwestern United States to prevent increased disease if this becomes a risk in the spring and fall.

Nevertheless, it seems unlikely that persons living, working, or playing in a rural or suburban environment will be able to entirely avoid virus exposure. Furthermore, in many areas of the Americas populations at risk are too poor to construct the appropriate housing to avoid rodent exposure or are engaged in agricultural occupations that will always bring them into contact with potentially infective rodents.

## VACCINES

Hantavirus vaccine development faces some formidable tasks. There is no animal model of HPS or HFRS to measure attenuation or to study possible immunopathological interactions with vaccines. In the absence of a realistic experimental analogue, one can nevertheless obtain a measure of protection by measuring antigen or RNA accumulation in some hosts as a surrogate (28, 139). With Hantaan virus, monoclonal antibodies can either neutralize virus or mediate immune enhancement (182). Initial efforts to develop inactivated or vectored vaccines for Hantaan and Seoul viruses have met with some success but require further evaluation and refinement (22, 139, 184). These vaccines would not be expected to be protective against arvicoline- or sigmodontine-associated viruses.

It is impractical to develop vaccines against each of the known HPS agents. However, cross-protection among the sigmodontine rodent viruses is a theoretical possibility. If a single immunogen could be used for special at-risk populations and for situations with unusually intense virus circulation, immunoprophylaxis of HPS could be practiced much as it is for meningococcal disease with selective vaccination. A cross-protective immunogen is not without some basis in our current knowledge of hantavirus immunology. For example, Seoul virus and Hantaan virus differ by up to 23% at the amino acid level in their glycoprotein precursor (GPC), the precursor of the viral surface glycoproteins G1 and G2 that would presumably be targets for protective antibodies (139). Antibodies elicited to either virus neutralize the other, often to appreciable titers, using antisera obtained from laboratory animals (140); humans receiving inactivated Seoul or Hantaan virus vaccines develop neutralizing antibodies to Hantaan virus, and these same vaccines protect immature rabbits and gerbils against antigen accumulation after Hantaan virus challenge (22, 184). In mice, there is an active $CD8^+$ T-lymphocyte response which is cross-reactive in tests of lysis in vitro or in protection of mice from challenge (5). Furthermore, in immunized experimental animals, Hantaan virus GPC vectored by vaccinia virus protects against either Hantaan or Seoul virus challenge whether antigen accumulation or infection is measured (28). Cross-protection has been absent or minimal when Puumala and Hantaan viruses are used; these two agents differ by 46% of the amino acids in GPC.

If we compare the 10 sigmodontine-derived hantaviruses for which the M segment RNA sequence is available, GPC differs by a maximum of 27% among them when deduced amino acid sequences are compared (111a). The known pathogenic North American viruses differ among themselves by less than 21%, and the South American Laguna Negra, Oran, Lechiguanas, and HU39694 viruses differ by only 14%. Functionally, neutralizing antibodies from a Black Creek Canal virus convalescent human had a homologous titer of 1:320 but still neutralized SNV at 1:40; rat antisera with a homologous titer of 1:160 also neutralized SNV at 1:10 in cell culture (28). The converse showed similar cross-neutralization. The limited data from epitopes recognized by human cytotoxic T cells also suggest there will be cross-reactive as well as specific epitopes (42). The laboratory studies needed to define the cross-protective activity of the immunogens and to identify the important epitopes are difficult, but possible.

## FUTURE EXPECTATIONS

Clearly we can expect to find more hantaviruses. Many of them will come from rodents of the subfamily Sigmodontinae, thus being candidates for causing HPS. I imagine that some of the sigmodontine associated viruses that are not yet associated with any human disease (Table 1) will be found to be human pathogens. It is likely that we will find less-pathogenic viruses in this group, but that remains to be proven.

Pathogenic viruses will often be encountered when local or regional epidemics occur because of climatic and ecological changes that affect rodent populations. The epidemiology will reflect the individual distribution and behavior of the particular rodent species involved. I believe that we will eventually conclude that Andes virus has the additional property of occasional interhuman spread, but that is a personal speculation and remains to be proven. Increasingly we will begin to recognize the importance of sporadic HPS cases in South America as more national and regional laboratories become able to perform IgM and IgG ELISAs with the readily available, cross-reactive antigens such as those from SNV and Laguna Negra virus (Table 2).

The early indications that renal failure may be associated with Bayou (17, 85) and Black Creek Canal (16, 82) viruses seem to be borne out as additional human Bayou virus infections are found (64, 157). We must remember that our surveillance for these viruses is based on pulmonary disease and not on other possible features of these infections, so it is possible that we are missing any number of cases presenting, for example, as renal disease. It seems unlikely that the picture of HPS described for SNV is confined to the viruses from *Peromyscus* species because a number of the cases associated with the South American viruses are so characteristic of SNV-caused HPS. For example, the first two Juquitiba virus fatalities diagnosed were classic HPS (35, 76, 113, 164), as were most Argentine Andes virus cases.

It has been suggested that there is a spectrum from HFRS to HPS, and each virus falls somewhere on that line. I personally doubt it, although I am willing to be convinced otherwise when we understand more about the pathogenesis of HFRS and the infections by sigmodontine-derived hantaviruses. Respiratory failure and renal failure are complicated events, each of which can have differing pathogenetic mechanisms. We know, for example, that there is much more macrophage infection by Hantaan virus in necropsied HFRS patients than in SNV HPS fatalities (186). Renal involvement in HFRS is seen in a setting of massive retroperitoneal changes that may also influence intrarenal circulation, whereas in HPS the permeability increases are virtually confined to the thoracic cavity (39, 114, 187). All HFRS patients have increased vascular permeability in the lung (99), yet frank pulmonary edema is exceedingly rare in the absence of overhydration (31).

We certainly have a lot of work ahead to understand the clinical pictures of the different virus infections we are faced with in South America. In addition to the sigmodontine-associated hantaviruses, we have to ask if the arvicoline-associated hantaviruses cause mild HFRS in the Americas as Puumala virus does in Europe and why we do not find substantial numbers of HFRS cases associated with Seoul virus infection in the Americas. The latter may well be a consequence of lesser contact with *R. norvegicus* than in Asia and poor recognition of cases that do occur. Milder cases of HFRS may resemble gastroenteritis with mild acute renal failure or the renal failure may be incorrectly attributed to antibiotic nephropathy or post-hypotensive "high-output renal failure" (122, 126). Could there be even more distantly related clinical syndromes caused by hantaviruses? In favor are the findings of abbreviated or unusual clinical forms of HFRS that can resemble primary central nervous system or hepatic disease and against is the observation that hantaviruses as different (Figure 2) as the Murinae-associated Hantaan, Seoul, and Dobrava viruses and the Arvicolinae-associated Puumala virus cause a disease readily recognized as HFRS. Pancreatitis is also a consideration.

We should expect more and better information on the pathogenesis of these syndromes, and it could bring welcome improvements in treatment. The identification of cytokines as important in pathogenesis (144, 145) may not bring immediate therapeutic measures, as has been the frustration with septic shock, but perhaps a treatment acting lower on the effector cascade can be developed. These same cytokines are also involved in inflammation, repair, and fibrosis of many tissues so the ongoing studies looking for sequelae of HPS are particularly important, even though patients may seem well when they leave the hospital (58).

## CONCLUSIONS

HPS is a disease of the Americas and is increasingly recognized in South America, where it is an important public health problem. The phylogenetic group of hantaviruses that cause HPS are maintained in nature and transmitted to humans by rodents of the family Muridae and subfamily Sigmodontinae. The diversity of this rodent taxon suggests that there will be variation in the epidemiology and clinical presentation of HPS according to the individual causative virus, although to date the syndrome has been recognizable as HPS, and the epidemiology can be largely understood by patterns of rodent-human interactions. Interhuman transmission of hantaviruses is thought not to occur, but a single well-defined episode with person-to-person spread of Andes virus requires further study of this agent.

**Acknowledgments.** I thank my colleagues who have taught me so much about hantaviruses and who have made this such an exciting field in which to work. This includes people all over the world and particularly the late Joel Dalrymple. Stuart Nichol, Sergei Morzunov, Jim Mills, Ali Khan, Joni Carson, Tim Doyle, and Bill Terry were particularly helpful in developing this review.

**Bibliographic Note.** Some of the data referred to in this paper are in press and will be available by the time this review appears. Much of the newer information was presented at the Fourth International Conference on HFRS and Hantaviruses, 5 to 7 March 1998, in Atlanta, Ga. The abstracts of the meeting are available on the "All About Hantavirus" web page, http://www.cdc.gov/ncidod/diseases/hanta/hps/index.htm. Several rodent ecology papers and a synthesis of U.S. findings will be published in *Emerging Infectious Diseases*, Fall 1998. An excellent source of general information on hantaviruses with an emphasis on research and laboratory aspects is the *Manual of Hemorrhagic Fever with Renal Syndrome and Hantavirus Pulmonary Syndrome* by Connie Schmaljohn, Charlie Calisher, and Ho Wang Lee, in press (due to be published in the fall of 1998). The Pan American Health Organization is also publishing a multilingual practical compendium for those who must deal with HPS: *Hantaviruses in the Americas*: *Guidelines for Diagnosis, Treatment, Prevention, and Control* (scheduled for fall 1998).

## REFERENCES

1. **Abbott, K. D., and T. G. Ksiazek.** 1998. Long-term hantavirus persistence in rodent populations in central arizona, p. 58. *In Abstracts of the Fourth International Conference on HFRS and Hantaviruses.*
2. **Armstrong, L. A., R. T. Bryan, J. Sarisky, et al.** 1995. Mild hantaviral disease caused by Sin Nombre virus in a four-year-old child. *Pediatr. Infect. Dis. J.* **14:**1108–1110.

3. **Armstrong, L. R., S. R. Zaki, M. J. Goldoft, R. L. Todd, A. S. Khan, R. F. Khabbaz, T. G. Ksiazek, and C. J. Peters.** 1995. Hantavirus pulmonary syndrome associated with entering or cleaning rarely used, rodent-infested structures. *J. Inf. Dis.* **172:**1166.

4. **Armstrong, L. R., R. F. Khabbaz, J. E. Childs, et al.** 1994. Occupational exposure to Hantavirus in mammalogists and rodent workers. *Am. J. Trop. Med. Hyg.* **51**(Suppl.):94.

5. **Asada, H., K. Balachandra, M. Tamura, K. Kondo, and K. Yamanishi.** 1989. Cross-reactive immunity among different serotypes of virus causing haemorrhagic fever with renal syndrome. *J. Gen. Virology* **70:**819–825.

6. **Avšic-Zupanc, T., M. Petrovec, T. Trilar, B. Krystufek, M. Poljak, and K. Prosenc.** Distribution and genetic heterogeneity of multiple hantaviruses circulating in slovenia, abstr., p. 77. *In Abstracts of the Fourth International Conference on HFRS and Hantaviruses.*

7. **Bharadwaj, M., J. Botten, N. Torrez-Martinez, and B. Hjelle.** 1997. Rio Mamore virus: genetic characterization of a newly recognized hantavirus of the pygmy rice rat, *Oligoryzomys microtis,* from Bolivia. *Am. J. Trop. Med. Hyg.* **57:**368–374.

8. **Bond, C. W., B. Irvine, H. M. Alterson, R. Van Horn, and R. Douglass.** 1998. Longitudinal incidence of hantavirus infection in deer mice, p. 116. *In Abstracts of the Fourth International Conference on HFRS and Hantaviruses.*

9. **Bryan, R. T., T. J. Doyle, R. L. Moolenaar, A. K. Pflieger, A. S. Khan, T. G. Ksiazek, and C. J. Peters.** 1997. Hantavirus pulmonary syndrome. *Semin. Pediatr. Infect. Dis.* **8:**44–49.

9a. **Burt, W. H., and R. P. Grossenheider.** 1980. *A Field Guide to the Mammals,* 3rd ed. Houghton Mifflin Co., New York, N.Y.

10. **Butler, J. C., and C. J. Peters.** 1994. Hantaviruses and hantavirus pulmonary syndrome. *Clin. Inf. Dis.* **19:**387–395.

11. **Centers for Disease Control and Prevention.** 1997. Case definitions for infectious conditions under public health surveillance. *Morbid. Mortal. Weekly Rep.* **46(RR-10):**16.

12. **Centers for Disease Control and Prevention.** 1993. Hantavirus infection—Southwestern United States: interim recommendations for risk reduction. *Morbid. Mortal. Weekly Rep.* **42(RR-11):** 1–12.

13. **Centers for Disease Control and Prevention.** 1994. Hantavirus pulmonary syndrome—northeastern United States. *Morbid. Mortal. Weekly Rep.* **43:**548–551.

14. **Centers for Disease Control and Prevention.** 1994. Laboratory management of agents associated with Hantavirus pulmonary syndrome: Interim biosafety guidelines. *Morbid. Mortal. Weekly Rep.* **43(RR-7):**1–7.

15. **Centers for Disease Control and Prevention.** 1995. *Methods for Trapping and Sampling Small Mammals for Virologic Testing.* Centers for Disease Control and Prevention, Atlanta, Ga.

16. **Centers for Disease Control and Prevention.** 1994. Newly identified hantavirus—Florida. *Morbid. Mortal. Weekly Rep.* **43:**99, 105.

17. **Centers for Disease Control and Prevention.** 1993. Update: hantavirus disease–United States. *Morbid. Mortal. Weekly Rep.* **42:**612–614.

18. **Centers for Disease Control and Prevention.** 1997. Hantavirus pulmonary syndrome—Chile, 1997. *Morbid. Mortal. Weekly Rep.* **46:**949–951.

19. **Chaparro, J. J., J. Vega, W. Terry, J. L. Vera, B. Barra, R. Meyer, C. J. Peters, A. S. Khan, and T. G. Ksiazek.** Assessment of person-to-person transmission of hantavirus pulmonary syndrome in a Chilean hospital setting. *J. Hosp. Infect.,* in press.

20. **Chapman, L. E., G. Mertz, A. S. Khan, D. C. Hart, C. J. Peters, E. Koster, T. G. Ksiazek, P. E. Rollin, L. Wilson, K. F. Baum, A. T. Pavia, J. C. Christenson, S. Allen, P. J. Rubin, D. Goad, and the Ribavirin Study Group.** 1994. Open label intravenous ribavirin for hantavirus pulmonary syndrome, abstr. H-111. *In Abstracts of the 34th Interscience Conference on Antimicrobial Agents and Chemotherapy.* American Society for Microbiology, Washington, D.C.

21. **Cheek, J., R. Bryan, and G. Glass.** Geographic distribution of high-risk, HPS areas in the U.S. southwest, p. 68. *In Abstracts of the Fourth International Conference on HFRS and Hantaviruses.*

22. **Chen, H.-X.** 1997. Cooperative Group on the ninth five years National Medical Scientific Study 96-906-03-13. Evaluation on the efficacy of vaccines against HFRS and study on their antibody dependent immunization enhancement and immunological strategy. *Chin. J. Prevent. Med.* **8:** 321–330.

23. **Childs, J. E., G. E. Glass, G. W. Korch, and J. W. LeDuc.** 1989. Effects of hantaviral infection on survival, growth and fertility in wild rat (*Rattus norvegicus*) populations of Baltimore, Maryland. *J. Wild. Dis.* **25:**469–476.

24. **Childs, J. E., G. E. Glass, G. W. Korch, and J. W. LeDuc.** 1998. The ecology and epizootiology of hantaviral infections in small mammal communities of Baltimore: a review and synthesis. *Bull. Soc. Vector Ecol.* **13:**113–122.

25. **Childs, J. E., J. W. Krebs, T. G. Ksiazek, G. O. Maupin, K. L. Gage, P. E. Rollin, P. S. Zeitz, J. Sarisky, R. E. Enscore, J. C. Butler, J. E. Cheek, G. E. Glass, and C. J. Peters.** 1995. A household-based, case-control study of environmental factors associated with hantavirus pulmonary syndrome in the southwestern United States. *Am. J. Trop. Med. Hyg.* **52:**393–397.

26. **Childs, J. E. T. G. Ksiazek, C. F. Spiropoulou, J. W. Krebs, S. Morzunov, G. O. Maupin, K. L. Gage, P. E. Rollin, J. Sarisky, R. E. Enscore, J. K. Frey, C. J. Peters, and S. T. Nichol.** 1994. Serologic and genetic identification of *Peromyscus maniculatus* as the primary reservoir for a new hantavirus in the southwestern United States. *J. Infect. Dis.* **169:**1271–1280.

27. **Chizhikov, V. E., C. F. Spiropoulou, S. P. Morzunov, M. C. Monroe, C. J. Peters, and S. T. Nichol.** 1995. Complete genetic characterization and analysis of isolation of Sin Nombre virus. *J. Virol.* **69:**8132–8136.

28. **Chu, Y. K., G. B. Jennings, and C. S. Schmaljohn.** 1995. A vaccinia virus-vectored Hantaan virus vaccine protects hamsters from challenge with Hantaan and Seoul viruses but not Puumala virus. *J. Virol.* **69(10):**6417–6423.

29. **Chu, Y-K., G. Jennings, A. Schmaljohn, F. Elgh, B. Hjelle, H. W. Lee, et al.** 1995. Cross-neutralization of hantaviruses from immune serum from experimentally-infected animals and from hemorrhagic fever with renal syndrome and hantavirus pulmonary syndrome patients. *J. Infect. Dis.* **172:**1581–1584.

30. **Chu, Y-K., C. Rossi, J. LeDuc, H. W. Lee, C. S. Schmaljohn, and J. M. Dalrymple.** 1994. Serological relationships among viruses in the Hantavirus genus, family Bunyaviridae. *Virology* **198:**196–204.

31. **Clement, J., P. McKenna, and P. Colson.** 1994. Hantavirus pulmonary syndrome (HPS) in New England and Europe. *N. Engl. J. Med.* **331:**545–546. (Letter.)

32. **Clement, J., P. McKenna, G. van der Groen, A. Vaheri, and C. J. Peters.** 1998. Hantaviruses, p. 331–351. *In* S. R. Palmer, E. J. L. Soulsby, and D. I. H. Simpson (ed.), *Zoonoses: Biology, Clinical Practice, and Public Health Control.* Oxford University Press, Oxford, United Kingdom.

33. **Comisión Conjunta de Centers for Disease Control and Prevention, Pan American Health Organization and ANLIS-Argentina.** 1997. Informe Final de las Actividades Realizadas por Comisión Conjunta—Centers for Disease Control and Prevention de Estados Unidos de América, Ministerion de Salud, Organización Panamericana de la Salud y ANLIS, Argentina-en Relación a la infección por Hantavirus en Chile. *Rev. Chil. Infect.* **14:**123–134.

34. **Cortes, J., M. L. Cacace, A. Seijo, M. N. Parisi, and L. T. Ayala.** 1994. Distress respiratorio del adulto en Oran, Salta. Presented in the 11th Simposio Internacional de Infectología Pediátrica, Córdoba, Argentina, 9 to 11 May 1994.

35. **Da Silva, M. V., M. J. Vasconcelos, N. T. R. Hidalgo, A. P. R. Veiga, M. Canzian, P. C. F. Marotto, and Y. C. P. Lima.** 1997. Hantavirus pulmonary syndrome, report of the first three cases in São Paulo, Brazil. *Rev. Inst. Med. Trop. S. Paulo* **39(4):**231–234.

35a. **de Souza, Luiza.** Personal communication.

36. **Douglass, R. J., and R. Van Horn.** 1998. Ecology of deer mice in western and central Montana, p. 123. *In Abstracts of the Fourth International Conference on HFRS and Hantaviruses.*

37. **Douglass, R. J., and D. White.** 1998. Ecology of deer mice in peridomestic settings, p. 56. *In Abstracts of the Fourth International Conference on HFRS and Hantaviruses.*

38. **Doyle, T. J., D. B. Coultas, J. C. Young, A. S. Khan, C. J. Peters, and R. T. Bryan** Etiology of respiratory distress in patients testing negative for hantavirus pulmonary syndrome. Submitted for publication.

39. **Duchin, J. S., F. T. Koster, C. J. Peters, G. L. Simpson, B. Tempest, S. R. Zaki, T. G. Ksiazek, P. E. Rollin, S. Nichol, E. T. Umland, R. L. Moolenaar, S. E. Reef, K. R. Nolte, M. M. Gallaher, J. C. Butler, R. F. Breiman, and the Hantavirus Study Group.** 1994. Hantavirus pulmonary

syndrome: a clinical description of 17 patients with a newly recognized disease. *N. Engl. J. Med.* **330:**949–955.

40. **Dunnum, J. L., T. L. Yates, K. H. Abbott, C. H. Calisher, B. J. Frey, K. K. Lamke, C. A. Parmenter, P. J. Polechla, and D. S. Tinnin.** 1998. The need for long-term monitoring in understanding epizootic events, p. 124. *In Abstracts of the Fourth International Conference on HFRS and Hantaviruses.*

41. **Elliott, L. H., T. G. Ksiazek, P. E. Rollin, C. F. Spiropoulou, S. Morzunov, M. Monroe, C. S. Goldsmith, C. D. Humphrey, S. R. Zaki, J. W. Krebs, G. Maupin, K. Gage, J. E. Childs, S. T. Nichol, and C. J. Peters.** 1994. Isolation of Muerto Canyon virus, causative agent of hantavirus pulmonary syndrome. *Am. J. Trop. Med. Hyg.* **51:**102–108.

42. **Ennis, F. A., J. Cruz, C. F. Spiropoulou, D. Waite, C. J. Peters, S. T. Nichol, H. Kariwa, and F. T. Koster.** 1997. Hantavirus pulmonary syndrome: CD8+ and CD4+ cytotoxic T lymphocytes to epitopes on Sin Nombre virus nucleocapsid protein isolated during acute illness. *Virology* **238:** 380–390.

42a. **Enria, D.** Personal communication.

43. **Enria, D., P. Padula, E. L. Segura, N. Pini, A. Edelstein, C. Riva Posse, and M. C. Weissenbacher.** 1996. Hantavirus pulmonary syndrome in Argentina: Possibility of person-to-person transmission. *Medicina* (B. Aires) **58:**709–711.

44. **Enria, D., M. Bowen, J. N. Mills, W. J. Shieh, D. Bausch, and C. J. Peters.** Arenaviruses. *In* R. L. Guerrant, D. H. Walker, and P. F. Weller (ed.), *Tropical Infectious Diseases*: *Principles, Pathogens, & Practice,* in press. W. B. Saunders, New York, N.Y.

45. **Espinosa, M. A., C. Lucero, P. Alvarez, I. Durán, C. Mansilla, M. Tapia, A. S. Khan, W. Terry.** 1998. Hantavirus infection in children, p. 106. *In Abstracts of the Fourth International Conference on HFRS and Hantaviruses.*

46. **Espinoza, R., P. Vial, L. M. Noriega, A. Johnson, S. T. Nichol, P. E. Rollin, R. Wells, S. Zaki, E. Reynolds, and T. G. Ksiazek.** 1998. Hantavirus pulmonary syndrome in a Chilean patient with recent travel in Bolivia. *Emerg. Infect. Dis.* **4:**93–94.

47. **Feldmann, H., A. Sanchez, S. Morzunov, C. F. Spiropoulou, P. E. Rollin, T. G. Ksiazek, C. J. Peters, and S. T. Nichol.** 1993. Utilization of autopsy RNA for the synthesis of the nucleocapsid antigen of a newly recognized virus associated with hantavirus pulmonary syndrome. *Virus Res.* **30:**351–367.

48. **Ferrer, J. F., C. Jonsson, N. Esteban, D. Galligan, M. A. Bosombrio, M. Peralta-Ramos, M. Bharadwaj, N. Torrez-Martinez, J. Callahan, A. Segovia, and B. Hjelle.** 1998. Epidemiological features of SNV-related hantavirus infection in high prevalence Gran Chaco indian populations, p. 144. *In Abstracts of the Fourth International Conference on HFRS and Hantaviruses.*

49. **Frampton, J. W., S. Lanser, C. R. Nichols, and P. J. Ettestad.** 1995. Sin Nombre virus infection in 1959. *Lancet* **346:**781–782. (Letter.)

50. **Franze-Fernandez, M. T., N. Lopez, and C. Rossi.** 1997. Caracterisation genetique du virus Andes, un hantavirus emergeant en Argentine. *Annales de l'Institut Pasteur* **8:**251–256.

50a. **Fulhorst, C. F.** Personal communication.

51. **Fulhorst, C. F., M. C. Monroe, R. A. Salas, G. Duno, A. Utrera, T. G. Ksiazek, S. T. Nichol, N. M. C. de Manzione, D. Tovar, and R. B. Tesh.** 1997. Isolation, characterization, and geographic distribution of Caño Delgadito virus, a newly discovered South American hantavirus (family Bunyaviridae). *Virus Res.* **51:**159–171.

52. **Gavrilovskaya, I. N., N. S. Apekina, A. D. Bernshtein, V. T. Demina, N. M. Okulova, Y. A. Myasnikov, and M. P. Chumakov.** 1990. Pathogenesis of hemorrhagic fever with renal syndrome virus infection and mode of horizontal transmission of Hantavirus in bank voles. *Arch. Virol.* **Suppl.** **1:**57–62.

53. **Gilson, G. J., J. A. Maciulla, B. G. Nevils, L. E. Izquierdo, M. S. Chatterjee, and L. B. Curet.** 1994. Hantavirus pulmonary syndrome complicating pregnancy. *Am. J. Obstet. Gynecol.* **171:**550–554.

54. **Glass, G. E., J. E. Childs, G. W. Korch, and J. W. LeDuc.** 1998. Association of intraspecific wounding with hantaviral infection in wild rats (*Rattus norvegicus*). *Epidemiol. Infect.* **101:**459–472.

55. **Glass, G. E., J. S. Johnson, G. A. Hodenbach, C. L. DiSalvo, C. J. Peters, J. E. Childs, and J. N. Mills.** 1997. Experimental evaluation of rodent exclusion methods to reduce hantavirus transmission to humans in rural housing. *Am. J. Trop. Med. Hyg.* **56:**359–364.

56. **Glass, G. E., W. Livingstone, J. Mills, W. Hlady, J. Fine, P. Rollin, P. Ksiazek, C. Peters, J. Childs.** Black Creek Canal virus infection in Sigmodon hispidus in southern Florida. *Am. J. Trop. Med. Hyg.,* in press.

57. **Glass, G. E., A. J. Watson, J. W. LeDuc, and J. E. Childs.** 1994. Domestic cases of hemorrhagic fever with renal syndrome in the United States. *Nephron* **68:**48–51.

58. **Goade, D. E., F. T. Koster, G. J. Mertz, G. Hjelle, and the Hantavirus Survivors Follow-up Study Group.** Preliminary evidence for pulmonary dysfunction in survivors of hantavirus pulmonary syndrome, abstr., p. 35. *In Abstracts of the Fourth International Conference on HFRS and Hantavirus.*

59. **Hallin, G. W., S. Q. Simpson, R. E. Crowell, D. S. James, F. T. Koster, G. J. Mertz, and H. Levy.** 1996. Cardiopulmonary manifestations of hantavirus pulmonary symptoms. *Crit. Care Med.* **24:**252–258.

60. **Henderson, W. W., M. C. Monroe, S. C. St Jeor, W. P. Thayer, J. E. Rowe, C. J. Peters, and S. T. Nichol.** 1995. Naturally occurring Sin Nombre virus genetic reassortants. *Virology* **214:**602–610.

61. **Hinrichsen, S., A. Medeiros de Andrade, J. Clement, H. Leirs, P. McKenna, P. Matthys, and G. Neild.** 1993. Evidence of hantavirus infection in Brazilian patients from Recife with suspected leptospirosis. *Lancet* **341:**50.

62. **Hjelle, B., B. Anderson, N. Torrez-Martinez, W. Song, W. L. Gannon, and T. L. Yates.** 1995. Prevalence and geographic genetic variation of hantaviruses of New World harvest mice (*Reithrodontomys*): identification of a divergent genotype from a Costa Rican *Reithrodontomys mexicanus*. *Virology* **207:**452–459.

63. **Hjelle, B., F. Chavez-Giles, N. Torrez-Martinez, et al.** 1994. Genetic identification of a novel hantavirus of the harvest mouse Reithrodontomys megalotis. *J. Virology* **68:**6751–6754.

64. **Hjelle, B., D. Goade, N. Torrez-Martinez, M. Lang-Williams, J. Kim, R. L. Harris, and J. A. Rawlings.** 1996. Hantavirus pulmonary syndrome, renal insufficiency, and myositis associated with infection by Bayou hantavirus. *Clin. Infect. Dis.* **23:**495–500.

65. **Hjelle, B., S. Jenison, N. Torrez-Martinez, B. Herring, S. Quan, A. Polito, S. Pichuantes, T. Yamada, C. Morris, F. Elgh, H. W. Lee, H. Artsob, and R. Dinello.** 1997. Rapid and specific detection of Sin Nombre virus antibodies in patients with hantavirus pulmonary syndrome by a strip immunoblot assay suitable for field diagnosis. *J. Clin. Microbiol.* **35:**600–608.

66. **Hjelle, B., J. Krolikowski, N. Torrez-Martinez, F. Chavez-Giles, C. Vanner, and E. Laposata.** 1995. Phylogenetically distinct hantavirus implicated in a case of hantavirus pulmonary syndrome in the northeastern United States. *J. Med. Virol.* **46:**21–27.

67. **Hjelle, B., S-W. Lee, W. Song, et al.** 1995. Molecular linkage of hantavirus pulmonary syndrome to the white-footed mouse, *Peromyscus leucopus*: genetic characterization of the M genome of New York virus. *J. Virol.* **69:**8137–8141.

68. **Hjelle, B., C. E. Spiropoulou, N. Torrez-Martinez, S. Morzunov, C. J. Peters, and S. T. Nichol.** 1994. Detection of Muerto Canyon virus RNA in peripheral blood mononuclear cells from patients with hantavirus pulmonary syndrome. *J. Infect. Dis.* **170:**1013–1017.

69. **Hjelle, B., N. Torrez-Martinez, and F. T. Koster.** 1996. Hantavirus pulmonary syndrome-related virus from Bolivia. (Letter.). *Lancet* **57:**347.

70. **Hjelle, B., N. Torrez-Martinez, F. T. Koster, M. Jay, M. S. Ascher, T. Brown, P. Reynolds, P. Ettestad, R. E. Voorhees, J. Sarisky, R. E. Enscore, L. Sands, D. G. Mosley, C. Kioski, R. T. Bryan, and C. M. Sewell.** 1996. Epidemiologic linkage of rodent and human hantavirus genomic sequences in case investigations of hantavirus pulmonary syndrome. *J. Infect. Dis.* **173:**781–786.

71. **Hoddenbach, G., J. Johnson, and C. DiSalvo.** 1997. *Mechanical Rodent-Proofing Techniques.* National Park Service Public Health Program, U.S. Department of the Interior, Washington, D.C.

72. **Horwitz, I., L. Thompson, V. Luchsinger, R. Lagos, E. Villagra, and R. Espinoza.** 1997. Infección por hantavirus: orientaciones generales para el diagnóstico y manejo de pacientes hospitalizados por sospecha o confirmación de síndrome pulmonar por hantavirus. *Rev. Chil. Infect.* **14:**74–82.

73. **Howard, M., T. Doyle, F. Koster, S. R. Zaki, A. S. Khan, C. J. Peters, and R. T. Bryan.** 1998. Hantavirus pulmonary syndrome in pregnancy, p. 108. *In Abstracts of the Fourth International Conference on HFRS and Hantaviruses.*

74. **Huggins, J. W., C. M. Hsiang, T. M. Cosgriff, M. Y. Guang, J. I. Smith, Z. O. Wu, J. W. LeDuc, Z. M. Zheng, J. M. Meegan, Q. N. Wang, D. D. Oland, X. E. Gui, P. H. Gibbs, G. H. Yuan, and T. M. Zhang.** 1991. Prospective, double-blind, concurrent, placebo-controlled clinical trial of intravenous ribavirin therapy of hemorrhagic fever with renal syndrome. *J. Infect. Dis.* **164:** 1119–1127.

75. **Hutchinson, K. L., P. E. Rollin, and C. J. Peters.** Pathogenesis of a North American hantavirus, Black Creek Canal virus, in experimentally infected *Sigmodon hispidus. Am. J. Trop. Med. Hyg.,* in press.

76. **Iversson, L. B., M. J. Vasconcelos, V. C. Pedroso de Lima, M. D. B. Rosa, A. P. A. Travassos da Rosa, E. S. T. da Rosa, P. E. Rollin, C. J. Peters, L. E. Pereira, E. Nassar, G. Katz, L. H. Matida, M. A. Zaparoli, and J. J. B. Ferreira.** 1994. Doença human por hantavirus na área rural do município de Juquitiba, Área Metropolitana de São Paulo, Brasil. Presented at the *XXX Congresso da Sociedade Brasileira de Medicina Tropical,* Bahia, Brazil, 6 to 11 March 1994.

77. **Iversson, L. B., A. P. A. Travassos da Rosa, M. D. B. Rosa, A. V. Lomar, M. D G. M. Sasaki, and J. W. LeDuc.** 1994. Human infection by Hantavirus in southern and southeastern Brazil. *Rev. Ass. Med. Brasil* **40(2):**85–92.

78. **Jay, M., M. S. Ascher, B. B. Chomel, M. Madon, D. Sesline, B. A. Enge, B. Hjelle, T. G. Ksiazek P. E. Rollin, P. H. Kass, and K. Reilly.** 1997. Seroepidemiologic studies of hantavirus infection among wild rodents in California. *Emerging Infect. Dis.* **3(2):**183–190.

79. **Jenison, S., T. Yamada, C. Morris, et al.** 1994. Characterization of human antibody responses to Four Corners hantavirus infections among patients with hantavirus pulmonary syndrome. *J. Virol.* **68:**3000–3006.

80. **Johnson, A. M., M. D. Bowen, T. G. Ksiazek, R. J. Williams, R. T. Bryan, J. N. Mills, C. J. Peters, and S. T. Nichol.** 1997. Laguna Negra virus associated with HPS in western Paraguay and Bolivia. *Virology* **238:**115–127.

81. **Ketai, L. H., M. R. Williamson, R. J. Telepak, H. Levy, F. T. Koster, K. B. Nolte, and S. E. Allen.** 1994. Hantavirus pulmonary syndrome: radiographic findings in 16 patients. *Radiology* **191:** 665–668.

82. **Khan, A. S., M. Gaviria, P. E. Rollin, W. G. Hlady, T. G. Ksiazek, L. R. Armstrong, R. Greenman, E. Ravkov, M. Kolber, H. Anapol, E. D. Sfakianaki, S. T. Nichol, C. J. Peters, and R. F. Khabbaz.** 1996. Hantavirus pulmonary syndrome in Florida: association with the newly identified Black Creek Canal virus. *Am. J. Med.* **100:**46–48.

83. **Khan, A. S., R. F. Khabbaz, L. R. Armstrong, R. C. Holman, S. P. Bauer, J. Graber, T. Strine, G. Miller, S. Reef, J. Tappero, P. E. Rollin, S. T. Nichol, S. R. Zaki, R. T. Bryan, L. E. Chapman, C. J. Peters, and T. G. Ksiazek.** 1996. Hantavirus pulmonary syndrome: the first 100 U.S. cases. *J. Infect. Dis.* **173:**1297–1303.

84. **Khan, A. S., T. G. Ksiazek, S. R. Zaki, S. T. Nichol, P. E. Rollin, C. J. Peters, R. F. Khabbaz J. E. Cheek, L. A. Shireley, S. L. McDonough, T. K. Welty, and D. Kuklinski.** 1995. Fatal hantavirus pulmonary syndrome in an adolescent. *Pediatrics* **95:**276–280.

85. **Khan, A. S., C. S. Spiropoulou, S. Morzunov, S. R. Zaki, M. A. Kohn, S. R. Nawas, L. McFarland, and S. T. Nichol.** 1995. A fatal illness associated with a new hantavirus in Louisiana. *J. Med. Virol.* **46:**281–286.

86. **Koster, F. T., and S. A. Jenison.** 1988. Hantaviruses, p. 2140–2147. *In* S. L. Gorbach, J. G. Bartlett, N. R. Blacklow (ed.), *Infectious* Diseases, 2nd ed. W. B. Saunders, Philadelphia, Pa.

86a. **Ksiazek, T. G.** Personal communication.

87. **Ksiazek, T. G., S. T. Nichol, J. N. Mills, M. G. Groves, A. Wozniak, S. McAdams, M. Monroe, A. Johnson, M. L. Martin, C. J. Peters, and P. E. Rollin.** 1997. Isolation, genetic diversity, and geographic distribution of Bayou virus (Bunyaviridae: Hantavirus). *Am. J. Trop. Med. Hyg.* **57:** 445–448.

88. **Ksiazek, T. G., C. J. Peters, P. E. Rollin, S. Zaki, S. Nichol, C. Spiropoulou, S. Morzunov, H. Feldmann, A. Sanchez, A. S. Khan, B. W. J. Mahy, K. Wachsmuth, and J. C. Butler.** 1995.

Identification of a new North American hantavirus that causes acute pulmonary insufficiency. *Am. J. Trop. Med. Hyg.* **52**:117–123.

89. **Lazaro, M. E., A. M. Resa, S. C. Levis, C. Y. Riva Posse, L. Zamengo, J. C. Merceob, I. Rojo, F. Bruzzo, and D. Enria.** Distres respiratorio del adulto en El Bolson, Río Negro, Presented at the I Congreso Argentino de Zoonosis and I Congreso Latinoamericano de Zoonosis, Buenos Aires, Argentina, 14 to 17 August 1995.

90. **LeDuc, J. W., G. A. Smith, F. P. Pinheiro, P. Vasconcelos, E. Rosa, and J. I. Maiztegui.** 1985. Isolation of a Hantaan-related virus from Brazilian rats and serologic evidence of its widespread distribution in South America. *Am. J. Trop. Med. Hyg.* **34**:810–815.

91. **LeDuc, J. W., G. A. Smith, J. E. Childs, F. P. Pinheiro, J. I. Maiztegui, B. Niklasson, A. Antoniadis, D. M. Robinson, M. Khin, K. E. Shortridge, M. T. Wooster, M. R. Elwell, P. L. T. Ilberty, D. Koech, E. S. T. Rosa, and L. Rosen.** Global survey of antibody to Hantaan-related viruses among peridomestic rodents. *Bull. W. H. O.* **64**:139–144.

92. **Lee, H. W.** 1982. Korean hemorrhagic fever. *Prog. Med. Virol.* **28**:96–113.

93. **Lee, H. W., P. W. Lee, L. J. Baek, C. K. Song, and I. W. Seong.** 1981. Intraspecific transmission of Hantaan Virus, Etiologic agent of Korean hemorrhagic fever, in the rodent *Apodemus agrarius*. *Am. J. Trop. Med. Hyg.* **30**:1106–1112.

94. **Levis, S. C., G. E. Calderon, N. Pini, T. G. Ksiazek, C. J. Peters, and D. A. Enria.** Síndrome pulmonar por hantavirus (SPH): resultados preliminares de estudios orientados a establecer los potenciales reservorios en la Argentina. Presented at the V Congreso Argentino de Virologia, Tandil, Argentina, 24 to 27 April 1996.

95. **Levis, S. C., J. E. Rowe, S. Morzunov, D. A. Enria, and S. S. Jeor.** 1997. New hantaviruses causing hantavirus pulmonary syndrome in central Argentina. *Lancet* **349**:998–999. (Letter.)

96. **Levis, S., A. M. Briggiler, M. Cacass, C. J. Peters, T. G. Ksiazek, J. Cortes, M. E. Lazaro, A. Resa, P. E. Rollin, F. P. Pinheiro, and D. Enria.** Emergence of hantavirus pulmonary syndrome in Argentina, abstr. 441. *In Abstracts of the 44th Annual Meeting of the American Society of Tropical Medicine and Hygiene.*

97. **Levis, S., S. Morzunov, J. Rowe, D. Enria, N. Pini, G. Calderon, M. Sabattini, and S. St. Jeor.** 1998. Genetic diversity and epidemiology of hantaviruses in Argentina. *J. Infect. Dis.* **177**:529–538.

97a. **Levis, S., and J. Mills.** Unpublished data.

98. **Li, D., A. L. Schmaljohn, K. Anderson, and C. S. Schmaljohn.** 1995. Complete nucleotide sequences of the M and S segments of two hantavirus isolates from California: evidence for reassortment in nature among viruses related to hantavirus pulmonary syndrome. *Virology* **206**:973–983.

99. **Linderholm, M., T. Sandström, O. Rinnström, S. Groth, A. Blomberg, and A. Tärnvik.** Pulmonary function in hemorrhagic fever with renal syndrome (HFRS), p. 38. *In Abstracts of the Fourth International Conference on HFRS and Hantaviruses.*

100. **Lopez, N., P. Padula, C. Rossi, M. E. Lazaro, and M. T. Franze-Fernandez.** 1996. Genetic identification of a new hantavirus causing severe pulmonary syndrome in Argentina. *Virology* **220**:223–226.

101. **Lopez, N., P. Padula, C. Rossi, S. Miguel, A. Edelstein, E. Ramirez, and M. T. Franze-Fernandez.** 1997. Genetic characterization and phylogeny of Andes virus and variants from Argentina and Chile. *Virus Res.* **50**:77–84.

102. **Lundkvist, A., M. Hukic, J. Horling, M. Gilljam, S. Nichol, and B. Niklasson.** 1997. Puumala and Dobrava viruses cause hemorrhagic fever with renal syndrome in Bosnia-Herzegovina: evidence of highly cross-neutralizing antibody responses in early patient sera. *J. Med. Virol.* **53**:51–59.

103. **Lyubsky, S., I. Gavrilovskaya, B. Luft, and E. Mackow.** 1996. Histopathology of *Peromyscus leucopus* naturally infected with pathogenic NY-1 hantaviruses: pathologic markers of HPS viral infection in mice. *Laboratory Investigation* **74**:627–633.

104. **Maiztegui, J. I., J. L. Becker, and J. W. LeDuc.** 1983. Actividad del virus de la fiebre hemorrágica de Corea o virus muroide en ratas del puerto de la ciudad de Buenos Aires. *Medicina* (Buenos Aires) **43**:871.

105. **Mills, J. N., J. M. Johnson, T. G. Ksiazek, B. A. Ellis, P. E. Rollin, T. L. Yates, M. O. Mann, R. M. Johnson, M. L. Campbell, J. Miyashiro, M. Patrick, M. Zyzak, D. Lavender, M. G.**

Novak, K. Schmidt, C. J. Peters, and J. E. Childs. 1998. A survey of hantavirus antibody in small-mammal populations in selected U.S. national parks. *Am. J. Trop. Med. Hyg.* **58:**525–532.

106. Mills, J. N., T. L. Yates, J. E. Childs, R. R. Parmenter, T. G. Ksiazek, P. E. Rollin, and C. J. Peters. 1995. Guidelines for working with rodents potentially infected with hantavirus. *J. Mammal.* **76:**716–722.

107. Mills, J. N., T. G. Ksiazek, B. A. Ellis, P. E. Rollin, S. T. Nichol, T. L. Yates, W. L. Gannon, C. E. Levy, D. M. Engelthaler, T. Davis, D. T. Tanda, J. W. Frampton, C. R. Nichols, C. J. Peters, and J. E. Childs. 1997. Patterns of association with host and habitat: antibody reactive with Sin Nombre virus in small mammals in the major biotic communities of the southwestern United States. *Am. J. Trop. Med. Hyg.* **56:**273–284.

108. Moolenaar, R. L., C. Dalton, H. B. Lipman, E. T. Umland, M. Gallaher, J. S. Duchin, L. Chapman, S. R. Zaki, T. G. Ksiazek, P. E. Rollin, S. T. Nichol, J. E. Cheek, J. C. Butler, and R. F. Breiman. 1995. Clinical features that differentiate hantavirus pulmonary syndrome from three other acute respiratory illnesses. *Clin. Infect. Dis.* **21:**643–649.

109. Morzunov, S. P., J. E. Rowe, T. G. Ksiazek, C. J. Peters, S. C. St Jeor, and S. T. Nichol. 1998. Genetic analysis of the diversity and origin of hantaviruses in *Peromyscus leucopus* mice in North America. *J. Virol.* **72:**57–64.

110. Morzunov, S. P., V. Feldmann, C. F. Spiropoulou, V. A. Semenova, P. E. Rollin, T. G. Ksiazek, C. J. Peters, and S. T. Nichol. 1995. A newly recognized virus associated with a fatal case of hantavirus pulmonary syndrome in Louisiana. *J. Virol.* **69:**1980–1983.

111. Murua, R., L. E. Gonzalez, M. Gonzalez, and Y. C. Joffre. 1996. Efectos del florecimiento del arbusto *Chusquea quila* Kunth (Poaceae) sobre la demografía de poblaciones de roedores de los bosques templados fríos del sur Chileno. *Bol. Soc. Biol.* (Concepción) **67:**37–42.

111a. Nichol, S. Personal communication.

112. Nichol, S., C. Spiropoulou, S. Morzunov, P. Rollin, G. Ksiazek, H. Feldmann, A. Sanchez, G. Childs, S. Zaki, and C. J. Peters. 1993. Genetic identification of a Hantavirus associated with an outbreak of acute respiratory illness. *Science* **262:**914–917.

113. Nichol, S. T., T. G. Ksiazek, P. E. Rollin, and C. J. Peters. 1996. Hantavirus pulmonary syndrome and newly described hantaviruses in the United States, p. 269–280. *In* R. M. Elliott (ed.), *The Bunyaviridae.* Plenum Press, New York, N.Y.

114. Nolte, K. B., R. M. Feddersen, K. Foucar, S. R. Zaki, F. T. Koster, D. Madar, T. L. Merlin, P. J. McFeeley, E. T. Umland, and R. E. Zumwalt. 1995. Hantavirus pulmonary syndrome in the United States: a pathological description of a disease caused by a new agent. *Hum. Pathol.* **26:**110–120.

115. O'Connor, C., J. P. Hayes, and S. C. St. Jeor. 1997. Sin Nombre virus does not impair respiratory function of wild deer mice. *J. Mammal.* **78:**661–668.

115a. Padula, P. J. Unpublished data.

116. Padula, P. J., A. Edelstein, S. D. L. Miguel, N. M. López, C. M. Rossi, and R. D. Rabinovich. 1998. Brote epidémico del síndrome pulmonar por hantavirus en la Argentina: evidencia molecular de la transmisión persona a persona del virus Andes. *Medicina* (Buenos Aires) **58**(Suppl. 1):27–36.

117. Padula, P. J., A. Edelstein, S. D. L. Miguel, N. M. López, C. M. Rossi, and R. D. Rabinovich. 1998. Hantavirus pulmonary syndrome (HPS) outbreak in Argentina: molecular evidence for person-to-person transmission of Andes virus. *Virology* **241:**323–330.

117a. Padula, P. J. Personal communication.

118. Pan American Health Organization. *Hantaviruses in the Americas: Guidelines for Diagnosis, Treatment, Prevention, and Control,* in press. Pan American Health Organization, Washington, D.C.

119. Parisi, M. N., E. Tiano, D. Enria, M. Sabattine, and J. Maiztegui, Actividad de un hantavirus en pacientes de la zona endémica de fiebre hemorrágica argentina. Presented at the XIV Reunión Científica Anual de la Sociedad Argentina de Virología, Buenos Aires, Argentina, 10 to 11 December 1992.

120. Parisi, M. D. N., D. A. Enria, N. C. Pini, and M. S. Sabattini. 1996. Retrospective detection of clinical infections caused by hantavirus in Argentina. *Medicina* (Buenos Aires) **56**(1):1–13.

121. **Parmenter, R. R., and R. Vigil.** 1993. *The HARDS Epidemic in the Southwest: an Assessment of Autumn Rodent Densities and Population Demographics in Central and Northern New Mexico, October 1993.* Department of Biology, University of New Mexico, Albuquerque.

122. **Peters, C. J., J. N. Mills, C. Spiropoulou, S. R. Zaki, and P. E. Rollin.** Hantaviruses. *In* R. L. Guerrant, D. H. Walker, and P. F. Weller (ed.), *Tropical Infectious Diseases: Principles, Pathogens, & Practice,* in press. The W. B. Saunders Co., Philadelphia, Pa.

123. **Peters, C. J., P. B. Jahrling, and A. S. Khan.** 1996. Management of patients infected with high-hazard viruses: scientific basis for infection control. *Arch. Virol.* **Suppl. 11:**1–28.

124. **Peters, C. J., and J. W. LeDuc.** 1996. Viral hemorrhagic fevers: persistent problems, persistent in reservoirs, p. 211–233. *In* B. W. J. Mahy, and R. W. Compans (ed.), *Immunobiology and Pathogenesis of Persistent Virus Infections.* Harwood Academic Publishers GmbH, Chur, Switzerland.

125. **Peters, C. J., and S. R. Zaki.** 1998. Viral hemorrhagic fever: an overview. *In* R. L. Guerrant, D. H. Walker, P. F. Weller (ed.), *Tropical Infectious Diseases: Principles, Pathogens, & Practice,* in press. The W. B. Saunders Co., Philadelphia, Pa.

126. **Peters, C. J.** 1997. Pathogenesis of viral hemorrhagic fevers, p. 779–799. *In* N. Nathanson, R. Ahmed, F. Gonzalez-Scarano, D. Griffin, K. V. Holmes, F. Murphy, and H. L. Robinson (ed.), *Viral Pathogenesis.* Lippincott-Raven Publishers, Philadelphia, Pa.

127. **Pinheiro, F. P., A. P. A. Travassos da Rosa, R. B. Freitas, J. F. S. Travassos da Rosa, and P. F. C. Vasconcelos.** 1986. Aspectos clínico-epidemiológicos, p. 395, 401–402. *In Instituto Evandro Chagas—50 Anos de Contribução as Ciências Biológicas e á Medicina Tropical: 1936–1986.* Ministerio da Saúde-Fundaçao Servicos de Saúde Pública, Belém, Brazil.

128. **Pini, N., A. Resa, G. Laime, G. Lecot, T. Ksiazek, S. Levis, and D. Enria.** 1998. Hantavirus infection in children in Argentina. *Emerg. Infect. Dis.* **4:**85–87.

129. **Plyusnin, A., O. Vapalahti, and A. Vaheri.** 1996. Hantaviruses: genome structure, expression and evolution. *J. Gen. Virol.* **77:**2677–2687.

129a. **Qian, D. Y., Y. S. Ding, G. F. Chen, J. J. Ding, Y. X. Chen, T. F. Lu, Z. X. Wang, and R. A. Smego, Jr.** 1990. A placebo-controlled clinical trial of prednisone in the treatment of early hemorrhagic fever. *J. Infect. Dis.* **162:**1213–1214. (Letter.)

130. **Ravkov, E. V., P. E. Rollin, T. G. Ksiazek, C. J. Peters, and S. T. Nichol.** 1995. Genetic and serologic analysis of Black Creek Canal virus and its association with human disease and *Sigmodon hispidus* infection. *Virology* **210:**482–489.

131. **Ravkov, E. V., S. T. Nichol, and R. W. Compans.** 1997. Polarized entry and release in epithelial cells of Black Creek Canal virus, a New World hantavirus. *J. Virol.* **71:**1147–1154.

132. **Rawlings, J., N. Torrez-Martinez, S. Neill, G. Moore, B. Hicks, S. Pichuantes, et al.** 1996. Cocirculation of multiple hantaviruses in Texas, with characterization of the S genome of a previously-undescribed virus of cotton rats (*Sigmodon hispidus*). *Am. J. Trop. Med. Hyg.* **55:**672–679.

133. **Rodriguez, L. L., J. H. Owens, C. J. Peters, and S. T. Nichol.** 1998. Genetic reassortment among viruses causing hantavirus pulmonary syndrome. *Virology* **242:**99–106.

134. **Rollin, P. E., T. G. Ksiazek, L. H. Elliott, E. Ravkov, M. L. Martin, S. Morzunov, W. Livingstone, M. Monroe, G. Glass, S. Ruo, A. S. Khan, J. E. Childs, S. T. Nichol, and C. J. Peters.** 1995. Isolation of Black Creek Canal virus, a new hantavirus from *Sigmodon hispidus* in Florida. *J. Med. Virol.* **46:**35–39.

135. **Rowe, J. E., S. C. St. Jeor, J. Riolo, E. W. Otteson, M. C. Monroe, W. W. Henderson, T. G. Ksiazek, P. E. Rollin, and S. T. Nichol.** 1995. Coexistence of several novel hantaviruses in rodents indigenous to North America. *Virology* **213:**122–130.

136. **Ruedas, L. A., T. L. Yates, M. L. Campbell, K. H. Abbott, C. H. Calisher, J. L. Dunnum, J. Mills, T. G. Ksiazek, C. A. Parmenter, C. J. Peters, and P. J. Polechla.** 1998. Effects of hantavirus infection on natural populations of rodents (*Muridae peromyscus*), p. 134. *In Abstracts of the Fourth International Conference on HFRS and Hantaviruses.*

136a. **Ruo, S., and C. J. Peters.** Unpublished data.

137. **Sayer, W. J., G. M. Entwisle, B. T. Uyeno, and R. C. Bignall.** 1955. Cortisone therapy of early epidemic hemorrhagic fever: a preliminary report. *Ann. Intern. Med.* **42:**839.

138. **Schmaljohn, A. L., D. Li, D. L. Negley, D. S. Bressler, M. J. Turell, G. W. Korch, M. S. Ascher, and C. S. Schmaljohn.** 1995. Isolation and initial characterization of a newfound hantavirus from California. *Virology* **206:**963–972.

139. **Schmaljohn, C.** 1994. Prospects for vaccines to control viruses in the family Bunyaviridae. *Rev. Med. Virol.* **4:**185–196.

140. **Schmaljohn, C., S. Hasty, J. Dalrymple, J. LeDuc, H. W. Lee, C. von Bonsdorff, M. Brummer-Korvenkontio, A. Vaheri, T. Tsai, H. Regnery, D. Goldgaber, and P. W. Lee.** 1985. Antigenic and genetic properties of viruses linked to hemorrhagic fever with renal syndrome. *Science* **227:**1041–1044.

141. **Schmaljohn, C. S., and B. Hjelle.** 1997. Hantaviruses: a global disease problem. *Emerg. Infect. Dis.* **3:**95–104.

142. **Schmaljohn, C. S., C. Calisher, and H. W. Lee.** *Manual of Hemorrhagic Fever with Renal Syndrome and Hantavirus Pulmonary Syndrome,* in press. Ui-Sul Munwhasa, Seoul, Republic of Korea.

143. **Simonsen, L., M. J. Dalton, R. F. Breiman, T. Hennessy, F. T. Umland, C. M. Sewell, P. E. Rollin, T. G. Ksiazek, and C. J. Peters.** 1995. Evalution of the magnitude of the 1993 hantavirus outbreak in the southwestern United States. *J. Infect. Dis.* **172:**729–733.

144. **Simpson, S. Q., V. Mapel, F. T. Koster, J. Montoya, D. E. Bice, and A. J. Williams.** 1995. Evidence for lymphocyte activation in the hantavirus pulmonary syndrome. *Chest* **108:**97S.

145. **Simpson, S. Q., V. Mapel, F. T. Koster, J. Montoya, D. E. Bice, and A. J. Williams.** 1996. Evidence for tumor necrosis factor activation in the hantavirus pulmonary syndrome. *Crit. Care Med.* **24:**A26.

146. **Song, J. W., L. J. Baek, I. N. Gavrilovskaya, E. R. Mackow, B. Hjelle, and R. Yanagihara.** 1996. Sequence analysis of the complete S genomic segment of a newly identified hantavirus isolated from the white-footed mouse (*Peromyscus leucopus*): phylogenetic relationship with other sigmodontine rodent-borne hantaviruses. *Virus Genes* **12:**249–256.

147. **Song, J. W., L. J. Baek, J. W. Nagle, D. Schlitter, and R. Yanagihara.** 1996. Genetic and phylogenetic analyses of hantaviral sequences amplified from archival tissues of deer mouse (*Peromyscus maniculatus nubiterrae*) captured in the eastern United States. *Arch. Virol.* **141:**959–967.

148. **Spiropoulou, C., S. Morzunov, H. Feldman, A. Sanchez, C. J. Peters, and S. T. Nichol.** 1994. Genome structure and variability of a virus causing hantavirus pulmonary syndrome. *Virology* **200:**715–723.

149. **Steier, K. J., and R. Clay,** 1993. Hantavirus pulmonary syndrome (HPS): report of first case in Louisiana. *J. Am. Osteopath. Assoc.* **93:**1286–1289.

150. **Sundstrom, J. B., S. Mahanty, D. F. Spiropoulou, D. Bressler, and P. E. Rollin.** 1998. Comparison of the direct effects of Sin Nombre (SNV) and Hantaan (HTN) virus infection on the activation of human lung microvascular endothelial cells (HMVEC-L) in vitro, p. 44. *In Abstracts of the Fourth International Conference on HFRS and Hantaviruses.*

151. **Tamura, M., S. Ogino, T. Matsunaga, et al.** 1991. Experimental labyrinthitis in guinea pigs caused by a hantavirus. *ORL* **53:**1–5.

152. **Tapia, M.** 1997. Síndrome pulmonar por hantavirus. *Rev. Chil. Enferm. Respir.* **13:**103–110.

153. **Tapia, M., C. Mansilla, H. Villalón, B. Vallejos, J. L. Vera, N. Gallegos, S. Zaki, W. Shieh, and A. S. Khan.** Hantavirus pulmonary syndrome: clinical description of thirteen cases in the XIth region of Aysén, Chile, p. 36. *In Abstracts of the Fourth International Conference on HFRS and Hantaviruses.*

154. **Tappero, J. W., A. S. Khan, R. W. Pinner, J. D. Wenger, J. M. Graber, L. R. Armstrong, R. C. Holman, T. G. Ksiazek, R. F. Khabbaz, and the *Hantavirus* Task Force.** 1996. Utility of emergency, telephone-based national surveillance for *Hantavirus* pulmonary syndrome. *JAMA* **275:**398–400.

154a. **Tesh, R. B., and D. M. Watts.** Personal communication.

155. **Theiler, M., and W. G. Downs.** 1973. *The Arthropod-Borne Viruses of Vertebrates.* Yale University Press, New Haven, Conn.

156. **Toro, J., J. Vega, J. Mills, et al.** An outbreak of hantavirus pulmonary syndrome, Chile 1997. *Emerg. Infect. Dis.,* in press.

157. **Torrez-Martinez, N., M. Bharadwaj, D. Goade, J. Delury, D. Moran, B. Hicks, B. Nix, J. L. Davis, and B. Hjelle.** 1998. Bayou virus-associated hantavirus pulmonary syndrome in eastern Texas: identification of the rice rat, *Oryzomys palustris*, as reservoir host. *Emerg. Infect. Dis.* **4:** 105–111.

158. **Torrez-Martinez, N., and B. Hjelle.** 1995. Enzootic of Bayou hantavirus in rice rats (*Oryzomys palustris*) in 1993. *Lancet* **346:**780–781. (Letter.)

159. **Traub, R., and C. L. Wisseman.** 1978. Korean hemorrhagic fever. *J. Infect. Dis.* **138:**267–272.

160. **Tsai, T. F., Y. W. Tang, S. L. Hu, K. L. Ye, G. L. Chen, and Y. X. Xu.** 1984. Hemagglutination-inhibiting antibody in hemorrhagic fever with renal syndrome. *J. Infect. Dis.* **150:**895–1215.

161. **Tsai, T. F.** 1987. Hemorrhagic fever with renal syndrome: mode of transmission to humans. *Lab. Anim. Sci.* **37:**428–430.

162. **Tsai, T. F., S. P. Bauer, D. R. Sasso, S. G. Whitfield, J. B. McCormick, C. T. Caraway, L. M. McFarland, H. Bradford, and T. Kurata.** 1985. Serological and virological evidence of a hantaan virus-related enzootic in the United States. *J. Infect. Dis.* **152:**126–136.

163. **Valderamma, R., J. Vega, and W. Terry.** Community serological survey of infection by hantavirus in the XI region, Aysen, Chile, p. 155. *In Abstracts of the Fourth International Conference on HFRS and Hantaviruses.*

164. **Vasconcelos, M., V. Lima, L. Iversson, M. Rosa, A. Travassos da Rosa, E. Travassos da Rosa, L. Pereira, E. Nassar, G. Katz, L. Matida, M. Zaparoli, J. Ferreira, and C. Peters.** 1997. Hantavirus pulmonary syndrome in the rural area of Juquitiba, São Paulo Metropolitan Area, Brazil. *Rev. Inst. Med. Trop.* (S. Paulo) **39:**237–238.

165. **Vasconcelos, P. F. C., E. S. Travassos da Rosa, A. P. A. Travassos da Rosa, and J. F. S. Travassos da Rosa.** 1992. Evidence of circulating hantaviruses in Brazilian Amazonia through high prevalence of antibodies in residents of Manaus, Brazil. *Ciencia e Cultura* **44:**162–163.

166. **Vasilenko, V., I. Golivljova, Å. Lundkwist, O. Vapalahti, H. Henttonen, A. Plyusnin, and A. Vaheri.** 1998. Studies on the distribution of hantaviruses in Estonia, 1990–1997, p. 57. *In Abstracts of the Fourth International Conference on HFRS and Hantaviruses.*

167. **Vitek, C. R., R. F. Breiman, T. G. Ksiazek, P. E. Rollin, J. C. McLaughlin, E. T. Umland, et al.** 1996. Evidence against person-to-person transmission of hantavirus to health care workers. *Clin. Infect. Dis.* **22:**824–826.

168. **Weissenbacher, M., M. S. Merani, V. L. Hodara, et al.** 1990. Hantavirus infection in laboratory and wild rodents in Argentina. *Medicina* (Buenos Aires) **50:**43–46.

169. **Weissenbacher, M. C., E. Cura, E. L. Segura, et al.** 1996. Serological evidence of human hantavirus infection in Argentina, Bolivia, and Uruguay. *Medicina* (Buenos Aires) **56:**17–22.

170. **Weissenbacher, M. C., H. W. Lee, E. Cura, and E. L. Segura.** Anti-Hantaan antibody prevalence among Argentinian laboratory workers and general population. Presented at the Pacific Science Association 16th Congress, Seoul, Republic of Korea, 20 to 30 August 1987.

171. **Wells, R. M., S. Sosa Estani, Z. E. Yadon, D. Enria, P. Padula, N. Pini, J. N. Mills, C. J. Peters, E. L. Segura, and the Hantavirus Pulmonary Syndrome Study Group for Patagonia.** 1997. An unusual hantavirus outbreak in southern Argentina: person-to-person transmission? *Emerg. Infect. Dis.* **3:**171–174.

172. **Wells, R. M., S. S. Sosa Estani, Z. E. Yadon, D. Enria, P. Padula, N. Pini, M. Gonzalez Della Valle, J. N. Mills, and C. J. Peters.** Hantaviral antibodies in health care workers and other residents of southern Argentina. Submitted for publication.

173. **Wells, R. M., J. Young, R. J. Williams, L. R. Armstrong, K. Busico, A. S. Khan, T. G. Ksiazek, P. E. Rollin, S. R. Zaki, S. T. Nichol, and C. J. Peters.** 1997. Hantavirus transmission in the United States. *Emerg. Infect. Dis.* **3:**361–365.

174. **Williams, R. J., R. T. Bryan, J. N. Mills, R. E. Palma, I. Vera, F. Velasquez, E. M. Baez, W. E. Schmidt, R. E. Figueroa, C. J. Peters, S. R. Zaki, A. S. Khan, and T. G. Ksiazek.** 1997. An outbreak of hantavirus pulmonary syndrome in western Paraguay. *Am. J. Trop. Med. Hyg.* **57:** 274–282.

175. **Wolfe, J. L.** 1982. Oryzomys palustris. *Mamm. Species* **176:**1–5.

176. **Xiao, S. Y., J. LeDuc, K. C. Yong, and C. Schmaljohn.** 1994. Phylogenetic analyses of virus isolates in the genus Hantavirus, family Bunyaviridae. *Virology* **198:**205–217.

177. **Yadon, Z. E.** 1998. Epidemiología del síndrome pulmonar por hantavirus en la Argentina (1991–1997). *Medicina* (Buenos Aires) **58**(Supp. 1):25–26.

178. **Yadon, Z. E., S. Sosa Estani, R. Wells, J. N. Mills, K. Busico, P. Padula, D. Enria, C. J. Peters, and E. L. Segura, and Hantavirus Pulmonary Syndrome Study Group for Patagonia.** Evidence of person-to-person transmission of hantavirus pulmonary syndrome (HPS) during an outbreak in the Patagonia region of Argentina, a case control study. Submitted for publication.

179. **Yanagihara, R., H. L. Amyx, and D. C. Gajdusek.** 1985. Experimental infection with Puumala virus, the etiologic agent of Nephropathia epidemica in bank voles (*Clethrionomys glareolus*). *J. Virol.* **55**:34–38.

180. **Yanagihara, R.** 1990. Hantavirus infection in the United States: epizootiology and epidemiology. *Rev. Infect. Dis.* **12**:449–457.

181. **Yang, L. L.** Hantavirus: an integrated multi-faceted communication campaign. Presented at the American Public Health Association 125th Annual Meeting and Exposition, Indianapolis, Ind., 9 to 13 November 1997.

182. **Yao, J. S., J. Arikawa, H. Kariwa, K. Yoshimatsu, I. Takashima, and N. Hashimoto.** 1992. Effect of neutralizing monoclonal antibodies on Hantaan virus infection of the macrophage P399D1 cell line. *Jpn. J. Vet. Res.* **40**:87–97.

182a. **Yates, T., T. Ksiazek, and S. T. Nichol.** Personal communication.

183. **Yates, T., T. Ksiazek, R. Parmenter, P. Rollin, S. Nichol, J. Dunnum, R. Baker, C. Parmenter, and C. Peters.** Hantavirus outbreaks and rodent ecology: the role of El Niño. p. 61. *In Abstracts of the Fourth International Conference on HFRS and Hantaviruses.*

184. **Yu, Y., X. Yiao, and G. Dong.** 1989. Comparative studies of the immunogenicity of different types of HFRS inactivated vaccines made in China. *JE and HFRS Bulletin* **3**:65–68.

184a. **Zaki, S. R.** Unpublished data.

184b. **Zaki, S. R.** Personal communication.

184c. **Zaki, S. R., and W. J. Shieh.** Personal communication.

185. **Zaki, S. R., A. S. Khan, R. A. Goodman, L. R. Armstrong, P. W. Greer, L. M. Coffield, T. G. Ksiazek, P. E. Rollin, C. J. Peters, and R. F. Khabbaz.** 1996. Retrospective diagnosis of hantavirus pulmonary syndrome, 1978–1993. *Arch. Pathol. Lab. Med.* **120**:134–139.

186. **Zaki, S. R.** 1997. Hantavirus-associated diseases, p. 125–136. *In* D. H. Connor, F. W. Chandler, D. A. Schwartz, H. J. Manz, and E. E. Lack (ed.), *The Pathology of Infectious Diseases*. Appleton and Lange, Norwalk, Conn.

187. **Zaki, S. R., P. W. Greer, L. M. Coffield, C. S. Goldsmith, K. B. Nolte, K. Foucar, R. M. Feddersen, R. E. Zumwalt, G. L. Miller, A. S. Khan, P. E. Rollin, T. G. Ksiazek, S. T. Nichol, B. W. J. Mahy, and C. J. Peters.** 1995. Hantavirus pulmonary syndrome: pathogenesis of an emerging infectious disease. *Am. J. Pathol.* **146**:552–579.

188. **Zaparoli, M. A., L. B. Iversson, M. D. Rosa, et al.** 1995. Investigation on case-contacts of human disease caused by hantavirus in Juquitiba, State of São Paulo, Brazil. *Am. J. Trop. Med.* **53**:232–233. (Abstract.)

189. **Zeitz, P. S., J. C. Butler, J. E. Cheek, M. C. Samuel, J. E. Childs, L. A. Shands, R. E. Turner, R. E. Voorhees, J. Sroisky, P. E. Rollin, T. G. Ksiazek, L. Chapman, S. E. Reef, K. K. Komatsu, C. Dalton, J. W. Krebs, G. O. Maupin, C. M. Sewell, R. F. Breiman, and C. J. Peters.** 1995. A case-control study of hantavirus pulmonary syndrome during an outbreak in the southwestern United States. *J. Infect. Dis.* **171**:864–870.

190. **Zeitz, P. S., J. M. Graber, R. A. Voorhees, C. Kioski, L. A. Shands, T. G. Ksiazek, S. Jenison, and R. F. Khabbaz.** 1997. Assessment of occupational risk for hantavirus infection in Arizona and New Mexico. *J. Occup. Environ. Med.* **39**:463–467.

*Emerging Infections 2*
Edited by W. M. Scheld, W. A. Craig, and J. M. Hughes
© 1998 ASM Press, Washington, D.C.

*Chapter 3*

# Emergence Mechanisms in Yellow Fever and Dengue

## Scott B. Halstead

Emerging infectious diseases have been defined as "diseases of infectious origin whose incidence in humans has increased within the past two decades or threatens to increase in the near future" (6). This definition embraces diseases which are clearly cyclic. Most lists of emerging diseases include microorganisms of many genera which are transmitted endemically or enzootically but whose transmission is governed by herd immunity and in some instances by weather phenomena. From a public health perspective any increase in disease incidence, no matter what the cause, must be of concern. However, from the standpoint of a microbiologist searching for coherent mechanisms which underlie emergence phenomena, herd immunity and weather-based epidemiological events do not convey the novelty implicit in the word "emergence." I propose, therefore, to define emerging infectious diseases as those diseases which increase or threaten to increase due to genetic changes or to stable changes in microbial trafficking.

This review considers what is known and unknown about the mechanisms which govern the emergence of yellow fever and the dengue viruses. These viruses use each of the emergence mechanisms just described.

## YELLOW FEVER

Yellow fever and dengue viruses are members of the family *Flaviviridae*, all transmitted to humans principally by the bite of *Aedes aegypti* mosquitoes. The fact that these viruses occupy precisely the same epidemiological niche but exhibit extraordinarily different behaviors adds interest to this examination of the underlying epidemiological and ecological mechanisms which contribute to epidemic disease.

*Scott B. Halstead* • Medical Science and Technology Division, Office of Naval Research, 800 N. Quincy Street, Arlington, VA 22217-5660.

## History in the Americas

In what is certainly one of the more important events in the history of infectious diseases, at a date unknown but likely the early 1600s, yellow fever virus "emerged" from West Africa to the West Indies (56). The domesticated West African *A. aegypti* undoubtedly infested many of the sailing vessels which plied the trade in human beings to supply sugar plantation workers to the British, French, Spanish, and Dutch colonies in the Caribbean. On occasion, the human cargo and crew offered a combustible mixture of yellow fever-infected, -immune, and -susceptible individuals, allowing epidemics to continue during the 2- to 3-month transit of the Atlantic Ocean. It is also possible that viral transmission aboard ship terminated prior to landfall but infected female mosquitoes survived to escape the ship when it docked.

Yellow fever virus became endemically established in its urban transmission cycle in the larger Caribbean ports. World trade soon introduced yellow fever to many of the towns and cities on the coasts of North and South America and the banks of the Mississippi and Amazon rivers. Another remarkable event occurred silently and unheralded: yellow fever virus escaped from its *Aedes aegypti*-human urban cycle to a forest cycle, infecting a huge range of South American subhuman primates and adopting its transmission to several species of *Hemagogus* mosquitoes. Studies have shown that epizootics of yellow fever in monkeys travel up and down the vast tropical forests in the river basins which drain South America east of the Andean Cordillera. In nature and in the laboratory, American subhuman primates experience a high fatality rate when infected with wild-type yellow fever virus (56, 63–66).

At the beginning of the 20th century, the urban yellow fever mosquito vector was identified, and effective mosquito control methods designed and implemented (56). As early as 1934, urban yellow fever was eradicated from the Western Hemisphere (56). And by 1960, *A. aegypti* had been eradicated from 13 large countries occupying 85% of the Central and South American land mass (39). Despite this show of competence, by the 1970s *A. aegypti* began to reinvade the Americas, and by 1990 it had virtually attained its previous range. From the late 1800s, yellow fever virus repeatedly emerged from its sylvatic cycle to infect human beings, principally adults with occupational exposure to the forests or forest fringe areas (40, 56). Over the past decade, more than 2000 cases have been reported from Bolivia, Brazil, Colombia, Ecuador, and Peru. In 1995, the largest jungle yellow fever epidemic in history recorded 422 cases with 213 deaths; in 1996, there were 155 cases and 80 deaths (40).

Despite the present abundance of *A. aegypti*, human beings infected with jungle yellow fever virus have not initiated urban outbreaks. This satisfactory result might be attributed to the use of yellow fever vaccine, although investigations of jungle yellow fever cases have consistently revealed low yellow fever vaccination rates in the at-risk frontier populations who often live in towns infested by *A. aegypti*.

## History in Africa

Yellow fever virus in Africa causes a wider spectrum of illness than in the Americas. In African adults, yellow fever is often a relatively mild disease. Case fatality rates are relatively lower than the terrifyingly high rates common in American outbreaks (40). These differences were sufficient to motivate the Rockefeller Foundation in 1926 to establish laboratories in Lagos, Nigeria, and Accra, Ghana (56). The African patient, Asibi, who yielded the prototype yellow fever virus strain parent to the 17D vaccine, had a mild, self-limited disease. Almost immediately thereafter, three Rockefeller researchers infected with the Asibi strain acquired yellow fever and died (56).

In 1960, a major epidemic occurred in Ethiopia. And in the past three decades, particularly the last 10 years, large yellow fever epidemics have been reported from Gambia, Senegal, Nigeria, and Cameroon (38–40, 50). In 1986, a classical urban *Aedes aegypti*-transmitted epidemic was centered in Ibadan.

Yellow fever is maintained in Africa in two sylvatic cycles. One is a West African cycle in which virus is transmitted among a wide range of subhuman primate species by *Aedes furcifer-taylori* or *Aedes luteocephalus* and other species of Stegomyia. Virus in this cycle is transmitted by these species to humans and then from human to human in rural and urban areas by *A. aegypti*. This species in Africa occupies a wider range of habitats and has a broader host-feeding preference than outside Africa. The other is an East and Central African cycle in which the virus is transmitted among subhuman primates by *Aedes africanus* and from monkeys to humans by *Aedes simpsoni*. Virus from this cycle produced the large 1960 Ethiopian outbreak and the smaller 1990 and 1996 outbreaks in Kenya (38–40). African monkeys have sufficiently high viremias to sustain transmission, but usually infection is clinically inapparent. The genetic resistance of African subhuman primates and the evolution of two distinct sylvatic cycles are consistent with the extremely long duration of yellow fever virus circulation in Africa. Despite the long-term presence of *A. aegypti* on the coast of East Africa, at no time has the virus escaped from Central Africa to cause coastal outbreaks of yellow fever (56).

Interestingly, yellow fever epizootics and epidemics in West Africa appear 1 year following a heavy rainy season which is correlated with El Niño southern oscillation (ENSO) events (40).

## Predicted Emergence Events

Based upon abundant evidence, historical and recent, yellow fever virus has moved out of the West African sylvatic cycle to cause urban outbreaks in West Africa and the Americas. Assuming all yellow fever viruses retain the capacity to be transmitted by *A. aegypti*, it can be confidently predicted that (i) a similar phenomenon should occur in South America because *A. aegypti* has been widely reestablished and (ii) yellow fever virus should break out of its African zoonotic cycles to invade the East African coast and from there the vast receptive areas of Asia.

## Genetic Emergence Mechanisms

A succession of genetic studies on yellow fever viruses have concluded that there are at least two or three genotypes in circulation: type I in Central Africa, type IIA in West Africa, and type IIB in the Americas (Fig. 1) (7). The yellow

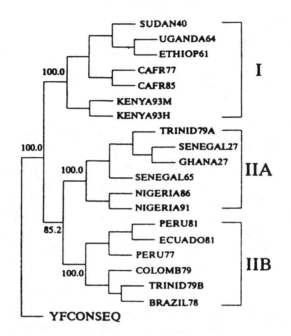

**Figure 1.** Phylogram derived from the nucleotide sequences of the E gene of yellow fever viruses illustrating the evolutionary relationships of genotype I, IIA, and IIB viruses. The numbers at the forks indicate the number of times the monophyletic group consisting of viruses to the right of the fork occurred among the 100 trees. (Reprinted with permission from reference 7.)

fever viruses with the greatest genetic distance from others are those transmitted in the Central African sylvatic cycle (7, 11, 33). A relatively close genetic relationship between genotypes IIA and IIB is consistent with the hypothesized West African origin of American yellow fever viruses which have adapted to a new set of vertebrate hosts and mosquito vectors (7, 11). In addition to genetic differences, many phenotypic differences also exist between types IIA and IIB (10, 12, 14, 27). Remarkably little work has been done, however, to define phenotypic differences between type I and II viruses. In fact, there is little evidence that yellow fever viruses from the East African and South American sylvatic cycles are capable of being transmitted by *A. aegypti*. Public health planning requires a definitive answer.

## MICROBIAL TRAFFICKING

The invasion of Asia by yellow fever has been the emergence event most widely predicted and feared during this century (13, 56). Many explanations have been put forward to explain the failure of this dreaded event to occur.

(i) Asian *A. aegypti* was not competent to transmit yellow fever. Several studies have furnished evidence that relatively high yellow fever viremias were required to infect Asian mosquitoes and that the percentage of infected mosquitoes capable of transmitting to experimental hosts was rather low (1, 37, 57). But when *A.*

*aegypti* strains from South America, Africa, and Asia were compared under similar conditions, the African strains (collected from sites of known urban transmission) demonstrated even lower levels of vector competence (36).

(ii) It has been postulated that infection by one or more dengue viruses might provide partial human herd immunity, reducing the chance of yellow fever transmission (56). As evidence of this, it has been observed that British troops "seasoned" in India or Indian plantation workers, both presumably immune to dengue viruses, suffered lower yellow fever case-fatality rates than did Caucasians who did not have this earlier immunological experience (2). These epidemiological observations received partial experimental confirmation through the studies of Theiler and Anderson who observed that dengue-immune monkeys had lower titers of yellow fever viremia than did susceptible controls (58). An immunological barrier hypothesis seems epidemiologically implausible. In West Africa, urban yellow fever epidemics are established in the face of considerable specific immunity and a high prevalence of antibodies to other flaviviruses. In areas where dengue is endemic, more than one-half of children under the age of 5 are totally susceptible to flaviviruses. It seems extremely unlikely that yellow fever transmission could be completely suppressed in such populations.

By process of elimination, the most compelling hypotheses to explain the absence of yellow fever in coastal East Africa and Asia are (i) the inability of genotype I viruses to be transmitted in the urban cycle and (ii) failure of type IIA viruses to reach the East Coast. The genotype I transmission cycle appears to have served historically as a geographic barrier to the passage of genotype IIA viruses through Africa from West to East Coast. Genotype IIA viruses are the only proven urban-competent strains. The Asian emergence event has not happened because of the failure of IIA yellow fever virus to transit the Cape of Good Hope to East Africa and/or to Asia. This is compatible with the historically low volume of trade between West Africa and Indian Ocean ports. With the advent of air transportation, this ancient barrier is gone.

### Emergence Events—America

Since the eradication of urban yellow fever in 1934, the reintroduction of yellow fever into urban areas of the Americas from jungle yellow fever cases has been repeatedly predicted. A few putative occurrences have been reported, but urban outbreaks have not occurred. One must ask whether jungle-*Hemagogus*-adapted IIB viruses have lost their ability to be transmitted by *A. aegypti*. In the 1940s, Waddell and Taylor demonstrated that South American yellow fever strains were capable of being serially transmitted among subhuman primates by *A. aegypti* (63–66). However, the proper experiment has not been done. It would compare the competence of American *A. aegypti* strains to transmit type IIA and IIB urban and sylvatic yellow fever viruses. Fortunately for the world but unfortunately for the experiment, American urban yellow fever strains do not exist.

### CONCLUSIONS

The following conclusions are offered. (i) The emergence of yellow fever in countries on the Indian Ocean or elsewhere in Asia is biologically possible and requires only the introduction of the West African type IIA virus. This event becomes increasingly likely with the increase in human trafficking between West Africa and the rest of the world. In this regard, reports of the involvement of Nigerians in global drug trafficking is worrisome. (ii) In the Americas, because of a paucity of relevant evidence the probability of the emergence of urban yellow fever is difficult to assess. (iii) There is an urgent need to study the transmission potential of type IIB and type I yellow fever viruses for *A. aegypti*.

## DENGUE HEMORRHAGIC FEVER

### History

From clinical reports, dengue hemorrhagic fever/dengue shock syndrome (DHF/DSS) can be identified in the medical literature in northeastern Australia in 1897 and continuing for the next fifteen years (26). Another major epidemic which featured DHF-like cases was that in Greece in 1928 which left serological evidence of dengue 1 and 2 virus transmission among survivors (25). In the modern era, DHF/DSS was recognized from 1950 in Bangkok, where cases of thrombocytopenia and vascular permeability were recognized by chart review (20). This disease seemingly "spread" to the Philippines, where cases were first reported in 1954, and then over a 15-year period to Vietnam, Burma, Singapore, Malaysia, and Indonesia (22). In the mid-1980s DHF/DSS spread to southern China and Hainan Island (44). In the same era in which urban yellow fever almost disappeared, dengue virus transmission is virtually ubiquitous in the tropics.

The virological attributes of all Asian DHF/DSS epidemics have been the same: (i) multiple types of dengue viruses circulated simultaneously or sequentially and (ii) patients with carefully defined DHF/DSS have secondary-type dengue antibody responses or (if they were less than 1 year old) primary-type responses (21, 25). In all prospective seroepidemiological studies, DHF/DSS cases have been documented only with secondary dengue infections (4, 51, 52, 59).

Importantly, in the American tropics in the 1970s and on the Indian subcontinent until 1988, three or four types of dengue viruses circulated simultaneously or sequentially without resulting in substantial numbers of DHF/DSS cases (5, 67). Then in 1981, DHF/DSS struck Cuba (18, 32). This epidemic was caused by a dengue 2 (DEN-2) virus, which infected a population partially immune to dengue 1. Virtually all classical DHF/DSS cases were in children with secondary dengue infections; severe disease syndromes seen in adults were also significantly associated with secondary infections (3, 31).

From about 1987 in the American tropics, DHF/DSS outbreaks have been reported annually from Venezuela, Colombia, Brazil, Guyana, and French Guiana as well as in Puerto Rico and Nicaragua (43, 45).

Next, in 1988, from the Maldive Islands and Sri Lanka and then from southern India to northern India, epidemics of DHF/DSS were reported (42, 55, 62).

Finally, in 1990, a classic sharp epidemic of DHF/DSS occurred on Tahiti. This was associated with secondary DEN-3 infections on a background of recent DEN-1 and more remote DEN-2 infections (15). By contrast, earlier sequential epidemics of DEN-1 during World War II, followed by DEN-3 in 1964 to 1969, DEN-2 in 1971, and DEN-1 again in 1974 and in 1988 and 1989 had not produced epidemic DHF/DSS (6, 9, 23).

## DHF/DSS Risk Factors

Below are listed the various host and virus factors which convert a benign and self-limited disease, dengue fever, to a severe and often fatal syndrome, DHF/DSS:

1. Infection parity. The overriding risk factor for DHF/DSS in individuals over the age of 1 year is history of one prior dengue infection (21).
2. Passively acquired dengue antibody. Dengue antibody acquired transplacentally places infants at high risk to DHF/DSS during a first dengue infection during the first year of life (21, 35).
3. Enhancing antibodies. Dengue virus infection-enhancing antibody activity in undiluted serum is strongly correlated with DHF/DSS in individuals who experience a subsequent secondary dengue infection (29, 30).
4. Absence of protective antibodies. Low levels of cross-reactive neutralizing antibody protect, but DHF/DSS occurs in their absence (30).
5. Viral strain. DHF/DSS is associated with secondary infections with dengue viruses of Asian origin (8, 47, 48).
6. Age. DHF/DSS is usually associated with children. From the epidemiologically unique 1981 Cuban DHF/DSS epidemic, it was determined that the modal age of greatest susceptibility to dengue shock syndrome is 8 to 10 years (32).
7. Sex. Careful studies have shown that shock cases and deaths occur more frequently in female than male children (21).
8. Race. In the 1981 Cuban epidemic, blacks had lower hospitalization rates for DHF/DSS than did whites or Asians (19).
9. Nutritional status. Many anecdotal reports and one formal study have shown that moderate to severe protein-calorie malnutrition reduces risk to DHF/DSS in dengue-infected children (60).
10. Preceding host conditions. Menstrual periods and peptic ulcers are risk factors for the severe bleeding in adults which occurs during some dengue infections (46, 61).

## PATHOGENESIS MECHANISMS IN DHF/DSS

Figure 2 summarizes current concepts of the mechanisms which result in DHF/DSS. In common with other infectious diseases, dengue is characterized by afferent and efferent phases. Afferent events are those phenomena which impact on the

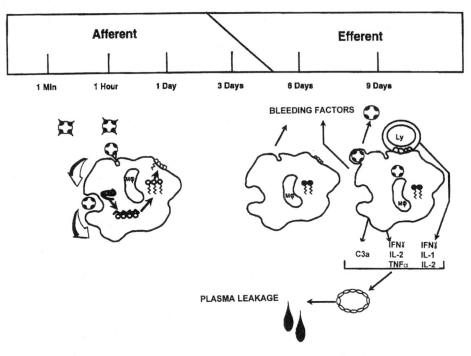

**Figure 2.** Illustration of postulated immunopathogenic events during the two stages of dengue infection. Across the top are shown times after infectious mosquito bite. Cells shown are of the mononuclear phagocyte lineage. C3a, complement breakdown product; IFNγ, interferon gamma; TNFα, tumor necrosis factor alpha; IL, interleukin; Ly, lymphocyte. (Reprinted with permission from reference 17.)

survival of microorganisms and their ability to enter cells and replicate. Efferent events are those phenomena which cause illness. These may be due to the direct pathogenic action of the microorganism or due to an immune response directed against antigens on the surface of virus-infected cells. In either phase, risk factors may operate to enhance disease severity.

## Afferent Phenomena

### Enhancing Antibodies

In the case of viruses, attachment to appropriate target cells and successful entry into the cell are crucial. It is likely that the important afferent events in dengue occur within seconds, perhaps minutes or hours, after virus is introduced into subcutaneous tissues by a mosquito proboscis and that non-neutralizing antibodies providing even a minimal advantage in target cell-seeking may enhance the infected cell mass and affect clinical outcome.

In the infant infection model, most of the mothers had been infected prior to the birth of the 12 studied infants with two or more different dengue viruses including the serotype which subsequently caused severe disease in the infants. It was estimated that DHF/DSS occurred during a short window in the life of each infant when maternal dengue-2 neutralizing antibodies were metabolically degraded below a titer of 1:10, measured in a LLC-MK2 plaque reduction assay (29). Thus, the age when an infant experiences DHF/DSS is related directly to the level of antibody acquired from the mother (29). Only a handful of cases from this extremely important pathogenic group has ever been studied, and only DEN-2 viruses have been recovered from infant DHF/DSS.

In the second-infection model, infection-enhancing antibodies are raised to antigens shared between the first and second infecting serotypes. The role of enhancing antibodies in humans was shown in a Bangkok study in which preinfection blood samples were collected from 40 school children who subsequently experienced a secondary dengue infection, mostly due to DEN-2 (30). All children were observed by school teachers and visiting nurses for illness episodes. During their secondary dengue infections, 33 children had no school absenteeism while 7 were hospitalized with an illness compatible with DHF/DSS. When undiluted preinfection serums were examined undiluted for dengue antibodies in a human monocyte assay, five of seven hospitalized children were circulating DEN-2 infection-enhancing antibodies.

## Absence of Protective Antibody

In the prospective epidemiological study just described, 30 of 33 asymptomatic children circulated DEN-2 neutralizing antibodies acquired from an earlier infection with a different dengue serotype (30). DEN-2 had been established as the most likely cause of secondary infections in Bangkok during 1980 (4).

It is not understood how or why these heterotypic neutralizing antibodies are raised. Explanations include the possibility that dengue envelope structure comes in two varieties, with or without epitopes closely similar to serotype-specific neutralizing epitopes of another virus (for example, DEN-1 viruses may or may not express DEN-2-like epitopes). From a study by Kliks et al. (30), it can be predicted that viruses which carry cross-reactive epitopes will be more abundant than viruses without such epitopes.

An alternate explanation is that dengue serotypes and genotypes are antigenically relatively homogeneous. It is the human immune system which responds differently to the available antigenic repertoire. This could express itself, for example, as "low" or "high" antibody-responders. High antibody responders might then raise protective concentrations of neutralizing antibodies to heterospecific antigens, while low responders would produce biologically insignificant amounts of these same neutralizing antibodies. Both groups, however, produce dengue infection-enhancing antibodies. Consistent with this hypothesis were data from children with DHF/DSS in the Rayong study who had very low levels of neutralizing antibodies in their pre-second dengue infection sample (52).

## Viral Strains

Dengue 1, 2, and 3 viruses circulate in more than one distinct genotypic grouping (34, 47, 48). The most distant of all the genetic groups are DEN-2 viruses recovered from a West African zoonotic cycle which involves subhuman primates and is transmitted by *A. africanus* and *A. furcifer-taylori* mosquitoes. There is no evidence of human infection with this genotype, nor is it known if it can be transmitted to humans by *A. aegypti*.

## First Infections

The first dengue infection generates enhancing or cross-neutralizing antibodies which critically determine the outcome of the second infection. Consistent with evidence suggesting that first infections determine the outcome of a second infection are data that all DEN viruses obtained from mild or severe secondary infection patients from the same epidemic are genetically identical (8, 49). That is, within a single geographic entity and time frame, dengue disease severity is not determined independently by viral strain

## Second Infections

A macro-observation has been made across the globe and over time that DHF/DSS occurs at epidemic proportions only when the second serotype is of Southeast Asian origin (8, 47, 48). As previously described, during the period from 1950 to 1980, a genetically distinct DEN-2 which failed to produce DHF/DSS in DEN-3 immunes circulated in the American tropics. At the same time, in India all four DEN serotypes circulated simultaneously or sequentially until the late 1980s without producing DHF/DSS. Even in areas where DHF/DSS is endemic, some dengue virus serotypes have circulated for prolonged periods without causing DHF/DSS. This was noted in the Rayong study, where secondary DEN-1 infections were far more numerous than secondary DEN-2 infections but yielded no DHF/DSS cases. It was with considerable surprise that secondary DEN-1 infections were found to be pathogenic while secondary DEN-2 were not in a prospective study in 1995 and 1996 in Yogyakarta, Indonesia (16). A similar switch from nonpathogenic to pathogenic dengue strains has been noted in Thailand with DEN-3. In the 1960s and 1970s, DEN-3 produced mild or inapparent second dengue infections in Thailand, but this changed abruptly in 1983 with the emergence of DEN-3 DHF/DSS cases. The origin of this virus is unknown, but in the 1970s DEN-3 was often associated with DHF/DSS in Indonesia (17). The genotypes of these viruses have not been studied extensively.

Why do secondary dengue infections differ in clinical outcome? Could this simply reflect the distribution of heterotypic and nonheterotypic antigens on the infecting virus pairs or a deeper biological behavior? The simplest explanation is that all secondary dengue infections are controlled by the presence or absence of heterotypic neutralizing antibodies. There is preliminary contradictory evidence from a small study in which dengue viruses from severely ill individuals replicated to higher titers in cultures of human mononuclear phagocytes in the presence of enhancing antibodies than did viruses from mildly ill children (41).

## Efferent Phenomena

### Viral Strains

In classical dengue fever, viral infection is followed by a 4- to 5-day "silent" incubation period which in turn is succeeded by the abrupt onset of myalgia, headache, fever, and lack of appetite. These are followed over the next several days by gastrointestinal disturbances, changing taste perception, and such signs as fever, diaphoresis, flushing face, early macular rash, neutropenia, bone marrow depression, thrombocytopenia, hemorrhagic diathesis, lymphadenopathy, bradycardia, and certain central nervous signs such as anxiety and depression (53, 54). Such efferent phenomena might be mediated by one or more cytokines released by dengue virus-infected cells or to cytokines generated as a result of virus replication (Fig. 2). Differences in dengue fever epidemics, such as those which have occurred on Pacific Islands over the past 30 years, are best explained by dengue virus strain variation (17). It is not yet clear whether intrinsic biological behavior governs the "DHF-genic" and "DHF-non-genic" dengue virus strains described above.

## Age, Sex, Race, and Nutritional Status

The role of these host factors in modulating dengue disease has been described (23, 25). The role of race in modulating DHF/DSS requires emphasis. The 1981 Cuban DHF/DSS outbreak documented a reduced risk of blacks for shock syndrome compared with whites (19). A retrospective seroepidemiological study provided evidence that blacks and whites were equally infected with DEN-1 and DEN-2 serotypes. In this study, blacks were underrepresented in hospital populations by as much as fivefold (19). It may be speculated that a dengue resistance gene exists which, in turn, may be related to a postulated (but as yet undocumented) yellow fever resistance gene. Yellow fever has been enzootic in Africa for millennia and is a lethal disease at all ages and over a prolonged period. Genetically resistant individuals would have a survival advantage. Currently, no DHF/DSS has been reported from Africa where three serotypes are known to circulate. A possibility which must be considered is that in Africa DHF/DSS expression is completely suppressed.

## Preceding Host Conditions

Other efferent phenomena which may result in severe dengue disease are pre-existing pathologies. Best documented is the severe gastrointestinal bleeding which accompanies dengue infections (primary or secondary) in individuals with peptic ulcer disease (61). Severe menorrhagia during dengue infections has also been described (46, 53, 54). It is presumed that a dengue hemorrhagic diathesis results in hemorrhage in individuals with open mucosal lesions. Blood loss may be catastrophic and life threatening. The mechanism of hemorrhage in dengue is unknown.

## Emergence Mechanisms

### Increased Microbial Trafficking

There can be no doubt that the fundamental reason for the emergence of DHF/DSS first in Southeast Asia and now throughout the globe is due to the vast increase in dengue virus transmissions resulting from the 20th century population explosion, the growth and deterioration of tropical cities, and the increasing movement of people within and between countries, particularly by air.

### Genetic Change

For DEN-2 there is compelling evidence that secondary DHF/DSS occurs only with a genotype which was first isolated in Southeast Asia and has been present there for the entire period of the modern DHF/DSS epidemic. DHF/DSS does not occur with secondary infections by a genetically distinct DEN-2 virus first recovered in the Caribbean in 1954, although this phenomenon has hardly been studied. All four serotypes cause DHF/DSS, but there is evidence that viruses which do and do not cause this syndrome cocirculate, appearing and disappearing over time.

Before speculating, as some have (28, 68), that the emergence of newly "virulent" genetic variants is the result of dengue virus "hypertransmission," it would be well to remember that exactly the same dengue syndrome apparently accompanied an earlier era of "hypertransmission" over 100 years ago. It must be concluded that positive and negative DHF/DSS-capable dengue virus variants are and have been in circulation for a very long time. Their recent emergence to endemicity may be a function of the remarkable steady acceleration of the global viral circulation system over the past four decades.

## CONCLUSIONS

Host resistance factors may permanently restrict the penetrance of DHF/DSS into Africa and may already have reduced predicted rates of DHF/DSS morbidity and mortality in the Americas through the widespread distribution of African dengue resistance genes. Except for the Cuban outbreak, no population-based studies of dengue have been conducted in the American hemisphere. As a result, neither the impact of virus genotype nor that of host resistance or risk factors on the patterns of dengue disease can be adequately assessed.

Documentation of a genetic marker for DHF/DSS-capable and noncapable viruses should not be interpreted to mean that the extensive documentation of the second-infection phenomenon is to be set aside or that inherent dengue virus virulence has been established. Far from it: what these new observations mean is that dengue pathogenesis has proven to be exceedingly complex and increasingly enigmatic. Without carefully integrated studies on viral and host factors conducted on a global scale, there can be little hope that we will soon understand emergence mechanisms for this fascinating but increasingly dangerous group of microorganisms.

## REFERENCES

1. **Aitken, T. H. G., W. G. Downs, and R. E. Shope.** 1977. *Aedes aegypti* strain fitness for yellow fever virus transmission. *Am. J. Trop. Med. Hyg.* **26:**985–1989.
2. **Ashcroft, M. T.** 1979. Historical evidence of resistance to yellow fever acquired by residence in India. *Trans. R. Soc. Trop. Med. Hyg.* **73:**247–248.
3. **Bravo, J. R., M. G. Guzman, and G. P. Kouri.** 1987. Why dengue haemorrhagic fever in Cuba? 1. Individual risk factors for dengue haemorrhagic fever/dengue shock syndrome (DHF/DSS). *Trans. R. Soc. of Trop. Med. Hyg.* **81:**816–820.
4. **Burke, D. S., A. Nisalak, D. E. Johnson, and R. M. Scott.** 1988. A prospective study of dengue infections in Bangkok. *Am. J. Trop. Med. Hyg.* **8:**172–180.
5. **Carey, D. E., R. M. Myers, and R. Reuben.** 1966. Studies on dengue in Vellore, South India. *Am. J. Trop. Med. Hyg.* **15:**580–587.
6. **Centers for Disease Control and Prevention.** 1994. *Addressing Emerging Infectious Disease Threats: a Prevention Strategy for the United States.* U.S. Department of Health and Human Services, Public Health Service, Atlanta, Ga.

7. **Chang, G.-J., B. C. Cropp, R. M. Kinney, D. W. Trent, and D. J. Gubler.** 1995. Nucleotide sequence variation of the envelope protein gene identifies two distinct genotypes of yellow fever virus. *J. Virol.* **69:**5773–5780.

8. **Chungue, E., V. Deubel, O. Cassar, M. Laille, and P. M. Martin.** 1993. Molecular epidemiology of dengue 3 virus and genetic relatedness among dengue 3 strains isolated from patients with mild or severe form of dengue fever in French Polynesia. *J. Gen. Virol.* **74:**1765–2770.

9. **Chungue, E., O. Cassar, M. T. Drouet, M. G. Guzman, M. Laille, L. Rosen, and V. Deubel.** 1995. Molecular epidemiology of dengue-1 and dengue-4 viruses. *J. Gen. Virol.* **76:**1877–1884.

10. **Clarke, D. H.** 1960. Antigenic analysis of certain group B arthropod-borne viruses by antibody absorption. *J. Exp. Med.* **111:**21–32.

11. **Deubel, V., J. P. Digoutte, T. P. Monath, and M. Girard.** 1986. Genetic heterogeneity of yellow fever virus strains from Africa and the Americas. *J. Gen. Virol.* **76:**209–213.

12. **Deubel, V., J. J. Schlesinger, J. P. Digoutte, and M. Girard.** 1987. Comparative immunochemical and biological analysis of African and South American Yellow fever viruses. *Arch. Virol.* **94:**331–338.

13. **Dudley, S. F.** 1934. Can yellow fever spread into Asia? *J. Trop. Med. Hyg.* **37:**273–278.

14. **Fitzgeorge, R., and C. J. Bradish.** 1980. The *in vivo* differentiation of strains of yellow fever virus in mice. *J. Gen. Virol.* **46:**1–13.

15. **Glaziou, P., E. Chungue, P. Gesta, O. Soulignac, J. P. Couter, P. Plichat, J. F. Roux, and L. Poli.** 1992. Dengue fever and dengue shock syndrome in French Polynesia. *S.E. Asian J. Trop. Med. Pub. Health.* **23:**531–532.

16. **Graham, R.** 1997. Personal communication.

17. **Gubler, D. J.** 1997. Dengue and dengue hemorrhagic fever: its history and resurgence as a global public health problem, p. 1–22. *In* D. J. Gubler and G. Kuno (ed.), *Dengue and Dengue Hemorrhagic Fever.* CAB International, New York, N.Y.

18. **Guzman, M. G., D. J. Kouri, J. M. Bravo, S. Sales, M. Vazquez, R. Santos, R. Villaescusa, P. Basanta, G. Indan, and J. M. Ballestes.** 1984. Dengue haemorrhagic fever in Cuba. II Clinical investigations. *Trans. R. Soc. Trop. Med. Hyg.* **78:**239–241.

19. **Guzman, M. G., G. P. Kouri, J. M. Bravo, S. Soler, L. Vazquez, and L. Morier.** 1990. Dengue hemorrhagic fever in Cuba, 1981: a retrospective seroepidemiologic study. *Am. J. Trop. Med. Hyg.* **42:**179–184.

20. **Halstead, S. B., and C. Yamarat.** 1965. Recent epidemics of hemorrhagic fever in Thailand. Observations related to pathogenesis of a "new" dengue disease. *Am. J. Public Health* **55:**1386–1395.

21. **Halstead, S. B., S. Nimmannitya, and S. N. Cohen.** 1970. Observations related to pathogenesis of dengue hemorrhagic fever. IV. Relation of disease severity to antibody response and virus recovered. *Yale J. Biol. Med.* **42:**311–328.

22. **Halstead, S. B.** 1980a. Dengue haemorrhagic fever, a public health problem and a field for research. *Bull. W. H. O.* **58:**1–21.

23. **Halstead, S. B.** 1980b. Immunological parameters of togavirus disease syndromes, p. 107–173. *In* R. W. Schlesinger (ed), *The Togaviruses, Biology, Structure, Replication.* Academic Press, New York, N.Y.

24. **Halstead, S. B., and G. Papaevangelou.** 1980. Transmission of dengue 1 and 2 viruses in Greece in 1928. *Am. J. Trop. Med. Hyg.* **29:**635–637.

25. **Halstead, S. B.** 1988. Pathogenesis of dengue: challenges to molecular biology. *Science* **239:**476–481.

26. **Hare, F. E.** 1898. The 1897 epidemic of dengue in North Queensland. *Australasian Med. Gaz.* **98:**107.

27. **Henderson, B. E., P. P. Cheshire, G. B. Kirya, and M. Lule.** 1970. Immunological studies with yellow fever and selected African group B arboviruses in rhesus and vervet monkeys. *Am. J. Trop. Med. Hyg.* **19:**110–119.

28. **Holland, J. J.** 1996. Evolving virus plagues. *Proc. Natl. Acad. Sci. USA* **93:**545–546.

29. **Kliks, S., S. Nimmannitya, A. Nisalak, and D. S. Burke.** 1988. Evidence that maternal dengue antibodies are important in the development of dengue hemorrhagic fever in infants. *Am. J. Trop. Med. Hyg.* **38:**411–419.

30. **Kliks, S., A. Nisalak, W. E. Brandt, L. Wahl, and D. S. Burke.** 1989. Antibody-dependent enhancement of dengue virus growth in human monocytes as a risk factor for dengue hemorrhagic fever. *Am. J. Trop. Med. Hyg.* **40:**444–451.

31. **Kouri, G. P., M. G. Guzman, and J. R. Bravo.** 1987. Why dengue haemorrhagic fever in Cuba? 2. An integral analysis. *Trans. R. Soc. Trop. Med. Hyg.* **81:**821–823.

32. **Kouri, G. P., M. G. Guzman, and J. R. Bravo.** 1989. Dengue haemorrhagic fever/dengue shock syndrome: lessons from the Cuban epidemic. *Bull. W. H. O.* **67:**375–380.

33. **Lepiniec, L., L. Dalgarno, V. T. Huong, T. P. Monath, J. P. Digoutte, and V. Deubel.** 1994. Geographic distribution and evolution of yellow fever viruses based on direct sequencing of genomic cDNA fragments. *J. Gen. Virol.* **75:**417–423.

34. **Lewis, J. G., G. J. Chang, R. S. Lanciotti, R. M. Kinney, L. W. Mayer, and D. W. Trent.** 1993. Phylogenic relationships of dengue-2 viruses. *Virology* **197:**216–224.

35. **Martinez, E., M. G. Guzman, and M. Valdes.** 1993. Dengue fever and hemorrhagic dengue in infants with a primary infection. *Rev. Cub. Trop. Med.* **45:**97–101.

36. **Miller, B. M., T. P. Monath, W. J. Tabachnik, and V. I. Ezike.** 1989. Epidemic yellow fever caused by an incompetent mosquito vector. *Trop. Med. Parasitol.* **40:**396–399.

37. **Mitchell, C. J., B. M. Miller, and D. J. Gubler.** Vector competence of *Aedes albopictus* from Houston, Texas, for dengue serotypes 1 to 4, yellow fever and Ross River viruses. *J. Amer. Mosq. Contr. Assoc.* **3:**460–465.

38. **Monath, T. P.** 1989. Recent epidemics of yellow fever in Africa and the risk of future urbanization and spread, p. 37–44. *In* M. F. Uren, J. Blok, and L. H. Manderson (ed.), *Arbovirus Research in Australia.* Queensland Institute of Medical Research, Brisbane, Australia.

39. **Monath, T. P.** 1994. Yellow fever and dengue–the interactions of virus, vector and host in the re-emergence of epidemic disease. *Semin. Virol.* **5:**133–145.

40. **Monath, T. P.** 1997. Epidemiology of yellow fever: current status and speculations on future trends, p. 143–156. *In* J. F. Saluzzo and B. Dodet (ed.), *Factors in the Emergence of Arbovirus Diseases.* Elsevier, Paris, France.

41. **Morens, D. M., N. J. Marchette, M. C. Chu, and S. B. Halstead.** 1991. Growth in human peripheral blood leukocytes of dengue type 2 isolates correlates with severe and mild dengue disease. *Am. J. Trop. Med. Hyg.* **45:**644–651.

42. **Nimmannitya, S.** 1988. Personal communication.

43. **Pan American Health Organization.** 1979. *Dengue in the Caribbean in 1977.* Proceedings of a workshop held in Montego Bay, Jamaica, May 8–11, 1978, p 1–186. Scientific Publication No. 375, Pan American Health Organization, Washington, D.C.

44. **Qui, F. X., D. J. Gubler, J. C. Liu, and Q. Q. Chen.** 1993. Dengue in China: a clinical review. *Bull. W. H. O.* **71:**349–359.

45. **Ramirez-Ronda, C. H. and Garcia, C. D.** 1994. Dengue in the Western Hemisphere. *Infect. Dis. Clin. N. Am.* **8:**107–128.

46. **Rice, L.** 1923. Dengue fever. A clinical report of the Galveston epidemic of 1922. *Am. J. Trop. Med.* **3:**73–90.

47. **Rico-Hesse, R.** 1990. Molecular evolution and distribution of dengue viruses type 1 and 2 in nature. *Virology* **174:**479–493.

48. **Rico-Hesse, R., L. M. Harrison, R. A. Salas, D. Tovar, A. Nisalak, C. Ramos, J. Boshell, M. T. deMesa, R. M. Noguera, A. Travassos da Rosa.** 1997. Origins of dengue type 2 viruses associated with increased pathogenicity in the Americas. *Virology* **230:**244–251.

49. **Rico-Hesse, R.** 1997. Personal communication.

50. **Robertson, S. E., B. P. Hull, O. Tomori, O. Bele, J. W. LeDuc, and K. Esteves.** 1996. Yellow fever: a decade of reemergence. *JAMA* **276:**1157–1162.

51. **Russell, P. K., T. M. Yuill, A. Nisalak, S. Udomsakdi, D. J. Gould, and P. E. Winter.** 1968. An insular outbreak of dengue hemorrhagic fever. II. Virologic and serologic studies. *Am. J. Trop. Med. Hyg.* **17:**600–608.

52. **Sangkawibha, N., S. Rojansuphot, S. Ahandrik, S. Viriyaponse, S. Jatanasen, V. Salitul, B. Phanthumachinda, and S. B. Halstead.** 1984. Risk factors in dengue shock syndrome: a prospective epidemiologic study in Rayong, Thailand. *Am. J. Epidemiol.* **120:**653–669.

53. **Siler, J. F., M. W. Hall, and A. P. Hitchens.** 1926. Dengue: its history, epidemiology, mechanisms of transmission, etiology, clinical manifestations, immunity and prevention. *Phil. J. Sci.* **29:**1–304.

54. **Simmons, J. S., J. H. St. John, and F. H. K. Reynolds.** 1931. Experimental studies of dengue. *Phil. J. Sci.* **44:**1–247.

55. **Srivastava, V. K., S. Suri, A. Bhasin, L. Srivastava, and M. Bharadwaj.** 1990. An epidemic of dengue haemorrhagic fever and dengue shock syndrome in Delhi: a clinical study. *Paed.* **10:**329–334.

56. **Strode, G. K., J. C. Bugher, J. A. Kerr, H. H. Smith, K. C. Smithburn, R. M. Taylor, M. Theiler, A. J. Warren, and L. Whitman** (ed.). 1951. *Yellow Fever.* McGraw-Hill, New York, N.Y.

57. **Tabachnick, W. J., G. P. Wallis, T. H. G. Aitkin, B. R. Miller, G. D. Amato, L. Lorenz, J. R. Powell, and B. J. Beaty.** 1985. Oral infection of *Aedes aegypti* with yellow fever virus: geographic variation and genetic considerations. *Am. J. Trop. Med. Hyg.* **34:**1219–1224.

58. **Theiler, M., and C. R. Anderson.** 1974. The relative resistance of dengue-immune monkeys to yellow fever virus. *Am. J. Trop. Med. Hyg.* **24:**115–117.

59. **Thein, S., M. M. Aung, T. N. Shwe, M. Aye, A. Zaw, K. Aye, K. M. Aye, and J. Aaskov.** 1997. Risk factors in dengue shock syndrome. *Am. J. Trop. Med. Hyg.* **56:**566–572.

60. **Thisyakorn, U., and S. Nimmannitya.** 1993. Nutritional status of children with dengue hemorrhagic fever. *Clin. Infect. Dis.* **16:**295–297.

61. **Tsai, J. C., C. H. Kuo, and P. C. Chen.** 1991. Upper gastrointestinal bleeding in dengue fever. *Am. J. Gastroent.* **86:**33–35.

62. **Vitarana, T., and N. Jayasekara.** 1990. Dengue haemorrhagic fever outbreak in Sri Lanka. *S.E. Asian J. Trop. Med. Pub. Health* **21:**682.

63. **Waddell, M. B., and R. M. Taylor.** 1945. Studies on cyclic passage of yellow fever virus in South American mammals and mosquitoes: I. Marmosets (*Callithrix autira*) and Cebus monkeys (*Cebus versutus*) in combination with *Aedes aegypti* and *Haemagogus equinus*. *Am. J. Trop. Med.* **25:**225–230.

64. **Waddell, M. B., and R. M. Taylor.** 1946. Studies on cyclic passage of yellow fever virus in South American mammals and mosquitoes: II. Marmosets (*Callithrix penicillata* and *Leontocebus chrysomela*) in combination with *Aedes aegypti*. *Am. J. Trop. Med.* **26:**455–463.

65. **Waddell, M. B., and R. M. Taylor.** 1947. Studies on the cyclic passage of yellow fever virus in South American mammals and mosquitoes. III. Further observations on *Haemagogus equinus* as a vector of the virus. *Am. J. Trop. Med.* **27:**471–476.

66. **Waddell, M. B., and T. M. Taylor.** 1948. Studies on the cyclic passage of yellow fever virus in South American mammals and mosquitoes. IV. Marsupials (*Metachirus nudicaudatus* and *Marmosa*) in combination with *Aedes aegypti* as vector. *Am. J. Trop. Med.* **28:**87–100.

67. **Woodall, J. P., R. H. Lopez-Correa, G. E. Sather, and C. G. Moore.** 1981. The absence of epidemic dengue hemorrhagic fever from the Americas, p. 95–106. *In* S. Hotta (ed.), *Dengue Hemorrhagic Fever 1981. Proceedings of the First International Center for Medical Research Seminar.* International Center for Medical Research, Kobe, Japan.

68. **Zanotto, P. M., E. A. Gould, G. F. Gao, P. H. Harvey, and E. C. Holmes.** 1996. Population dynamics of flaviviruses revealed by molecular phylogenies. *Proc. Natl. Acad. Sci. USA* **93:**548–553.

*Emerging Infections 2*
Edited by W. M. Scheld, W. A. Craig, and J. M. Hughes
© 1998 ASM Press, Washington, D.C.

*Chapter 4*

# Human Herpesvirus 8 and Kaposi's Sarcoma

## Thomas J. Spira and Harold W. Jaffe

In this chapter, we will review the association between the recently recognized virus human herpesvirus 8 (HHV-8) and Kaposi's sarcoma (KS), the most common malignancy seen in persons with AIDS. Other malignancies associated with HHV-8 will also be reviewed. We hope to illustrate the use of epidemiologic methods to indicate an infectious agent as the cause of a disease of unknown etiology and the use of molecular biologic methods to identify infectious agents that may have remained undetectable by more conventional approaches.

### EPIDEMIOLOGY OF KS

In 1872, Moritz Kaposi, a dermatologist working in Vienna, described five men over age 40 and one boy with "idiopathic multiple pigmented sarcomas" of the skin (77). Since that time, the disease described by Kaposi has become known as "classical" KS, and epidemiologic studies have shown it to be primarily a disease of elderly men, particularly men of southern European (especially Italian) and Ashkenazi Jewish ancestry (49, 157). Classical KS has been rare in the United States; an estimated 300 to 400 cases occurred annually in this country during the mid-1970s (14). This form of KS is typically described as having an indolent clinical course, with lesions usually limited to skin, especially the skin of the lower legs or feet. Elderly men were said to die with rather than from KS. Persons with classical KS are at increased risk for a second malignancy, especially lymphomas (137).

A second epidemiologic form of KS was recognized in Africa. This endemic form of the disease occurs most commonly in equatorial Africa, especially in northeastern Zaire, western Uganda, and Tanzania; in the mid-1960s, it accounted for 8% of all cancers among Ugandan men (153). Like classical KS, endemic KS occurs more often among men than women, and its incidence increases with age.

*Thomas J. Spira and Harold W. Jaffe* • Division of AIDS, STD, and TB Laboratory Research, National Center for Infectious Diseases, Centers for Disease Control and Prevention (A-25), 1600 Clifton Road, Atlanta, GA 30333.

Children also may be affected. The clinical course of KS among Africans may be more aggressive than that seen among Americans or Europeans.

A third epidemiologic form of KS has been seen among persons with iatrogenic immunosuppression, most often organ transplant recipients. In the Cincinnati Transplant Tumor Registry, KS accounted for 3% to 4% of all tumors reported (128). The incubation period for KS following transplantation was relatively short, a median of 16 months versus 54 months for other tumors. In contrast to the other forms of KS, there is no clear male predominance in this form; rather, the sex distribution of cases is similar to that of transplant recipients. In about two-thirds of cases, the clinical course of disease is described as indolent; in some cases, complete remission of disease has been reported following cessation of immunosuppressive therapy.

A fourth epidemiologic form of KS occurs among human immunodeficiency virus (HIV)-infected persons. The occurrence of KS among young, previously healthy men who have sex with men (MSM) was one of the first indications of the AIDS epidemic in the United States (5), and KS in HIV-infected persons is an AIDS-defining condition. KS is by far the most common malignancy found in HIV-infected persons. Among the 612,000 Americans reported with AIDS through June 1997, almost 52,000 were reported to have KS (28). Since AIDS case reports largely reflect conditions present at the time of an initial AIDS diagnosis rather than conditions that develop subsequently, this estimate of KS rate is a minimum estimate. An analysis done in 1990 indicated that the incidence of KS among Americans with AIDS was about 20,000 times that seen in the general population and about 300 times that seen in other immunosuppressed patients (13). The course of KS among HIV-infected persons is often aggressive with multiple mucocutaneous lesions and with visceral disease involving the lungs and gastrointestinal system commonly occurring.

The proportion of HIV-infected persons who develop KS varies considerably among persons in different HIV transmission categories. In the United States, the KS risk is highest for men infected through homosexual contact, intermediate for persons infected through heterosexual contact and intravenous drug use, and lowest for persons with hemophilia infected through the use of contaminated clotting factors (13).

The HIV epidemic has also had a major impact on the occurrence of KS in endemic regions of Africa. For example, in the cancer registry maintained in Kampala, Uganda, KS was the most common cancer reported for men (48.6% of all cancers) and the second most common cancer for women (17.9% of all cancers) during the period 1989 to 1991. This represented a more than 10-fold increase in KS incidence since the 1950s (156). Among Ugandan children, the incidence of KS has also risen about 40-fold in the AIDS era. Of children with KS seen at the Uganda Cancer Institute from 1989 to 1994, 78% were HIV infected (159).

## THE CASE FOR AN INFECTIOUS CAUSE OF KS

Many epidemiologic aspects of KS suggest that it may have an infectious cause (10, 129, 130). One group of studies concerns risk factors for KS among MSM.

While the findings from these studies are not entirely consistent, they suggest that the KS risk for MSM is highest if they have multiple sex partners (7, 8, 74). Some studies indicate that sexual practices that lead to exposure to feces may additionally increase the KS risk (11). For MSM living in the United States, KS risk is highest for those living in areas of high AIDS incidence (13). For MSM living in the United Kingdom, KS risk is highest for those having sex partners from the United States or Africa (12).

Additional epidemiologic data come from studies of KS among women with heterosexually acquired HIV infection. In the United States, the highest KS rates for HIV-infected women are seen in women who were born in Haiti or have sex partners from Haiti, an area of high KS incidence. Women whose male partners are bisexual have an intermediate KS risk, while women who acquired HIV through sex with heterosexual men have the lowest risk (13). Similar findings from Europe among women with KS have confirmed an increasing risk for KS development in women infected via heterosexual intercourse, women infected through contact with bisexual men, and women originating from African or Caribbean countries (141). Finally, support for the infectious agent hypothesis comes from reports of KS among relatively young, HIV-uninfected MSM. These men, described mainly in New York City, have normal CD4$^+$ T-lymphocyte counts and a clinically indolent course of KS disease (57).

Taken together, these observations suggested that if there was an infectious cause of KS, its primary route of transmission might be sexual, although fecal-oral exposure might also play a role. This latter transmission route could be more important in developing parts of the world, such as Africa or Haiti, where sanitation may be poor. Whether KS in African children is the result of vertical (mother-to-child) or horizontal transmission of a "KS agent" is not clear. The occurrence of KS among HIV-uninfected MSM may represent the presence of the agent in the absence of HIV infection. Further, the paucity of KS cases among HIV-infected transfusion recipients, hemophiliacs, and injection drug users argues against this agent's being a blood-borne pathogen.

## DISCOVERY OF THE VIRUS

Even before the increased incidence of KS associated with HIV infection, researchers had been looking for a possible infectious agent as a cause of KS. Early seroepidemiologic studies examined cytomegalovirus as a possible cause (61). More recently, human T-cell lymphotropic virus type 1 has also been postulated as a possible etiology (88). However, there has been no convincing evidence that either of these two agents is involved in the pathogenesis of KS.

In 1994, Chang and Moore and collaborators employed a novel technique in the search for an etiologic agent for KS (34). This technique, representational difference analysis, compared DNA from Kaposi's skin lesions to normal uninvolved skin from the same individual. They applied the technique on samples from individuals with AIDS-associated KS. Viral sequences were demonstrated in all AIDS-KS lesions examined; the sequences were most closely related to the human herpesvirus Epstein-Barr virus (EBV) and a simian herpesvirus, herpesvirus saimiri (HVS), both of which are in the gamma herpesvirus subfamily in the genus *Rhadinovirus* (34). The virus, corresponding to the viral sequences found, was then isolated from a cell line derived from an individual with AIDS-related body-cavity-based lymphoma (BCBL), a rare AIDS-associated malignancy. While the virus was called Kaposi's sarcoma-associated herpesvirus (KSHV) by its discoverers to indicate its association with KS, its formal name is human herpesvirus 8. In this discussion, we use the terminology HHV-8, although both these terms are currently used.

## DETECTION OF HHV-8 BY PCR

Use of the PCR to detect HHV-8 DNA is one of the primary methods of determining HHV-8 infection. PCR has most frequently been performed with the original primer set described by Chang et al., which produced a 233-bp fragment. Some studies combined this primer set with a second primer set in a nested PCR assay. Although nested PCR can increase the sensitivity of the assay, it also has an increased potential for false positives due to contamination. PCR was first applied to KS lesion biopsies, and studies have found a rate of positivity ranging from 70 to 100% in all forms of KS: HIV-associated, classic, endemic African, and iatrogenic or transplant-associated (Table 1).

PCR-based studies have also examined the rate of positivity of KS biopsies based on the stage of the lesion. Nodular lesions, which appear later in the disease, have been shown to have a higher rate of positivity (87 to 91%) than the rates found in the earlier patch and plaque stages (40 to 50% and 50 to 67%, respectively) (100, 103).

Lymph nodes from HIV-infected individuals have also been tested. In lymph nodes from those with KS, rates of HHV-8 positivity ranging from 0 to 25% have been reported (15, 34, 140). In those without KS, 13% of biopsies from HIV-positive Italians with lymphadenopathy were found to be HHV-8 positive, while the rate of positivity in HIV-negative reactive lymphadenopathies was 9% (15). In a Taiwanese study of benign hyperplastic lymph nodes, none were HHV-8 positive (151), while an Italian study found a positivity rate of 18% in hyperplastic tonsils from normal individuals (99).

Studies of peripheral blood mononuclear cells (PBMCs) or peripheral blood lymphocytes (PBLs) from HIV-infected individuals with KS have shown an HHV-8 positivity rate ranging from 35 to 84% with a combined rate of 53% (Table 2). In HIV-infected individuals without KS, HHV-8 positivity rates in PBMCs/PBLs tend to be higher in MSM, 6 to 24%, compared with those with hemophilia, 7 to 10% (72). In HIV-negative individuals without KS, HHV-8 has usually been undetectable in PBMCs/PBLs by PCR.

HHV-8 has also been detected in plasma and serum, with rates of positivity usually higher in serum (0 to 16% vs. 11 to 46%). The higher rate in serum may be secondary to the release of cell-associated DNA during clotting and may not represent infectious virus (9, 86, 105, 158).

Additional PCR studies of HHV-8 have focused on other body fluids. A study of sputum from HIV-infected KS patients found only one patient with pulmonary

**Table 1.** HHV-8 PCR of KS tissue biopsies

| Type of PCR and reference | No. of biopsies positive for HHV-8/total | | | | | | |
|---|---|---|---|---|---|---|---|
| | HIV-associated KS | Non-KS control skin | Classic KS | Iatrogenic or transplant KS | KS in HIV-negative MSM | African KS | Normal control skin |
| One-step PCR | | | | | | | |
| 34 | 25/27 | | | | | | |
| 3 | 12/12 | 4/11 | 1/1 | | | | |
| 51 | 4/4 | | 5/5 | | | | |
| 71 | 12/12 | | 7/8 | | | | |
| 132 | 13/13 | | 13/18 | | | | |
| 140 | 25/25 | | 3/3 | | | 18/18 | |
| 35 | 22/24 | | | | | 17/20 | |
| 37 | | | | | 1/2 | 4/4 | |
| 54 | 6/6 | | | | | 3/9[a] | |
| 75 | 5/5 | | 12/12 | | | | |
| 79 | | | | 4/4 | | | |
| 105 | 28/28 | 6/26 | 7/8 | | 2/2 | 7/10 | |
| 120 | 27/41 | | 3/6 | 5/11 | | | |
| 159 | | | | | | 8/8 | |
| 2 | | | | 27/28 | | | |
| 46 | 5/11 | | | | | | |
| 55 | 53/54 | | | | 2/2 | | |
| 69 | 12/12 | 5/12 | | | | | |
| 85 | | | 16/18 | | | 24/49 | |
| 88 | 2/2 | 3/9 | 10/10 | 1/1 | | 3/3 | |
| 131 | 32/32 | 11/36[b] | | | | 6/6 | |
| 145 | 8/9 | 4/7 | | | | | |
| 155 | 3/4 | | 17/22 | | | | 0/5 |
| Total | 294/309 | 33/101 | 94/111 | 37/44 | 5/6 | 90/127 | 0/5 |
| (% positive) | (95.1) | (32.7) | (84.7) | (84.1) | (83.3) | (70.9) | (0) |
| Nested PCR | | | | | | | |
| 22 | 14/14 | | 16/17 | 8/8 | 1/1 | | |
| 26 | 9/9 | | 12/12 | 1/1 | | | |
| 48 | 14/14 | | 35/40 | | | | |
| 112 | | | | | | | 1/18 |
| 142 | 7/7 | | | | | | |
| 52 | 3/3 | | 6/6 | 3/3 | | | |
| 103 | 10/13 | | 16/23 | | | | |
| 155 | 4/4 | | 20/22 | | | | |
| Total | 61/64 | | 105/120 | 12/12 | 1/1 | | 1/18 |
| (% positive) | (95.3) | | (87.5) | (100) | (100) | | (5.6) |

[a]None of eight children were positive.
[b]Data for both HIV-infected and uninfected persons with KS in Uganda.

KS positive for HHV-8 (158). None of 24 HIV-infected patients without KS was HHV-8 positive. Saliva was found to be HHV-8 positive in 75% of HIV-infected MSM with KS (86). In HIV-infected individuals without KS the HHV-8 positivity rate ranged from 15 to 33% with the higher figure detected by nested PCR (16,

**Table 2.** HHV-8 PCR of peripheral blood mononuclear cells

| Reference | No. of positive samples/total | | | | | | |
|---|---|---|---|---|---|---|---|
| | HIV+KS+[a] | HIV−KS+[b] | HIV+KS−[c] | HIV−KS−[d] | HIV+, coagulation defect[e] | HIV−, coagulation defect[f] | HIV+, other[g] |
| 3 | 7/7 | 3/3 | | 0/14 | | | |
| 38 | 2/10 | | 0/9 | | | | |
| 90 | | 0/5 | | | | | |
| 140 | | | 0/13 | 0/12 | | | |
| 158[h] | 24/46 | | 11/143 | 0/134 | | | |
| 15 | | | 4/58 | 5/56 | | | |
| 23 | | 24/40 | | | | | |
| 56 | 6/7 | 0/2 | | 0/5 | | | |
| 72 | 34/98 | | 10/42 | 0/11 | 1/14 | | 1/8 |
| 92 | 10/11 | | 3/6[i] | | | | |
| | | | 1/45 | | | | |
| 105 | 46/99 | 0/2 | 0/64 | 0/163 | | | |
| 112[h] | | | | 1/14 | | | |
| 114[h] | | | 12/21[i] | | | | |
| 131 | 29/31 | 2/6 | 2/23[j] | | | 2/9 | |
| 18[h] | | | 9/33 | | | | |
| 47 | | | 10/96 | | | | |
| 68[h] | 10/15 | | 2/9 | | | | |
| 69 | 4/12 | 0/2 | | | | | |
| 86 | 17/24 | 1/1 | 2/20 | | | | |
| 125 | 11/21 | | 2/23 | | 0/19 | | |
| 135 | 7/10 | | 5/13 | | | | 0/10 |
| 145 | 4/8 | | | | | | |
| 155[h] | 2/4 | 2/4 | 3/30 | | | | |
| Total | 213/403 | 32/72 | 61/621 | 6/409 | 1/33 | 2/9 | 1/18 |
| (%) | (52.9) | (44.4) | (9.8)[k] | (0.2) | (3.0) | (22.2) | (5.6) |

[a]HIV infected with KS.
[b]HIV uninfected with KS.
[c]HIV infected without KS.
[d]HIV uninfected without KS.
[e]HIV infected with a coagulation defect.
[f]HIV uninfected with a coagulation defect.
[g]HIV infected, other.
[h]Nested PCR.
[i]Prior to the development of KS.
[j]None of 51 children were positive.
[k]Excluding data from individuals known to later develop KS. For this group, the total is 15 of 27 (55.6%) positive.

19, 86). In HIV-negative individuals, no HHV-8 DNA was detected, even by nested PCR (19, 86).

Nasal secretions, both cellular and fluid fractions (40 and 60%, respectively), have been found to be positive for HHV-8 in HIV-infected patients with KS (16). Bronchioalveolar lavage (BAL) fluid was HHV-8 positive in 40% of HIV-infected patients with pulmonary KS, but in only 20% of those with cutaneous KS. Among those persons, BAL cells were 58 and 0% positive, respectively. HIV-infected patients without KS had lower HHV-8 positivity rates, 3 and 7%, respectively (9).

Studies of semen from HIV-infected individuals with KS have found from 0 to 40% to be positive for HHV-8 (3, 47, 65, 68, 69, 86, 105, 155). HHV-8 rates in semen from HIV-infected individuals without KS have ranged from 0 to 33% positive, with several studies reporting no positive results (47, 65, 68, 86). Other studies have reported higher rates of viral detection of HHV-8 with nested PCR (91%), but these studies have been questioned because of the increased risk of contamination when nesting is used (96, 112). In addition, one study from Italy (112) has reported a 63% HHV-8 positivity rate in normal prostate tissue, but this finding has been contradicted by another study of similar tissue from men in both the United States and Italy which found none positive (152).

## SEROEPIDEMIOLOGY

If HHV-8, like many other human herpesviruses, were ubiquitous among American and European adults, questions would remain regarding the connection between HHV-8 and KS. Why is KS much more commonly seen in HIV-infected MSM than in other HIV-infected persons? Might HHV-8 simply be an opportunistic infection in HIV-immunosuppressed individuals, normally existing in a latent state with reactivation occurring because of immunosuppression?

To determine the prevalence of HHV-8 infection, seroepidemiologic studies have used a variety of methods. Tests to detect antibodies to HHV-8 include Western blot or immunoblot assays using lysates of HHV-8-infected BCBL cell lines, an indirect immunofluorescent antibody (IFA) assay (also using BCBL cell lines), and enzyme-linked immunoassays (ELISAs) against viral peptides or viral lysates (Table 3).

With most of the available tests, antibodies to HHV-8 have been detected in a majority of individuals with KS, including AIDS-associated KS, classic KS, endemic African KS, and iatrogenic KS (associated with iatrogenic immunosuppression or transplantation). IFA has been used to detect both latent and lytic HHV-8 antigens in BCBL cells. Latent nuclear antigens are expressed in all BCBL cells without any stimulation. Lytic cytoplasmic antigens representing replicative products of HHV-8 are detected in about 20 to 30% of cells induced with tetradecanoyl phorbol ester acetate (TPA). When the IFA assay for latent antigen was directly compared to that for lytic antigen on specimens from HIV-infected KS patients, the former had an HHV-8 positivity rate of 52%, and the latter of 96% (93). However, their respective positivity rates in normal blood donors were 0 and 20%. In a number of studies, HHV-8 seropositivity for KS patients has ranged from 52 to 100% with the IFA assay for latent antigen and from 65 to 100% with the IFA for lytic antigen (Table 3). Rates of HHV-8 seropositivity by IFA tended to be highest in persons with non-HIV-associated KS, such as those with classic or African endemic KS. Peptide ELISAs tended to be less sensitive than the IFA assays (33 to 84%), while immunoblot assays were comparable to IFA for latent antigen.

Rates of HHV-8 seropositivity in HIV-infected individuals without evident KS vary by HIV exposure category. Paralleling the higher incidence of KS in MSM, HHV-8 seropositivity rates in this group range from 23 to 55% (HIV-infected) and from 0 to 13% (HIV-uninfected) by the IFA latent antigen assay and from 13 to

**Table 3.** HHV-8 serology detected by IFA, immunoblot, and ELISA

| Method and reference | Antigen | HIV+KS+[a] | HIV−KS+[b] | HIV+KS−[c] | HIV−KS−[d] |
|---|---|---|---|---|---|
| Detected by IFA | | | | | |
| 58 | LANA[e] | 34/40 (MSM, USA) | | 12/40 (AIDS) | 0/122 (USA) |
| | | 10/14 (Italy) | 11/11 (Italy) | 0/20 (US hemophiliacs) | 4/107 (Italy) |
| | | 14/18 (Uganda) | 1/1 (Uganda) | 18/35 (Uganda) | 24/51 (Uganda) |
| 82 | LANA | 37/38 | 1/1 | 9/300 (hemophiliacs) | 0/18 (women) |
| | | | | 2/44 (recipients of HIV+ transfusions) | 0/50 (blood donors) |
| | | | | 13/37 (MSM) | 3/23 (MSM) |
| | | | | 13/46 (STD[h] patients) | 10/130 (STD patients) |
| | | | | 0/9 (heterosexuals) | 7/107 (heterosexuals) |
| | | | | | 2/141 (blood donors) |
| 93 | LANA | 47/91 (USA) | 28/28 (Africa) | 16/71 (MSM) | 0/44 (blood donors) |
| | | | | 0/33 (women) | 0/54 (women) |
| | | | | 0/13 (IVDUs[f]) | 0/263 (children) |
| | Lytic | 84/87 (USA) | 3/4 (USA) | 64/71 (MSM) | 9/44 (blood donors) |
| | | | 28/28 (Africa) | 7/33 (women) | 15/54 (women) |
| | | | | 3/13 (IVDUs) | 10/263 (children) |
| 110 | Lytic | 31/48 (USA) | | 7/54 | |
| 143 | LANA | 84/103 (USA/UK) | 17/18 (Greece) | 10/33 (MSM) | 0/117 (US blood donors) |
| | | | | 0/26 (hemophiliacs) | 4/150 (UK blood donors) |
| | | | | 0/38 (IVDUs) | 3/26 (Greek blood donors) |
| | | | | 18/34 (Uganda) | 9/17 (Ugandan blood donors) |
| | | | | 3/15 (women with STD) | 2/26 (women with STD) |
| 63 | LANA | | | 2/118 (US women) | 1/80 (US women) |
| | | | | 1/28 (Haitian women) | 8/63 (Haitian women) |
| | | | | 0/26 (infants) | 0/158 (infants) |
| 81 | LANA | | | 12/302 (US women) | 1/84 (US women) |

*(Table continues)*

**Table 3.** *Continued*

| Method and reference | Antigen | HIV+KS+[a] | HIV−KS+[b] | HIV+KS−[c] | HIV−KS−[d] |
|---|---|---|---|---|---|
| 86 | LANA | 21/24 | 1/1 | 11/20 | 0/10 |
| 145 | LANA | 7/7 | | 6/18 | 0/52 |
| | Lytic | 7/7 | | 6/18 | 0/52 |
| Detected by immunoblot | | | | | |
| 58 | LANA[e] | 32/40 (MSM, USA) | | 7/40 (MSM with AIDS) | 0/122 (USA) |
| | | 11/14 (Italy) | 11/11 (Italy) | 0/20 (hemophiliacs, USA) | 4/107 (Italy) |
| | | 16/18 (Uganda) | 1/1 (Uganda) | 25/35 (Uganda) | 29/41 (Uganda) |
| 110 | P40 peptide | 32/48 (USA) | | 7/54 | |
| Detected by ELISA | | | | | |
| 143 | orf65 recombinant protein | 46/57 (USA, UK) | 17/18 (Greece) | 5/16 (MSM) | 6/117 (US blood donors) |
| | | 14/17 (Uganda) | | 0/28 (hemophiliacs) | 3/174 (UK blood donors) |
| | | | | 2/38 (IVDUs) | 3/26 (Greek blood donors) |
| | | | | 16/34 (Uganda) | 6/17 (Ugandan blood donors) |
| 4 | orf26 recombinant protein | 23/69 (Germany) | | 7/30 (Germany) | 5/55 (Germany) |
| 43 | orf26 peptide-BSA[g] | 16/29 (MSM, USA) | | 3/9 (MSM, USA) | 6/30 (US blood donors) |
| | | | | 6/24 (hemophiliacs, USA) | |
| 36 | Whole virus lysate | 9/9 (USA) | | | 2/14 (USA) |

[a]HIV-infected with KS.
[b]HIV-uninfected with KS.
[c]HIV-infected without KS.
[d]HIV-uninfected with KS (OD > 0.4, greater than "low reactivity").
[e]Latency-associated nuclear antigen.
[f]Intravenous drug users.
[g]Peptide conjugated to bovine serum albumin.
[h]Sexually transmitted disease.
[i]KS+, 87 HIV+, breakdown of HHV-8-positive not given.

90% by the IFA lytic antigen assay. The peptide ELISA yielded a rate of 31% HHV-8 positive. Rates among persons in other HIV exposure categories are substantially lower: 0 to 3% for hemophiliacs and 0 to 4.5% for HIV-infected intravenous drug users by IFA latent antigen but 23% for HIV-infected intravenous drug users by IFA lytic antigen (123). With the protein ELISA, the HHV-8 rate for

HIV-infected hemophiliacs was 0 to 25% and 5% for HIV-infected intravenous drug users.

HHV-8 seropositivity rates for normal controls or blood donors vary both geographically and by the assay used. In the United States, rates are generally low: from 0 to 1.4% in adults (including adult and pregnant women) by the IFA latent antigen assay or 20% by the lytic antigen assay. Children are either negative by the IFA latent antigen assay or are positive by the lytic antigen assay at rates ranging from 2% in the 3- to 5-year-old age group, 8% in 6- to 10-year-olds, and 4% in 11- to 15-year-olds and rising to adult rates of 18% in the 16- to 20-year-old age group (93). HHV-8 rates among persons in countries with higher rates of KS, either classic or African endemic, are higher. For example, in Greece HHV-8 seroprevalence is reported to be 11.5%, while in Central Africa rates range from 11 to 53% with the IFA latent antigen assay to 32 to 82% with the lytic antigen assay (93, 143). With a protein ELISA, in Greece the rate is 12% while in Uganda it is 35% (143). In West Africa, HHV-8 rates range from 6 to 43% with the latent antigen assay and from 56 to 100% in the lytic antigen assay (although the highest rates were from studies of low numbers of individuals) (93).

## OTHER MALIGNANCIES

Since HHV-8 is a member of the gammaherpesvirus subfamily and other members of this subfamily have been associated with malignancies (e.g. EBV with nasopharyngeal carcinoma and certain B-cell lymphomas and HVS with T-cell lymphomas in squirrel monkeys), biopsy material from a variety of lymphoproliferative diseases has been examined for presence of HHV-8. Results from a number of studies have found only two diseases convincingly associated with HHV-8. The first of these is (BCBL) or primary effusion lymphoma (PEL). This lymphoma consists of primarily malignant lymphomatous effusions containing large-cell immunoblasts or anaplastic large cells. The malignant cells usually lack *c-myc* rearrangement. A tumor mass is usually absent, and the malignant cells remain localized to the body cavity of origin. The lymphoma cells are CD45-positive and have one or more activation antigens (CD30, CD38, CD71, HLA-DR, or epithelial membrane antigen). They lack T-cell or B-cell antigens but have evidence for clonal immunoglobulin gene rearrangements. They are often also EBV-positive. Most recent cases have been described in HIV-infected MSM, although BCBL/PEL also occurs in HIV-uninfected individuals (Table 4). The prognosis is poor, with an overall survival time after diagnosis in one series of 60 days (24, 30, 78, 87, 117). The levels of HHV-8 in the cells are often 40- to 80-fold higher than those found in KS tissue cells (29). While most cases are unassociated with a tumor mass, two cases associated with lymphoma of the bowel in HIV-infected men have been reported where both the tumor and the effusion contained HHV-8 (45). Other benign and malignant effusions are usually negative for HHV-8 (25, 31, 117).

In addition to BCBL/PEL, HHV-8 has been consistently found in lymph nodes of patients with HIV-associated multicentric Castleman's disease (MCD). Castleman's disease (CD) has two distinct histopathologic types: the more common hyaline vascular type, which presents as a tumor-like mass in the mediastinum or

**Table 4.** PCR of HHV-8-associated malignancies: body-cavity-based lymphoma/primary effusion lymphoma

| Reference | HIV infected | HIV uninfected |
|---|---|---|
| 6 | 5/5 | |
| 25 | 3/4 | 1/2 |
| 29 | 8/8 | |
| 34 | 3/3 | |
| 59 | 2/2 | |
| 78 | 7/7 | |
| 117 | | 2/2 |
| 126 | 3/3 | |
| 139 | | 2/2 |
| Total (%) | 31/32 (96.9) | 83.3 |

retroperitoneum, and the rarer plasma cell type with immune dysfunction, generalized lymphadenopathy, and constitutional symptoms. The plasma cell type, or MCD, is associated with HHV-8, while persons with the hyaline vascular type have been found to be HHV-8 negative (83). MCD may be accompanied by autoimmune phenomena, rashes, cytopenias, and infections and is associated with KS and non-Hodgkin's lymphoma (64, 83, 148). While most cases of HHV-8 in persons with MCD have been found in those with HIV infection, HHV-8 has also been detected in about half of MCD cases not associated with HIV infection, even in the absence of KS (Table 5). In HIV-associated cases, HHV-8 is found most commonly in MSM (122). While HHV-8 is most commonly detected in the lymph nodes of persons with MCD, it has also been found in peripheral blood in one case of HIV-negative MCD (148).

## OTHER DISEASES

Because of the association of HHV-8 with KS, which usually begins as a neoplasm involving the skin, a variety of other skin conditions have been studied to

**Table 5.** PCR of HHV-8-associated malignancies: MCD

| Reference | Type | HIV-infected | HIV-uninfected |
|---|---|---|---|
| 33 | Multicentric | | 3/5 |
| | Hyaline vascular type | | 0/6 |
| 60 | Multicentric | 3/4 | 1/3 |
| | Hyaline vascular type | | 0/3 |
| 40 | Multicentric | | 4/4 |
| | Hyaline vascular type | | 0/2 |
| 98 | Multicentric | | 0/5 |
| | Hyaline vascular type | | 0/7 |
| 144 | | | 0/4[a] |
| 148 | Multicentric | 14/14 | 7/17 |
| Total[b] (%) | | 17/18 (94.4) | 15/34 (44.1) |

[a]Children.
[b]Multicentric only.

determine if they are also associated with this virus. Some of these are conditions which (like KS) also involve a proliferation of endothelial cells (48) or which are also vascular lesions (75, 84, 106, 146). Other skin conditions examined include those found at increased incidence in immunocompromised individuals. With rare exceptions (73, 106, 119, 133), these skin lesions have all been negative for HHV-8 by PCR. These exceptions have been questioned by other reports of similar skin tumors in which no HHV-8 has been found (20, 21, 26, 48, 50, 91, 154).

In addition to BCBL/PEL and MCD, a variety of lymphoid proliferations have been studied to determine if any of these may also be associated with HHV-8. With few exceptions, no associations have been found (1, 27, 29, 31, 67, 95, 97, 100, 105, 116, 126, 127, 136, 151). In a recent report, HHV-8 was found by PCR in bone marrow dendritic cells of individuals with multiple myeloma and in such cells of some individuals with monoclonal gammopathy of undetermined significance, a precursor to multiple myeloma. The authors failed to find the virus in the malignant plasma cells or in bone marrow dendritic cells from normal donors (134). Others have found no increased incidence of HHV-8 seropositivity in multiple myeloma patients (102, 104).

A few other diseases have also been studied for a possible association with HHV-8 (Tables 4 and 5). Of these, HHV-8 has been found by PCR in 29 to 38% of normal brain and stillborn brain tissues as well as brain tissue from individuals from Italy with multiple sclerosis (108). Multiple sclerosis was studied because of reports of the association of HHV-6 with this condition. HHV-8 has also been found in a small number of individuals, both HIV-infected and -uninfected, with encephalitis (138). These persons were studied because of the association of other herpesviruses with encephalitis. In one individual with interstitial pneumonitis, studied because of the association of some herpesviruses with this condition, HHV-8 was found in pulmonary tissue (101). These findings require further confirmation.

## TROPISM AND TISSUE LOCALIZATION

Other gammaherpesviruses have been found to be tropic to either B-lymphocytes (EBV) or T-lymphocytes (HVS). HHV-8 has been found in purified peripheral blood B-lymphocytes (CD19$^+$/CD20$^+$) but not in purified T-suppressor/cytotoxic cells (CD8$^+$) from individuals with KS (3, 56, 66). Peripheral blood monocytes (CD14$^+$) and pleural fluid CD34$^+$ (an endothelial cell and hemopoietic stem cell marker) cells have also been found to contain HHV-8 genome (56). In one report (66), HHV-8 was found by in situ hybridization (ISH) in a minority of peripheral blood T-lymphocytes (0.1 to 2.2%), compared to B-lymphocytes (27 to 48%) from two patients followed over time. HHV-8 has also been found by ISH in cells of monocytoid origin in KS lesions (17). An examination of autopsy tissues from HIV-infected patients from Italy with KS detected HHV-8 in paravertebral sensory ganglia, lymphoid tissue, and bone marrow (39, 41).

HHV-8 has been transmitted from a BCBL cell line to purified CD19$^+$ umbilical cord B lymphocytes (109) and from early passage spindle cells from KS lesions to a human embryonal-kidney epithelial-cell line (293 cells) (56a). No success in propagation was achieved with a variety of endothelial cells (human umbilical vein, porcine, or human or porcine vascular smooth muscle primary cells) (56a).

KS tissue has been examined by using ISH to localize HHV-8 infected cells. Viral mRNA (both 0.7 and 1.1 kb) has been found in typical perivascular spindle cells as well as endothelial cells lining the vascular slits (17, 20, 70, 94, 124, 149, 150). The 0.7-kb transcript is seen at all stages of KS and in most cells, while the 1.1-kb transcript is seen primarily in late lesions and in only 10% of cells. The former is associated with latent infection, and the latter with lytic infection. Intra-nuclear inclusions have also been noted in spindle cells and mononuclear cells of KS lesion. Using transmission electron microscopy, the typical morphology and cytopathicity of herpesvirus has been found in both spindle cells and mononuclear cells (resembling lymphocytes) (124) (Fig. 1). Viral genomic DNA has been found to be in covalently closed, circular episomes characteristic of latent herpesviruses in KS lesions. Although linear forms characteristic of lytic infection were not found in lesions, they have been found in the PBMCs of some HHV-8 infected individuals (44).

## SENSITIVITY TO ANTIVIRALS

Several epidemiologic studies have examined the effect of antivirals active against herpesviruses on the development of KS. One showed a reduced risk for KS development among persons using foscarnet but not among those using acyclovir or ganciclovir (76). In another study, no effect was found for any of the three drugs (42). Both of these studies showed a slightly increased relative hazard

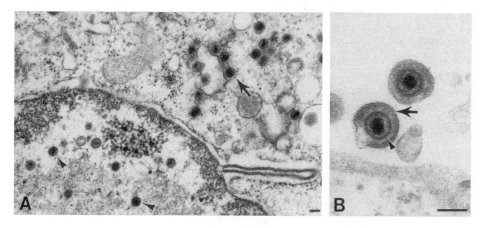

**Figure 1.** (A) Electron micrograph of HHV-8 grown in BCBL-1 cells, showing viral nucleocapsids (arrowheads) in the cell nucleus and cytoplasmic particles (arrow) budding upon the membranes of the Golgi apparatus. (B) Extracellular particles containing nucleocapsid (arrowhead) surrounded by a layer of tegument and enclosed in viral envelope (arrow). Bars, 100 nm. (Courtesy of C. Goldsmith [Centers for Disease Control and Prevention] and M. Offerman [Emory University School of Medicine].)

for KS with use of acyclovir (1.3 and 1.4, respectively). A third study found that both foscarnet and ganciclovir, but not acyclovir, reduced the risk for KS development (111). Another study also found a similar effect for foscarnet and ganciclovir, but it did not reach the level of significance (62). These results should be interpreted with caution, since all of the studies were retrospective analyses.

The development of cell lines productive for HHV-8 has led to studies of the susceptibility of the virus to antivirals. Two studies have shown HHV-8 to be highly sensitive to cidofovir, moderately sensitive to foscarnet and ganciclovir, and weakly sensitive or insensitive to acyclovir (80, 107). There was no inhibition of the episomal, or latent, form of the virus (107). Remission of KS has also been described in patients treated with foscarnet (115). While many of these agents are possibly feasible for use in short-term treatment, they are not practical for the long-term prophylaxis needed for KS. They must be given intravenously and also have significant toxicity. Other newer antivirals with activity against herpesviruses are being evaluated for treatment of KS and may also be useful for prophylaxis.

Interferon alpha, which is used for KS treatment, has also been found to have a slight inhibitory effect on the growth of KS-derived cells. It increased the expression of MHC-class I antigens and rendered the cells susceptible to interferon-primed natural killer cell cytotoxicity (89), but it has not been tested for any anti-HHV-8 effect. In one patient, thalidomide treatment for oral ulcers reportedly induced regression of KS lesions, disappearance of HHV-8 from blood, and a decrease in viral load in tumor tissue (147).

## PATHOGENESIS

Although evidence for the association of HHV-8 and KS, as well as BCBL/PEL and MCD, is increasing, the precise nature of the virus's involvement in the pathogenesis of these diseases is unknown. It appears that infection with the virus alone is not sufficient for the development of these conditions since small percentages of normal blood donors appear to be infected and the risks for development of these diseases is low in this population. Since HHV-8 viral genome can be detected in almost all persons with these diseases, the virus appears to be necessary but perhaps not sufficient for their development; other cofactors may be necessary.

Pertinent to KS, the tat protein of HIV has been found to induce proliferation of endothelial cells. Tat augments the proliferation induced by basic fibroblast growth factor (bFGF) (53). This, together with the immunosuppression caused by HIV, may promote KS development in persons with HIV infection. Although HHV-8 is not clearly a transforming virus, it is possible that some of the yet-to-be-identified viral gene products may have transforming capability. The virus does contain a number of homologs of human proteins which may affect cell proliferation and/or survival. These include a viral IL-6 homolog, homologs of the CC chemokine macrophage inflammatory protein $1\alpha$ (MIP-$1\alpha$), a bcl-2 homolog, a type D cyclin homolog, and a homolog of IL-8 receptor (113). KS spindle cells express high-affinity IL-6 receptor, and IL-6 increases the growth of cultured KS spindle cells. Viral IL-6 has been shown to support the growth of IL-6-dependent cell lines. Viral bcl-2 may also be capable of inhibiting apoptosis as does its human homolog.

Cytokines induced by HHV-8 infection and/or by HIV infection may also promote the development of KS. KS cells from HIV-infected individuals have been shown to produce angiogenic growth factors and cytokines such as fibroblast growth factor (FGF), tumor necrosis factor alpha, IL-6, vascular endothelial growth factor, and oncostatin M. These may act in an autocrine or paracrine manner to maintain KS. Only a small percentage of cells within a KS lesion appear to be lytically infected with HHV-8, but this may suffice to induce these growth factors to act on other noninfected cells (118, 121). Viral cyclin D and G protein-coupled receptor homologs, which are involved in controlling cellular growth and differentiation, may be involved in the development of both KS and BCBL/PEL (32).

## CONCLUSIONS

The epidemiology of KS first suggested a possible infectious etiology for this condition. During the past 4 years, a proliferation of studies have shown a clear association between HHV-8 and KS, BCBL/PEL, and MCD. Other conditions reported to be associated with HHV-8 require further confirmatory studies. With the discovery of this agent has come the opportunity to develop new interventions to prevent these malignancies in high-risk individuals. Knowledge about HHV-8 also may provide insights which may be useful to treat existing disease. However, many questions, such as the mode of transmission of the virus and its specific effect on disease pathogenesis, still remain.

### REFERENCES

1. **Adams, V., W. Kempf, M. Schmid, B. Muller, J. Briner, and G. Burg.** 1995. Absence of herpesvirus-like DNA sequences in skin cancers of non-immunosuppressed patients. *Lancet* **346:**1715–1716. (Abstract.)
2. **Alkan, S., D. S. Karcher, A. Ortiz, S. Khalil, M. Akhtar, and M. A. Ali.** 1997. Human herpesvirus-8/Kaposi's sarcoma-associated herpesvirus in organ transplant patients with immunosuppression. *Br. J. Haematol.* **96:**412–414.
3. **Ambroziak, J. A., D. J. Blackbourn, B. G. Herndier, R. G. Glogau, J. H. Gullett, A. R. McDonald, E. T. Lennette, and J. A. Levy.** 1995. Herpes-like sequences in HIV-infected and uninfected Kaposi's sarcoma patients. *Science* **268:**582–583. (Letter.)
4. **Andre, S., O. Schatz, J. R. Bogner, H. Zeichhardt, M. Stoffler-Meilicke, H. U. Jahn, R. Ullrich, A. K. Sonntag, R. Kehn, and J. Haas.** 1997. Detection of antibodies against viral capsid proteins of human herpesvirus 8 in AIDS-associated Kaposi's sarcoma. *J. Mol. Med.* **75:**145–152.
5. **Anonymous.** 1981. Kaposi's sarcoma and Pneumocystis pneumonia among homosexual men—New York City and California. *Morbid. Mortal. Weekly Rep.* **30:**305–308.
6. **Ansari, M. Q., D. B. Dawson, R. Nador, C. Rutherford, N. R. Schneider, M. J. Latimer, L. Picker, D. M. Knowles, and R. W. McKenna.** 1996. Primary body cavity-based AIDS-related lymphomas. *Am. J. Clin. Pathol.* **105:**221–229.
7. **Archibald, C. P., M. T. Schechtr, T. N. Le, K. J. Craib, J. S. Montaner, and M. V. O'Shaughnessy.** 1992. Evidence for a sexually transmitted cofactor for AIDS-related Kaposi's sarcoma in a cohort of homosexual men. *Epidemiology* **3:**203–209.
8. **Armenian, H. K., D. R. Hoover, S. Rubb, S. Metz, R. Kaslow, B. Visscher, J. Chmiel, L. Kingsley, and A. Saah.** 1993. Composite risk score for Kaposi's sarcoma based on a case-control and longitudinal study in the Multicenter AIDS Cohort Study (MACS) population. *Am. J. Epidemiol.* **138:**256–265.

9. **Benfield, T. L., K. K. Dodt, and J. D. Lundgren.** 1997. Human herpes virus-8 DNA in bronchoalveolar lavage samples from patients with AIDS-associated pulmonary Kaposi's sarcoma. *Scand. J. Infect. Dis.* **29**:13–16.

10. **Beral, V.** 1991. Epidemiology of Kaposi's sarcoma, p. 5–52. *In* V. Beral, H. W. Jaffe, and R. A. Weiss (ed.), *Cancer, HIV, and AIDS.* Cold Spring Harbor Laboratory, Cold Spring Harbor, N.Y.

11. **Beral, V., D. Bull, S. Darby, I. Weller, C. Carne, M. Beecham, and H. Jaffe.** 1992. Risk of Kaposi's sarcoma and sexual practices associated with faecal contact in homosexual or bisexual men with AIDS. *Lancet* **339**:632–635.

12. **Beral, V., D. Bull, H. Jaffe, B. Evans, N. Gill, H. Tillett, and A. J. Swerdlow.** 1991. Is risk of Kaposi's sarcoma in AIDS patients in Britain increased if sexual partners came from United States or Africa? *Br. Med. J.* **302**:624–625. (Erratum, **302**:752.)

13. **Beral, V., T. A. Peterman, R. L. Berkelman, and H. W. Jaffe.** 1990. Kaposi's sarcoma among persons with AIDS: a sexually transmitted infection? *Lancet* **335**:123–128.

14. **Biggar, R. J., J. Horm, J. F. Fraumeni, Jr., M. H. Greene, and J. J. Goedert.** 1984. Incidence of Kaposi's sarcoma and mycosis fungoides in the United States including Puerto Rico, 1973–81. *JNCI* **73**:89–94.

15. **Bigoni, B., R. Dolcetti, L. de Lellis, A. Carbone, M. Boiocchi, E. Cassai, and D. DiLuca.** 1996. Human herpesvirus 8 is present in the lymphoid system of healthy persons and can reactivate in the course of AIDS. *J. Infect. Dis.* **173**:542–549.

16. **Blackbourn, D. J., E. T. Lennette, J. Ambroziak, D. V. Mourich, and J. A. Levy.** 1998. Human herpesvirus 8 detection in nasal secretions and saliva. *J. Infect. Dis.* **177**:213–216. (Abstract.)

17. **Blasig, C., C. Zietz, B. Haar, F. Neipel, S. Esser, N. H. T. Brockmeyer, E. S. Colombini, B. Ensoli, and M. Sturzl.** 1997. Monocytes in Kaposi's sarcoma lesions are productively infected by human herpesvirus 8. *J. Virol.* **71**:7963–7968.

18. **Blauvelt, A., S. Sei, P. M. Cook, T. F. Schulz, and K. T. Jeang.** 1997. Human herpesvirus 8 infection occurs following adolescence in the United States. *J. Infect. Dis.* **176**:771–774.

19. **Boldogh, I., P. Szaniszlo, W. A. Bresnahan, C. M. Flaitz, M. C. Nichols, and T. Albrecht.** 1996. Kaposi's sarcoma herpesvirus-like DNA sequences in the saliva of individuals infected with human immunodeficiency virus. *Clin. Infect. Dis.* **23**:406–407.

20. **Boshoff, C., T. F. Schulz, M. M. Kennedy, A. K. Graham, C. Fisher, A. Thomas, J. O. McGee, R. A. Weiss, and J. J. O'Leary.** 1995. Kaposi's sarcoma-associated herpesvirus infects endothelial and spindle cells. *Nat. Med.* **1**:1274–1278.

21. **Boshoff, C., S. Talbot, M. Kennedy, J. O'Leary, T. Schulz, and Y. Chang.** 1996. HHV8 and skin cancers in immunosupressed patients. *Lancet* **347**:338–339. (Letter.) (Erratum **348**:138, 1996.)

22. **Boshoff, C., D. Whitby, T. Hatziioannou, C. Fisher, J. van der Walt, A. Hatzakis, and R. Weiss.** 1995. Kaposi's-sarcoma-associated herpesvirus in HIV-negative Kaposi's sarcoma. *Lancet* **345**:1043–1044. (Abstract.)

23. **Brambilla, L., V. Boneschi, E. Berti, M. Corbellino, and C. Parravicini.** 1996. HHV8 cell-associated viraemia and clinical presentation of Mediterranean Kaposi's sarcoma. *Lancet* **347**:1338. (Letter.)

24. **Carbone, A., and G. Gaidano.** 1997. HHV-8-positive body-cavity-based lymphoma: a novel lymphoma entity. *Br. J. Haematol.* **97**:515–522.

25. **Carbone, A., A. Gloghini, E. Vaccher, V. Zagonel, C. Pastore, P. Dalla Palma, F. Branz, G. Saglio, R. Volpe, U. Tirelli, and G. Gaidano.** 1996. Kaposi's sarcoma-associated herpesvirus DNA sequences in AIDS-related and AIDS-unrelated lymphomatous effusions. *Br. J. Haematol.* **94**:533–543.

26. **Cathomas, G., C. E. McGandy, L. M. Terracciano, P. H. Itin, G. De Rosa, and G. Gudat.** 1996. Detection of herpesvirus-like DNA by nested PCR on archival skin biopsy specimens of various forms of Kaposi sarcoma. *J. Clin. Pathol.* **49**:631–633.

27. **Cathomas, G., M. Tamm, C. E. McGandy, P. H. Itin, F. Gudat, G. Thiel, and M. J. Mihatsch.** 1997. Transplantation-associated malignancies: restriction of human herpes virus 8 to Kaposi's sarcoma. *Transplantation* **64**:175–178.

28. **Centers for Disease Control and Prevention.** 1998. Unpublished data.

29. Cesarman, E., Y. Chang, P. S. Moore, J. W. Said, and D. M. Knowles. 1995. Kaposi's sarcoma-associated herpesvirus-like DNA sequences in AIDS-related body-cavity-based lymphomas. *N. Engl. J. Med.* **332:**1186–1191.

30. Cesarman, E., and D. M. Knowles. 1997. Kaposi's sarcoma-associated herpesvirus: a lymphotropic human herpesvirus associated with Kaposi's sarcoma, primary effusion lymphoma, and multicentric Castleman's disease. *Semin. Diagn. Pathol.* **14:**54–66.

31. Cesarman, E., R. G. Nador, K. Aozasa, G. Delsol, J. W. Said, and D. M. Knowles. 1996. Kaposi's sarcoma-associated herpesvirus in non-AIDS related lymphomas occurring in body cavities. *Am. J. Pathol.* **149:**53–57.

32. Cesarman, E., R. G. Nador, F. Bai, R. A. Bohenzky, J. J. Russo, P. S. Moore, Y. Chang, and D. M. Knowles. 1996. Kaposi's sarcoma-associated herpesvirus contains G protein-coupled receptor and cyclin D homologs which are expressed in Kaposi's sarcoma and malignant lymphoma. *J. Virol.* **70:**8218–8223.

33. Chadburn, A., E. Cesarman, R. G. Nador, Y. F. Liu, and D. M. Knowles. 1997. Kaposi's sarcoma-associated herpesvirus sequences in benign lymphoid proliferations not associated with human immunodeficiency virus. *Cancer* **80:**788–797.

34. Chang, Y., E. Cesarman, M. S. Pessin, F. Lee, J. Culpepper, D. M. Knowles, and P. S. Moore. 1994. Identification of herpesvirus-like DNA sequences in AIDS-associated Kaposi's sarcoma. *Science* **266:**1865–1869.

35. Chang, Y., J. Ziegler, H. Wabinga, E. Katangole-Mbidde, C. Boshoff, T. Schulz, D. Whitby, D. Maddalena, H. W. Jaffe, R. A. Weiss, and P. S. Moore. 1996. Kaposi's sarcoma-associated herpesvirus and Kaposi's sarcoma in Africa. Uganda Kaposi's Sarcoma Study Group. *Arch. Intern. Med.* **156:**202–204.

36. Chatlynne, L. G., M. Handy, J. W. Said, H. P. Koeffler, M. H. Kaplan, J. E. Whitman, and D. Ablashi 1997. HHV-8 ELISA using whole virus lysate to detect KS antibodies in human sera, abstr. 193. *In Conference on Retroviruses and Opportunistic Infections.*

37. Chuck, S., R. M. Grant, E. Katongole-Mbidde, M. Conant, and D. Ganem. 1996. Frequent presence of a novel herpesvirus genome in lesions of human immunodeficiency virus-negative Kaposi's sarcoma. *J. Infect. Dis.* **173:**248–251. (Abstract.)

38. Collandre, H., S. Ferris, O. Grau, L. Montagnier, and A. Blanchard. 1995. Kaposi's sarcoma and new herpesvirus. *Lancet* **345:**1043. (Abstract.)

39. Corbellino, M., C. Parravicini, J. T. Aubin, and E. Berti. 1996. Kaposi's sarcoma and herpesvirus-like DNA sequences in sensory ganglia. *N. Engl. J. Med.* **334:**1341–1342. (Abstract.)

40. Corbellino, M., L. Poirel, J. T. Aubin, M. Paulli, U. Magrini, G. Bestetti, M. Galli, and C. Parravicini. 1996. The role of human herpesvirus 8 and Epstein-Barr virus in the pathogenesis of giant lymph node hyperplasia (Castleman's disease). *Clin. Infect. Dis.* **22:**1120–1121.

41. Corbellino, M., L. Poirel, G. Bestetti, M. Pizzuto, J. T. Aubin, M. Capra, C. Bifulco, E. Berti, H. Agut, G. Rizzardini, M. Galli, and C. Parravicini. 1996. Restricted tissue distribution of extralesional Kaposi's sarcoma-associated herpesvirus-like DNA sequences in AIDS patients with Kaposi's sarcoma. *AIDS Res. Hum. Retroviruses* **12:**651–657.

42. Costagliola, D., and M. Mary-Krause. 1995. Can antiviral agents decrease the occurrence of Kaposi's sarcoma? Clinical Epidemiology Group from Centres d'Information et de Soins de L'Immunodeficience Humaine. *Lancet* **346:**578. (Letter.)

43. Davis, D. A., R. W. Humphrey, F. M. Newcomb, T. R. O'Brien, J. J. Goedert, S. E. Straus, and R. Yarchoan. 1997. Detection of serum antibodies to a Kaposi's sarcoma-associated herpesvirus-specific peptide. *J. Infect. Dis.* **175:**1071–1079.

44. Decker, L. L., P. Shankar, G. Khan, R. B. Freeman, B. J. Dezube, J. Lieberman, and D. A. Thorley-Lawson. 1996. The Kaposi sarcoma-associated herpesvirus (KSHV) is present as an intact latent genome in KS tissue but replicates in the peripheral blood mononuclear cells of KS patients. *J. Exp. Med.* **184:**283–288.

45. DePond, W., J. W. Said, T. Tasaka, S. de Vos, D. Kahn, E. Cesarman, D. M. Knowles, and H. P. Koeffler. 1997. Kaposi's sarcoma-associated herpesvirus and human herpesvirus 8 (KSHV/HHV8)-associated lymphoma of the bowel. Report of two cases in HIV-positive men with secondary effusion lymphomas. *Am. J. Surg. Pathol.* **21:**719–724.

46. **Di Alberti, L., S. L. Ngui, S. R. Porter, P. M. Speight, C. M. Scully, J. M. Zakrewska, I. G. Williams, L. Artese, A. Piattelli, and C. G. Teo.** 1997. Presence of human herpesvirus 8 variants in the oral tissues of human immunodeficiency virus-infected persons. *J. Infect. Dis.* **175:**703–707.

47. **Diamond, C., M. L. Huang, D. H. Kedes, C. Speck, G. W. Rankin, Jr., D. C. Ganem, R. W. Coombs, T. M. Rose, J. N. Krieger, and L. Corey.** 1997. Absenced of detectable human herpesvirus 8 in the semen of human immunodeficiency virus-infected men without Kaposi's sarcoma. *J. Infect. Dis.* **176:**775–777.

48. **Dictor, M., E. Rambech, D. Way, M. Witte, and N. Bendsoe.** 1996. Human herpesvirus 8 (Kaposi's sarcoma-associated herpesvirus) DNA in Kaposi's sarcoma lesions, AIDS Kaposi's sarcoma cell lines, endothelial Kaposi's sarcoma simulators, and the skin of immunosuppressed patients. *Am. J. Pathol.* **148:**2009–2016.

49. **DiGiovanna, J. J., and B. Safai.** 1981. Kaposi's sarcoma. Retrospective study of 90 cases with particular emphasis on the familial occurrence, ethnic background and prevalence of other diseases. *Am. J. Med.* **71:**779–783.

50. **Dupin, N., I. Gorin, J. P. Escande, V. Calvez, M. Crandadam, J. M. Huraux and H. Agut.** 1997. Lack of evidence of any association between human herpesvirus 8 and various skin tumors from both immunocompetent and immunosuppressed patients. *Arch. Dermatol.* **133:**537. (Letter.)

51. **Dupin, N., M. Grandadam, V. Calvez, I. Gorin, J. T. Aubin, S. Havard, F. Lamy, M. Leibowitch, J. M. Huraux, J. P. Escande, and H. Agut.** 1995. Herpesvirus-like DNA sequences in patients with Mediterranean Kaposi's sarcoma. *Lancet* **345:**761–762. (Abstract.)

52. **Engelbrecht, S., F. K. Treurnicht, J. W. Schneider, H. F. Jordaan, J. G. Steytler, P. A. Wranz, and E. J. van Rensburg.** 1997. Detection of human herpes virus 8 DNA and sequence polymorphism in classical, epidemic, and iatrogenic Kaposi's sarcoma in South Africa. *J. Med. Virol.* **52:**168–172.

53. **Ensoli, B., R. Gendelman, P. Markham, V. Fiorelli, S. Colombini, M. Raffeld, A. Cafaro, H. K. Chang, J. N. Brady, and R. C. Gallo.** 1994. Synergy between basic fibroblast growth factor and HIV-1 Tat protein in induction of Kaposi's sarcoma. *Nature* **371:**674–680.

54. **Eto, H., N. O. Kamidigo, K. Murakami-Mori, S. Nakamura, K. Toriyama, and H. Itakura.** 1996. Short report: herpes-like DNA sequences in African-endemic and acquired immunodeficiency syndrome-associated Kaposi's sarcoma. *Am. J. Trop. Med. Hyg.* **55:**405–406.

55. **Flaitz, C. M., Y. T. Jin, M. J. Hicks, C. M. Nichols, Y. W. Wang, and I. J. Su.** 1997. Kaposi's sarcoma-associated herpesvirus-like DNA sequences (KSHV/HHV-8) in oral AIDS-Kaposi's sarcoma: a PCR and clinicopathologic study. *Oral. Surg. Oral. Med. Oral. Pathol. Oral. Radiol. Endod.* **83:**259–264.

56. **Flamand, L., R. A. Zeman, J. L. Bryant, Y. Lunardi-Iskandar, and R. C. Gallo.** 1996. Absence of human herpesvirus 8 DNA sequences in neoplastic Kaposi's sarcoma cell lines. *J. Acquired Immune Defic. Syndr. Hum. Retrovirol.* **13:**194–197.

56a. **Foreman, K. E., J. Friborg, Jr., W. P. Kong, C. Woffendin, P. J. Polverini, B. J. Nickoloff, and G. J. Nabel.** 1997. Propagation of a human herpesvirus from AIDS-associated Kaposi's sarcoma. *N. Engl. J. Med.* **336:**163–171.

57. **Friedman-Kien, A. E., B. R. Saltzman, Y. Z. Cao, M. S. Nestor, M. Mirabile, J. J. Li, and T. A. Peterman.** 1990. Kaposi's sarcoma in HIV-negative homosexual men. *Lancet* **335:**168–169. (Letter.)

58. **Gao, S. J., L. Kingsley, M. Li, W. Zheng, C. Parravicini, J. Ziegler, R. Newton, C. R. Rinaldo, A. Saah, J. Phair, R. Detels, Y. Chang, and P. S. Moore.** 1996. KSHV antibodies among Americans, Italians and Ugandans with and without Kaposi's sarcoma. *Nat. Med.* **2:**925–928.

59. **Gessain, A., J. Briere, C. Angelin-Duclos, F. Valensi, H. M. Beral, F. Davi, M. A. Nicola, A. Sudaka, N. Fouchard, J. Gabarre, X. Troussard, E. Dulmet, J. Audouin, J. Diebold, and G. de The.** 1997. Human herpes virus 8 (Kaposi's sarcoma herpes virus) and malignant lymphoproliferations in France: a molecular study of 250 cases including two AIDS-associated body cavity based lymphomas. *Leukemia* **11:**266–272.

60. **Gessain, A., A. Sudaka, J. Briere, N. Fouchard, M. A. Nicola, B. Rio, M. Arborio, X. Troussard, J. Audouin, J. Diebold, and G. de The.** 1996. Kaposi's sarcoma-associated herpesvirus (Human Herpesvirus Type 8) DNA sequences in multicentric Castleman's disease: Is there any

relevant association in non-human immunodeficiency virus-infected patients? *Blood* **87**:414–416. (Abstract.)

61. **Giraldo, G., F. M. Buonaguro, and E. Beth-Giraldo.** 1989. The role of opportunistic viruses in Kaposi's sarcoma (KS) evolution. *APMIS Suppl.* **8**:62–70.

62. **Glesby, M. J., D. R. Hoover, S. Weng, N. M. Graham, J. P. Phair, R. Detels, M. Ho, and A. J. Saah.** 1996. Use of antiherpes drugs and the risk of Kaposi's sarcoma: data from the Multicenter AIDS Cohort Study. *J. Infect. Dis.* **173**:1477–1480.

63. **Goedert, J. J., D. H. Kedes, and D. Ganem.** 1997. Antibodies to human herpesvirus 8 in women and infants born in Haiti and the USA. *Lancet* **349**:1368. (Letter.)

64. **Grandadam, M., N. Dupin, V. Calvez, I. Gorin, L. Blum, S. Kernbaum, D. Sicard, Y. Buisson, H. Agut, J. P. Escande, and J. M. Huraux.** 1997. Exacerbations of clinical symptoms in human immunodeficiency virus type 1-infected patients with multicentric Castleman's disease are associated with a high increase in Kaposi's sarcoma herpesvirus DNA load in peripheral blood mononuclear cells. *J. Infect. Dis.* **175**:1198–1201.

65. **Gupta, P., M. K. Singh, C. Rinaldo, M. Ding, H. Farzadegan, A. Saah, D. Hoover, P. Moore, and L. Kingsley.** 1996. Detection of Kaposi's sarcoma herpesvirus DNA in semen of homosexual men with Kaposi's sarcoma *AIDS* **10**:1596–1598. (Letter.)

66. **Harrington, W. J., Jr., O. Bagasra, C. E. Sosa, L. E. Bobroski, M. Baum, X. L. Wen, L. Cabral, G. E. Byrne, R. J. Pomerantz, and C. Wood.** 1996. Human herpesvirus type 8 DNA sequences in cell-free plasma and mononuclear cells of Kaposi's sarcoma patients. *J. Infect. Dis.* **174**:1101–1105.

67. **Henghold, W. B. II, S. F. Purvis, J. Schaffer, C. Z. Giam, and G. S. Wood.** 1997. No evidence of KSHV/HHV-8 in mycosis fungoides or associated disorders. *J. Invest. Dermatol.* **108**:920–922.

68. **Howard, M. R., D. Whitby, G. Bahadur, F. Suggett, C. Boshoff, M. Tenant-Flowers, T. F. Schulz, S. Kirk, S. Matthews, I. V. Weller, R. S. Tedder, and R. A. Weiss.** 1997. Detection of human herpesvirus 8 DNA in semen from HIV-infected individuals but not healthy semen donors. *AIDS* **11**:F15-9.

69. **Huang, Y. Q., J. J. Li, B. J. Poiesz, M. H. Kaplan, and A. E. Friedman-Kien.** 1997. Detection of the herpesvirus-like DNA sequences in matched specimens of semen and blood from patients with AIDS-related Kaposi's sarcoma by polymerase chain reaction in situ hybridization. *Am. J. Pathol.* **150**:147–153.

70. **Huang, Y. Q., J. J. Li, W. G. Zhang, D. Feiner, and A. E. Friedman-Mien.** 1996. Transcription of human herpesvirus-like agent (HHV-8) in Kaposi's sarcoma. *J. Clin. Invest.* **97**:2803–2806.

71. **Huang, Y. Q., J. L. Li, M. H. Kaplan, B. Poiesz, E. Katabira, W. C. Zhang, D. Feiner, and A. E. Friedman-Kien.** 1995. Human herpesvirus-like nucleic acid in various forms of Kaposi's sarcoma. *Lancet* **345**:759–761. (Abstract.)

72. **Humphrey, R. W., T. R. O'Brien, F. M. Newcomb, H. Nishihara, K. M. Wyvill, G. A. Ramos, M. W. Saville, J. J. Goedert, S. E. Straus, and R. Yarchoan.** 1996. Kaposi's sarcoma (KS)-associated herpesvirus-like DNA sequences in peripheral blood mononuclear cells: association with KS and persistence in patients receiving anti-herpesvirus drugs. *Blood* **88**:297–301.

73. **Inagi, R., H. Kosuge, H. Nishimoto, K. Yoshikawa, and K. Yamanishi.** 1996. Kaposi's sarcoma-associated herpesvirus (KSHV) sequences in premalignant and malignant skin tumors. *Arch. Virol.* **141**:2217–2223.

74. **Jacobson, L. P., A. Munoz, R. Fox, J. P. Phair, J. Dudley, G. I. Obrams, L. A. Kingsley, and B. F. Polk.** 1990. Incidence of Kaposi's sarcoma in a cohort of homosexual men infected with the human immunodeficiency virus type 1. The Multicenter AIDS Cohort Study Group. *J. Acquired Immune Defic. Syndr.* **3**(Suppl. 1):S24–S31.

75. **Jin, Y. T., S. T. Tsai, J. J. Yan, J. H. Hsiao, Y. Y. Lee, and I. J. Su.** 1996. Detection of Kaposi's sarcoma-associated herpesvirus-like DNA sequence in vascular lesions. A reliable diagnostic marker for Kaposi's sarcoma. *Am. J. Clin. Pathol.* **105**:360–363.

76. **Jones, J. L., D. L. Hanson, S. Y. Chu, J. W. Ward, and H. W. Jaffe.** 1995. AIDS-associated Kaposi's sarcoma. *Science* **276**:1078–1079 (Letter.)

77. **Kaposi, M.** 1872. Idiopathisches multiples Pigmentsarkom der Haut. *Arch. Dermatol. Syphilis* **4**:265–273.

78. **Karcher, D. S., and S. Alkan.** 1997. Human herpesvirus-8-associated body cavity-based lymphoma in human immunodeficiency virus-infected patients: a unique B-cell neoplasm. *Hum. Pathol.* **28:** 801–808.

79. **Kedda, M. A., L. Margolius, M. C. Kew, C. Swanepoel, and D. Pearson.** 1996. Kaposi's sarcoma-associated herpesvirus in Kaposi's sarcoma occurring in immunosuppressed renal transplant recipients. *Clin. Transplant.* **10:**429–431.

80. **Kedes, D. H., and D. Ganem.** 1997. Sensitivity of Kaposi's sarcoma-associated herpesvirus replication to antiviral drugs. Implications for potential therapy. *J. Clin. Invest.* **99:**2082–2086.

81. **Kedes, D. H., D. Ganem, N. Ameli, P. Bacchetti, and R. Greenblatt.** 1997. The prevalence of serum antibody to human herpesvirus 8 (Kaposi sarcoma-associated herpesvirus) among HIV-seropositive and high-risk HIV-seronegative women. *JAMA* **277:**478–481.

82. **Kedes, D. H., E. Operskalski, M. Busch, R. Kohn, J. Flood, and D. Ganem.** 1996. The seroepidemiology of human herpesvirus 8 (Kaposi's sarcoma-associated herpesvirus): distribution of infection in KS risk groups and evidence for sexual transmission. *Nat. Med.* **2:**918–924. (Erratum, **2:**1041.)

83. **Kemeny, L., R. Gyulai, M. Kiss, F. Nagy, and A. Dobozy.** 1997. Kaposi's sarcoma-associated herpesvirus/human herpesvirus-8: a new virus in human pathology. *J. Am. Acad. Dermatol.* **37:** 107–113.

84. **Kemeny, L., M. Kiss, R. Gyulai, A. S. Kenderessy, E. Adam, F. Nagy, and A. Dobozy.** 1996. Human herpesvirus 8 in classic Kaposi sarcoma. *Acta Microbiol. Immunol. Hung.* **43:**391–395.

85. **Kennedy, M. M., S. B. Lucas, R. R. Jones, D. D. Howells, S. J. Picton, E. E. Hanks, J. O. McGee, and J. J. O'Leary.** 1997. HHV8 and Kaposi's sarcoma: a time cohort study. *Mol. Pathol.* **50:**96–100.

86. **Koelle, D. M., M. L. Huang, B. Chandran, J. Vieira, M. Piepkorn, and L. Corey.** 1997. Frequent detection of Kaposi's sarcoma-associated herpesvirus (human herpesvirus 8) DNA in saliva of human immunodeficiency virus-infected men: clinical and immunologic correlates. *J. Infect. Dis.* **176:**94–102.

87. **Komanduri, K. V., J. A. Luce, M. S. McGrath, B. G. Herndier, and V. L. Ng.** 1996. The natural history and molecular heterogeneity of HIV-associated primary malignant lymphomatous effusions. *J. Acquired Immune Defic. Syndr. Hum. Retrovirol.* **13:**215–226.

88. **Lebbe, C., F. Agbalika, P. de Cremoux, M. Deplanche, M. Rybojad, E. Masgrau, P. Morel, and F. Calvo.** 1997. Detection of human herpesvirus 8 and human T-cell lymphotropic virus type 1 sequences in Kaposi sarcoma. *Arch. Dermatol.* **133:**25–30.

89. **Lebbe, C., P. de Cremoux, G. Millot, M. P. Podgorniak, O. Verola, R. Berger, P. Morel, and F. Calvo.** 1997. Characterization of in vitro culture of HIV-negative Kaposi's sarcoma-derived cells. In vitro responses to alfa interferon. *Arch. Dermatol. Res.* **289:**421–428.

90. **Lebbe, C., P. de Cremoux, M. Rybojad, C. Costa da Cunha, P. Morel, and F. Calvo.** 1995. Kaposi's sarcoma and new herpesvirus. *Lancet* **345:**1180. (Abstract.)

91. **Lebbe, C., R. Tatoud, P. Morel, F. Calvo, S. Euvrard, J. Kanitakis, M. Faure, and A. Claudy.** 1997. Human herpesvirus 8 sequences are not detected in epithelial tumors from patients receiving transplants. *Arch. Dermatol.* **133:**111. (Letter.)

92. **Lefrere, J. J., M. C. Meyohas, M. Mariotti, J. L. Meynard, M. Thauvin, and J. Frottier.** 1996. Detection of human herpesvirus 8 DNA sequences before the appearance of Kaposi's sarcoma in human immunodeficiency virus (HIV)-positive subjects with a known date of HIV seroconversion. *J. Infect. Dis.* **174:**283–287.

93. **Lennette, E. T., D. J. Blackbourn, and J. A. Levy.** 1996. Antibodies to human herpesvirus type 8 in the general population and in Kaposi's sarcoma patients. *Lancet* **348:**858–861.

94. **Li, J. J., Y. Q. Huang, C. J. Cockerell, and A. E. Friedman-Kien.** 1996. Localization of human herpes-like virus type 8 in vascular endothelial cells and perivascular spindle-shaped cells of Kaposi's sarcoma lesions by in situ hybridization. *Am. J. Pathol.* **148:**1741–1748.

95. **Lin, B. T., and L. M. Weiss.** 1997. Primary plasmacytoma of lymph nodes. *Hum. Pathol.* **28:** 1083–1090.

96. **Lin, J. C., S. C. Lin, E. C. Mar, P. E. Pellett, F. R. Stamey, J. A. Stewart, and T. J. Spira.** 1995. Is Kaposi's-sarcoma-associated herpesvirus detectable in semen of HIV-infected homosexual men? *Lancet* **346:**1601–1602.

97. **Loughran, T. P., Jr., L. Abbott, T. C. Gentile, J. Love, C. Cunningham, A. Friedman-Kien, Y. Q. Huang, and B. J. Poiesz.** 1997. Absence of human herpes virus 8 DNA sequences in large granular lymphocyte (LGL) leukemia. *Leuk. Lymphoma* **26:**177–180.

98. **Luppi, M., P. Barozzi, A. Maiorana, T. Artusi, R. Trovato, R. Marasca, M. Savarino, L. Ceccherini-Nelli, and G. Torelli.** 1996. Human herpesvirus-8 DNA sequences in human immunodeficiency virus-negative angioimmunoblastic lymphadenopathy and benign lymphadenopathy with giant germinal center hyperplasia and increased vascularity. *Blood* **87:**3903–3909.

99. **Luppi, M., P. Barozzi, A. Maiorana, G. Collina, M. G. Ferrari, R. Marasca, M. Morselli, E. Rossi, L. Ceccherini-Nelli, and G. Torelli.** 1996. Frequency and distribution of herpesvirus-like DNA sequences (KSHV) in different stages of classic Kaposi's sarcoma and in normal tissues from an Italian population. *Int. J. Cancer* **66:**427–431.

100. **Luppi, M., P. Barozzi, R. Marasca, M. G. Ferrari, and G. Torelli.** 1997. Human herpesvirus 8 strain variability in clinical conditions other than Kaposi's sarcoma. *J. Virol.* **71:**8082–8083. (Letter.)

101. **Luppi, M., and G. Torelli.** 1996. Human herpesvirus 8 and interstitial pneumonitis in an HIV-negative patient. *N. Engl. J. Med.* **335:**351–352. (Letter.)

102. **Mackenzie, J., J. Sheldon, G. Morgan, G. Cook, T. F. Schulz, and R. F. Jarrett.** 1997. HHV-8 and multiple myeloma in the UK. *Lancet* **350:**1144–1145. (Letter.)

103. **Maiorana, A., M. Luppi, P. Barozzi, G. Collina, R. A. Fano, and G. Torelli.** 1997. Detection of human herpes virus type 8 DNA sequences as a valuable aid in the differential diagnosis of Kaposi's sarcoma. *Mod. Pathol.* **10:**182–187.

104. **Marcelin, A. G., N. Dupin, D. Bouscary, P. Bossi, P. Cacoub, P. Ravaud, and V. Calvez.** 1997. HHV-8 and multiple myeloma in France. *Lancet* **350:**1144. (Letter.)

105. **Marchioli, C. C., J. L. Love, L. Z. Abbott, Y. Q. Huang, S. C. Remick, N. Surtento-Reodica, R. E. Hutchison, D. Mildvan, A. E. Friedman-Kien, and B. J. Poiesz.** 1996. Prevalence of human herpesvirus 8 DNA sequences in several patient populations. *J. Clin. Microbiol.* **34:**2635–2638.

106. **McDonagh, D. P., J. Liu, M. J. Gaffey, L. J. Layfield, N. Azumi, and S. T. Traweek.** 1996. Detection of Kaposi's sarcoma-associated herpesvirus-like DNA sequence in angiosarcoma. *Am. J. Pathol.* **149:**1363–1368.

107. **Medveczky, M. M., E. Horvath, T. Lund, and P. G. Medveczky.** 1997. In vitro antiviral drug sensitivity of the Kaposi's sarcoma-associated herpesvirus. *AIDS* **11:**1327–1332.

108. **Merelli, E., R. Bedin, P. Sola, P. Barozzi, G. L. Mancardi, G. Ficarra, and G. Franchini.** 1997. Human herpes virus 6 and human herpes virus 8 DNA sequences in brains of multiple sclerosis patients, normal adults and children. *J. Neurol.* **244:**450–454.

109. **Mesri, E. A., E. Cesarman, L. Arvanitakis, S. Rafii, M. A. Moore, D. N. Posnett, D. M. Knowles, and A. S. Asch.** 1996. Human herpesvirus-8/Kaposi's sarcoma-associated herpesvirus is a new transmissible virus that infects B cells. *J. Exp. Med.* **183:**2385–2390.

110. **Miller, G., M. O. Rigsby, L. Heston, E. Grogan, R. Sun, C. Metroka, J. A. Levy, S. J. Gao, Y. Chang, and P. Moore.** 1996. Antibodies to butyrate-inducible antigens of Kaposi's sarcoma-associated herpesvirus in patients with HIV-1 infection. *N. Engl. J. Med.* **334:**1292–1297.

111. **Mocroft, A., M. Youle, B. Gazzard, J. Morcinek, R. Halai, and A. N. Phillips.** 1996. Anti-herpesvirus treatment and risk of Kaposi's sarcoma in HIV infection. *AIDS* **10:**1101–1105.

112. **Monini, P., L. de Lellis, M. Fabris, F. Rigolin, and E. Cassai.** 1996. Kaposi's sarcoma-associated herpesvirus DNA sequences in prostate tissue and human semen. *N. Engl. J. Med.* **334:**1168–1172.

113. **Moore, P. S., C. Boshoff, R. A. Weiss, and Y. Chang.** 1996. Molecular mimicry of human cytokine and cytokine response pathway genes by KSHV. *Science* **274:**1739–1744.

114. **Moore, P. S., L. A. Kingsley, S. D. Holmberg, T. Spira, P. Gupta, D. R. Hoover, J. P. Parry, L. J. Conley, H. W. Jaffe, and Y. Chang.** 1996. Kaposi's sarcoma-associated herpesvirus infection prior to onset of Kaposi's sarcoma. *AIDS* **10:**175–180.

115. **Morfeldt, L., and J. Torssander.** 1994. Long-term remission of Kaposi's sarcoma following foscarnet treatment in HIV-infected patients. *Scand. J. Infect. Dis.* **26:**749–752.

116. **Morgello, S., M. Tagliati, and M. R. Ewart.** 1997. HHV-8 and AIDS-related CNS lymphoma. *Neurology* **48:**1333–1335.

117. **Nador, R. G., E. Cesarman, A. Chadburn, D. B. Dawson, M. Q. Ansari, J. K. Said, D. M. Knowles.** 1996. Primary effusion lymphoma: a distinct clinicopathologic entity associated with the Kaposi's sarcoma-associated herpes virus. *Blood* **88:**645–656.
118. **Neipel, F., J. C. Albrecht, and B. Fleckenstein.** 1997. Cell-homologous genes in the Kaposi's sarcoma-associated rhadinovirus human herpesvirus 8: determinants of its pathogenicity? *J. Virol.* **71:**4187–4192.
119. **Nishimoto, S., R. Inagi, K. Yamanishi, K. Hosokawa, M. Kakibuchi, and K. Yoshikawa.** 1997. Prevalence of human herpesvirus-8 in skin lesions. *Br. J. Dermatol.* **137:**179–184.
120. **Noel, J. C., P. Hermans, J. Andre, I. Fayt, T. Simonart, A. Verhest, J. Haot, and A. Burny.** 1996. Herpesvirus-like DNA sequences and Kaposi's sarcoma: relationship with epidemiology, clinical spectrum, and histologic features. *Cancer* **77:**2132–2136.
121. **O'Leary, J. J., M. M. Kennedy, and J. O. McGee.** 1997. Kaposi's sarcoma associated herpes virus (KSHV/HHV 8): epidemiology, molecular biology and tissue distribution. *Mol. Pathol.* **50:** 4–8.
122. **Oksenhendler, E., M. Duarte, J. Soulier, P. Cacoub, Y. Welker, J. Cadranel, D. Cazals-Hatem, B. Autran, J. P. Clauvel, and M. Raphael.** 1996. Multicentric Castleman's disease in HIV infection: a clinical and pathological study of 20 patients. *AIDS* **10:**61–67.
123. **Operskalski, E. A., M. P. Busch, J. W. Mosley, and D. H. Kedes.** 1997. Blood donations and viruses. *Lancet* **349:**1327. (Letter.)
124. **Orenstein, J. M., S. Alkan, A. Blauvelt, K. T. Jeang, M. D. Weinstein, and D. Ganem, B. Herndier.** 1997. Visualization of human herpesvirus type 8 in Kaposi's sarcoma by light and transmission electron microscopy. *AIDS* **11:**F35–45.
125. **Parry, J. P., and P. S. Moore.** 1997. Corrected prevalence of Kaposi's sarcoma (KS)-associated herpesvirus infection prior to onset of KS. *AIDS* **11:**127–128. (Letter.)
126. **Pastore, C., A. Gloghini, G. Volpe, J. Nomdedeu, E. Leonardo, U. Mazza, G. Saglio, A. Carbone, and G. Gaidano.** 1995. Distribution of Kaposi's sarcoma herpesvirus sequences among lymphoid malignancies in Italy and Spain. *Br. J. Haematol.* **91:**918–920.
127. **Pawson, R., D. Catovsky, and T. F. Schulz.** 1996. Lack of evidence of HHV-8 in mature T-cell lymphoproliferative disorders. *Lancet* **348:**1450–1451. (Letter.)
128. **Penn, I.** 1983. Kaposi's sarcoma in immunosuppressed patients. *J. Clin. Lab. Immunol.* **12:**1–10.
129. **Peterman, T. A., H. W. Jaffe, and V. Beral.** 1993. Epidemiologic clues to the etiology of Kaposi's sarcoma. *AIDS* **7:**605–611. (Editorial.)
130. **Peterman, T. A., H. W. Jaffe, and A. E. Friedman-Kien.** 1991. The aetiology of Kaposi's sarcoma, p. 23–37. *In* V. Beral, H. W. Jaffe, and R. A. Weiss (ed.), *Cancer, HIV, and AIDS.* Cold Spring Harbor Laboratory, Cold Spring Harbor, N. Y.
131. **Purvis, S. F., E. Katongole-Mbidde, J. L. Johnson, D. G. Leonard, N. Byabazaire, C. Luckey, H. E. Schick, R. Wallis, C. A. Elmets, and C. Z. Giam.** 1997. High incidence of Kaposi's sarcoma-associated herpesvirus and Epstein-Barr virus in tumor lesions and peripheral blood mononuclear cells from patients with Kaposi's sarcoma in Uganda. *J. Infect. Dis.* **175:**947–950.
132. **Rady, P. L., A. Yen, R. W. Martin III, I. Nedelcu, T. K. Hughes, and S. K. Tyring.** 1995. Herpesvirus-like DNA sequences in classic Kaposi's sarcomas. *J. Med. Virol.* **47:**179–183.
133. **Rady, P. L., A. Yen, J. L. Rollefson I. Orengo, S. Bruce, T. K. Hughes, and S. K. Tyring.** 1995. Herpesvirus-like DNA sequences in non-Kaposi's sarcoma skin lesions of transplant patients. *Lancet* **345:**1339–1340.
134. **Rettig, M. B., H. J. Ma, R. A. Vescio, M. Pold, G. Schiller, D. Belson, A. Savage, C. Nishikubo, C. Wu, J. Fraser, J. W. Said, and J. R. Berenson.** 1997. Kaposi's sarcoma-associated herpesvirus infection of bone marrow dendritic cells from multiple myeloma patients. *Science* **276:**1851–1854.
135. **Rizzieri, D. A., J. Liu, D. Miralles, and S. T. Traweek.** 1997. Kaposi's-sarcoma-associated herpesvirus is detected in peripheral blood mononuclear cells of HIV-infected homosexuals more often than in heterosexuals. *Cancer Sci. Am.* **3:**153–156.
136. **Royer, B., D. Cazals-Hatem, J. Sibilia, F. Agbalika, J. M. Cayuela, T. Soussi, F. Maloisel, J. P. Clauvel, J. C. Brouet, and X. Mariette.** 1997. Lymphomas in patients with Sjogren's syndrome are marginal zone B-cell neoplasms, arise in diverse extranodal and nodal sites, and are not associated with viruses. *Blood* **90:**766–775.

137. **Safai, B., V. Mike, G. Giraldo, E. Beth, and R. A. Good.** 1980. Association of Kaposi's sarcoma with second primary malignancies: possible etiopathogenic implications. *Cancer* **45**:1472–1479.

138. **Said, J. W., T. Tasaka, S. de Vos, and H. P. Koeffler.** 1997. Kaposi's sarcoma-associated herpesvirus/human herpesvirus type 8 encephalitis in HIV-positive and -negative individuals. *AIDS* **11**:1119–1122.

139. **Said, J. W., T. Tasaka, S. Takeuchi, H. Asou, S. de Vos, E. Cesarman, D. M. Knowles, and H. P. Koeffler.** 1996. Primary effusion lymphoma in women: report of two cases of Kaposi's sarcoma herpes virus-associated effusion-based lymphoma in human immunodeficiency virus-negative women. *Blood* **88**:3124–3128.

140. **Schalling, M., M. Ekman, E. E. Kaaya, A. Linde, and P. Biberfeld.** 1995. A role for a new herpes virus (KSHV) in different forms of Kaposi's sarcoma. *Nat. Med.* **1**:707–708.

141. **Serraino, D., S. Franceschi, L. Dal Maso, and C. La Vecchia.** 1995. HIV transmission and Kaposi's sarcoma among European women. *AIDS* **9**:971–973.

142. **Simonart, T., J. C. Noel, C. Liesnard, D. Parent, M. Heenen, F. Brancart, J. P. VanVooren, C. M. Farber, D. Blankaert, and J. Werenne.** 1996. Kaposi's sarcoma and herpesvirus 8: a word of caution: *Dermatology* **193**:272. (Letter.)

143. **Simpson, G. R., T. F. Schulz, D. Whitby, P. M. Cook, C. Boshoff, L. Rainbow, M. R. Howard, S. J. Gao, R. A. Bohenzky, P. Simmonds, C. Lee, A. de Ruiter, A. Hatzakis, R. S. Tedder, I. V. Weller, R. A. Weiss, and P. S. Moore.** 1996. Prevalence of Kaposi's sarcoma associated herpesvirus infection measured by antibodies to recombinant capsid protein and latent immunofluorescence antigen. *Lancet* **348**:1133–1138.

144. **Smir, B. N., T. C. Greiner, and D. D. Weisenburger.** 1996. Multicentric angiofollicular lymph node hyperplasia in children: a clinicopathologic study of eight patients. *Mod. Pathol.* **9**:1135–1142.

145. **Smith, M. S., C. Bloomer, R. Horvat, E. Goldstein, J. M. Casparian, and B. Chandran.** 1997. Detection of human herpesvirus 8 DNA in Kaposi's sarcoma lesions and peripheral blood of human immunodeficiency virus-positive patients and correlation with serologic measurements. *J. Infect. Dis.* **176**:84–93.

146. **Smoller, B. R., P. P. Chang, and O. W. Kamel.** 1997. No role for human herpes virus 8 in the etiology of infantile capillary hemangioma. *Mod. Pathol.* **10**:675–678.

147. **Soler, R. A., M. Howard, N. S. Brink, D. Gibb, R. S. Tedder, and D. Nadal.** 1996. Regression of AIDS-related Kaposi's sarcoma during therapy with thalidomide. *Clin. Infect. Dis.* **23**:501–503.

148. **Soulier, J., L. Grollet, E. Oksenhendler, P. Cacoub, D. Cazals-Hatem, P. Babinet, M. F. D'Agay, J. P. Clauvel, M. Raphael, L. Degos, and F. Sigaux.** 1995. Kaposi's sarcoma-associated herpesvirus-like DNA sequences in multicentric Castleman's disease. *Blood* **86**:1276–1280.

149. **Staskus, K. A., W. Zhong, K. Gebhard, B. Herndier, H. Wang, R. Renne, J. Beneke, J. Pudney, D. J. Anderson, D. Ganem, and A. T. Haase.** 1997. Kaposi's sarcoma-associated herpesvirus gene expression in endothelial (spindle) tumor cells. *J. Virol.* **71**:715–719.

150. **Sturzl, M., C. Blasig, A. Schreier, F. Neipel, C. Hohenadl, E. Cornali, G. Ascherl, S. Esser, N. H. Brockmeyer, M. Ekman, E. E. Kaaya, E. Tschachler, and P. Biberfeld.** 1997. Expression of HHV-8 latency-associated T0.7 RNA in spindle cells and endothelial cells of AIDS-associated, classical and African Kaposi's sarcoma. *Int. J. Cancer* **72**:68–71.

151. **Su, I. J., Y. S. Hsu, Y. C. Chang, and I. W. Wang.** 1995. Herpesvirus-like DNA sequence in Kaposi's sarcoma from AIDS and non-AIDS patients in Taiwan. *Lancet* **345**:722–723. (Letter.)

152. **Tasaka, T., J. W. Said, R. Morosetti, D. Park, W. Verbeek, M. Nagai, J. Takahara, and H. P. Koeffler.** 1997. Is Kaposi's sarcoma-associated herpesvirus ubiquitous in urogenital and prostate tissues? *Blood* **89**:1686–1689.

153. **Taylor, J. F., P. G. Smith, D. Bull, and M. C. Pike.** 1972. Kaposi's sarcoma in Uganda: geographic and ethnic distribution. *Br. J. Cancer* **26**:483–497.

154. **Tomita, Y., N. Naka, K. Aozasa, E. Cesarman, and D. M. Knowles.** 1996. Absence of Kaposi's-sarcoma-associated herpesvirus-like DNA sequences (KSHV) in angiosarcomas developing in body-cavity and other sites. *Int. J. Cancer* **66**:141–142. (Letter.)

155. **Viviano, E., F. Vitale, F. Ajello, A. M. Perna, M. R. Villafrate, F. Bonura, M. Arica, G. Mazzola, and N. Romano.** 1997. Human herpesvirus type 8 DNA sequences in biological samples of HIV-positive and negative individuals in Sicily. *AIDS* **11:**607–612.

156. **Wabinga, H. R., D. M. Parkin, F. Wabwire-Mangen, and J. W. Mugerwa.** 1993. Cancer in Kampala, Uganda, in 1989–91: changes in incidence in the era of *AIDS. Int. J. Cancer* **54:**26–36.

157. **Wahman, A., S. L. Melnick, F. S. Rhame, and J. D. Potter.** 1991. The epidemiology of classic, African and immunosuppressed Kaposi's sarcoma. *Epidemiol. Rev.* **12:**179–199.

158. **Whitby, D., M. R. Howard, M. Tenant-Flowers, N. S. Brink, A. Copas, C. Boshoff, T. Hatzioannou, F. E. Suggett, D. M. Aldam, A. S. Denton, R. F. Miller, I. V. D. Miller, R. A. Weiss, R. S. Tedder, and T. F. Schulz.** 1995. Detection of Kaposi sarcoma associated herpesvirus in peripheral blood of HIV-infected individuals and progression to Kaposi's sarcoma. *Lancet* **346:** 799–802.

159. **Ziegler, J. L., and E. Katongole-Mbidde.** 1996. Kaposi's sarcoma in childhood: an analysis of 100 cases from Uganda and relationship to HIV infection. *Int. J. Cancer* **65:**200–203.

*Emerging Infections 2*
Edited by W. M. Scheld, W. A. Craig, and J. M. Hughes
© 1998 ASM Press, Washington, D.C.

*Chapter 5*

# The Association of *Chlamydia pneumoniae* and Atherogenesis

## Michael Dunne

The disease responsible for the greatest number of deaths in the Western world still remains largely a mystery. The American Heart Association estimates that 60 million Americans live with the sequelae of atherosclerosis. Of those, 13 million have had a myocardial infarction, and approximately 500,000 will die each year (3a). Despite recent progress in understanding the various risk factors associated with atherosclerosis, such as hypertension, cigarette smoking, hypercholesterolemia and diabetes, only 50% of the overall risk has been explained (57).

The development of newer and more sophisticated diagnostic technologies has opened up many new avenues of investigation, leaving no field of medicine untouched. Our understanding of the etiology of disease has benefited from techniques such as increasingly more refined applications of the polymerase chain reaction, advances in digital subtractive hybridization, and the continually expanding library of monoclonal antibody reagents. Certainly we have obtained a greater insight into the infectious etiology of well-established disease states through the use of these tools. Recent advances have led us to understand that ulcer disease is a consequence of infection with *Helicobacter pylori*, that Kaposi's sarcoma may be due to infection with a herpesvirus, and that Whipple's disease is due to a fastidious gram-negative bacillus, *Tropheryma whippelii*. Not to be forgotten, only recently have we learned that the etiology of a progressively debilitating immunodeficiency syndrome is the result of infection with a previously unidentified human retrovirus. Given these stunning achievements, it is not surprising that a growing number of investigators are asking if a disease as common as atherosclerosis may have an infectious etiology.

The earliest indication that atherogenesis may be influenced by microorganisms came from work done with poultry. Marek's disease virus, a herpesvirus, has been shown to cause atherosclerosis in chickens (43). A potential association between human disease and cytomegalovirus (CMV) infection has also been explored (78).

*Michael Dunne* • Department of Clinical Research, Pfizer Central Research, Eastern Point Road, Groton, CT 06340.

Epidemiologic studies have implicated *H. pylori* and atherosclerosis, (54) though these results have not been universally supported (13). This review will attempt to frame the issues surrounding the association of atherosclerosis and infection with *Chlamydia pneumoniae*. The results of seroepidemiologic and histopathologic studies will be discussed in addition to data from animal experiments. In vivo and in vitro experiments regarding the cell biology of *C. pneumoniae* and the immune response it engenders will be explored, highlighting features pertinent to a possible role in the pathogenesis of atherosclerosis. Finally, results from two recent antibiotic intervention studies will be examined.

## IS PRIOR EXPOSURE TO *C. PNEUMONIAE* ASSOCIATED WITH HEART DISEASE?

There has been evidence that certain chlamydia species may have a tropism for cardiovascular tissue. A chlamydial infection was first associated with myocarditis as early as 1930, but the first series of patients with heart disease and a chlamydia infection was reported in 1967. Nine patients with pericarditis or myocarditis were noted to have elevated complement fixation titers to *Chlamydia psittaci* (64). A follow-up to this report was published 4 years later in which an additional 40 patients who again had pericarditis or myocarditis were found to have positive complement fixation tests to *C. psittaci*. Coronary artery disease was uncommon in these patients (63).

In 1988, Pekka Saikku et al. found that a higher percentage of young Finnish men with a history of either an acute myocardial infarction or angina had elevated *C. pneumoniae* IgG titers when compared to age-matched controls who did not have heart disease (58). Since that time more than a dozen seroepidemiologic studies have been performed; some are listed in Table 1. These studies, ranging in size from 90 to 1500 subjects, have been performed on a number of different populations in the United States and Europe. The serologic analyses have been performed

**Table 1.** Epidemiologic studies correlating risk of cardiovascular disease with exposure to *C. pneumoniae*

| Country (reference) | Yr | Cases/controls | Serology | Risk |
|---|---|---|---|---|
| Finland (58) | 1988 | 70/41 | IgG $\geq$ 1:32 | 3.8 |
| Finland (61) | 1992 | 103/103 | IgG $\geq$ 1:128 | 2.1[a] |
| United States (40) | 1993 | 297/297 | IgG $\geq$ 1:8 | 2.0[a] |
| United States (67) | 1993 | 171/120 | IgG $\geq$ 1:8 | 2.6[a] |
| Sweden (11) | 1995 | 60/60 | IgG $\geq$ 1:32 | 3.8 |
| United States (68) | 1995 | 461/95 | IgG $\geq$ 1:16 | 1.6 |
| Great Britain (14) | 1995 | 13/183 | IgG $\geq$ 1:64 | 7.4[a] |
| Great Britain (15) | 1995 | 47/341 | IgG $\geq$ 1:64 | 3.1[a] |
| Germany (19) | 1995 | 400/400 | IgG $\geq$ 1:128 | 1.8 |
| Netherlands (51) | 1995 | 34/148 | IgG | 4.0[a] |
| Great Britain (54) | 1995 | 80/308 | IgG $\geq$ 1:64 | 2.3[a] |
| Great Britain (23) | 1996 | 40/59 | IgG $\geq$ 1:64 | 4.2[a] |

[a]Adjusted for typical cardiovascular risk factors; for statistical methods, see references.

in a variety of laboratories, but most have used an IgG microimmunofluorescence assay. The titer cutoffs have varied between studies although the majority have used either 1:32 or 1:64 for the determination of excess risk. The odds ratios were determined predominantly by means of a Cox regression; however, not all studies accounted for the influence of other covariates known to be associated with atherosclerosis. Nonetheless, the data from these studies taken as a whole appear to suggest that, on a population basis, elevations in *C. pneumoniae* titers above 1:32 are associated with a three- to fourfold excess risk of developing clinical manifestations of atherosclerosis. This excess risk is similar to that associated with diabetes and hypertension (40).

While these seroepidemiologic studies suggest an association between exposure to *C. pneumoniae* and atherosclerosis, they are inherently unable to provide evidence of causality. It may be that the relationship between each of these is based on the nature of the host's immune response, in one case to an exogenous pathogen, in the other to endogenous phenomena associated with atherogenesis. It should also be noted that the antibody response to *C. pneumoniae* infection is not well understood. As in other biologic responses, some individuals do not mount a significant rise in antibody titer after exposure while others demonstrate persistently high titers long after clinical disease has resolved (2). As a consequence, these data are limited to implications on a population basis, as antibody-negative patients have been found to have evidence of active *C. pneumoniae* infection (56). Given these issues, the association between this organism and atherogenesis can build on a seroepidemiologic link but ultimately requires support from other lines of investigation.

## CAN *C. PNEUMONIAE* BE FOUND IN ATHEROSCLEROTIC PLAQUES WITHIN THE ARTERIAL WALL?

Intuitively, one would like to see evidence that a potential pathogen is intimately involved in the lesion responsible for clinical disease. Finding *Mycobacterium tuberculosis* within the granuloma or *Treponema pallidum* within the gumma is enough evidence in a clinical setting to direct a therapeutic intervention. Similarly, if one could identify *C. pneumoniae* within the atherosclerotic plaque, a tightening of the association would follow.

Since 1992 there have been at least 15 histopathologic studies which have attempted to identify *C. pneumoniae* within aortic, coronary, iliac, femoral, and carotid arteries or excised plaque removed from these vessels. Identification has been attempted by a combination of immunohistochemistry, using type-specific antibodies, polymerase chain reaction using primers specific for *C. pneumoniae*, electron microscopy looking for ultrastructrual features typical for organisms of the species of chlamydia, and occasionally, by culture of the plaque. Among the 15 studies listed in Table 2, specimens from a total of 574 patients were examined; the number of specimens in each particular study ranged from 7 to 114. Accepting any positive test as evidence of infection, 45% of these 574 patients with clinical evidence of atherosclerosis demonstrated *C. pneumoniae* within the plaque, with a range of 2 to 100% in each individual study. Culture of *C. pneumoniae* from human plaque has been successful on only two occasions (29, 59). This inability to isolate the

**Table 2.** Detection of *C. pneumoniae* in atherosclerotic plaques

| Country (reference) | Yr | No. of patients | % Positive | Tissue |
|---|---|---|---|---|
| South Africa (62) | 1992 | 7 | 100 | Coronary |
| South Africa (31) | 1993 | 36 | 42 | Coronary |
| United States (33) | 1995 | 49 | 45 | Coronary |
| United States (7) | 1995 | 38 | 53 | Coronary |
| United States (74) | 1996 | 58 | 2 | Coronary |
| United States (48) | 1996 | 114 | 79 | Coronary |
| United States (8) | 1995 | 18 | 39 | Coronary |
| Japan (52) | 1995 | 29 | 55 | Coronary |
| India (72) | 1995 | 40 | 10 | Coronary |
| United States | 1996 | 9 | 67 | Coronary |
| United States (32) | 1993 | 17 | 35 | Aorta |
| United Kingdom (50) | 1996 | 25 | 44 | Aorta, iliac, femoral |
| United States | 1997 | 23 | 48 | Popliteal, femoral |
| United States (22) | 1995 | 61 | 61 | Carotid |
| Germany (36) | 1996 | 50 | 14 | Carotid |
| Total | | 574 | 45 | |

organism from pathologic specimens may serve to weaken the case of any potential pathological association. It can be argued, however, that difficulty in culture of an organism from tissue is not atypical, especially in the setting of a chronic infection. *C. pneumoniae* has been difficult to grow under optimal circumstances, a problem compounded by the technical limitations in transfer of a small amount of clinical material into adequate media. In many of these studies, tissue was obtained after fixation, precluding the option of culture. The low frequency of recovery prevents culture from serving as supportive evidence but equally does not serve to disprove the association.

Other findings from these studies include the localization of *C. pneumoniae* within the smooth muscle cells and macrophages of the atheromatous lesions as well as within the foam cells of carotid artery plaques, confirming in vitro results demonstrating growth in cell culture (20, 30). The importance of these findings is that the organism is being found within the cells that are felt to be responsible for both the vasculopathy associated with atherosclerosis as well as the instability associated with acute plaque rupture.

These data now place the pathogen at the site of disease. A number of questions, however, still remain. Why are only half of the plaques positive? Perhaps there are situations in which *C. pneumoniae* does not need to be present for atherosclerosis to develop. Genetically altered animals with dyslipidemias have not been infected with *C. pneumoniae* but will develop atheroma. Perhaps the *C. pneumoniae* is simply being scavenged by locally activated macrophages and is an innocent bystander. While there may be situations in which this occurs, these "innocently" engulfed organisms would need to develop a persistent infection at the site to explain how 45% of patients with atherosclerosis have evidence of the organism, given that the annual infection rate of *C. pneumoniae* is in the range of 1 to 2% per year. If persistence develops, one has to wonder how "innocent" an infection this would represent.

There are also many examples of infectious diseases, such as tuberculoid leprosy, in which it is difficult to identify organisms within the lesion but the immune reaction is brisk. Technical considerations such as the size of the slice examined could also account for an underestimate of the presence of infection within an entire plaque.

Alternatively, evidence of *C. pneumoniae* by PCR could represent DNA remaining after a transient prior infection. While this possibility needs to be considered, exploratory experiments have shown that DNA, when within UV-irradiated organisms, is cleared within days, making it unlikely that this scenario would generate false positive findings (9). Clinical studies of *Chlamydia trachomatis* genital tract infections confirm these observations. Other technical issues with the performance of PCR assays are well known, and can never be completely excluded. Nevertheless, one would have to conclude that these technical difficulties were pervasive throughout the different laboratories and resulted in almost exclusively false positive as opposed to false negative results.

Immunocytochemistry was the most frequently positive test in these studies. While the antibodies chosen for these tests have a high degree of specificity, (2) there is always the potential for some cross-reactivity. In addition, observer bias may be introduced in assessing the results if all samples are not read in a blinded fashion. Even given these potential limitations, it seems implausible that they would account for more than a small amount of error and unlikely to result in reversal of the overall conclusion that these organisms can be seen within an atherosclerotic plaque.

The association now rests on two lines of investigation, seroepidemiologic and histopathologic. Taken together they strengthen each other. Even so, these data do not provide evidence that *C. pneumoniae*, while present within an atherosclerotic plaque, actually contributes to atherogenesis. To explore this possibility, it would be important to know whether infection in a susceptible host results in the generation of an atheroma. For this it is necessary to move to animal models of disease.

## CAN INFECTION WITH *C. PNEUMONIAE* STIMULATE ATHEROGENESIS?

In order to fill another of Koch's postulates, the potential pathogen when inoculated into a susceptible host should cause disease. Given that for this disease it is unlikely to see this postulate fulfilled in humans, evidence will need to come from animal models. Murine and rabbit models have traditionally been used to study atherosclerosis and recently have been adapted for study of *C. pneumoniae* pathogenesis (34).

At least three mouse strains have been tested so far. All of these strains are, to different extents, capable of developing atheromas under various circumstances. Among these strains, it has been relatively difficult to demonstrate that *C. pneumoniae* infection results in a vasculopathy in the C57B6 strain although the organism has been identified in aortic plaque after intranasal challenge (44, 73). There is limited experience with NIH/s mice. However, infection has resulted in persistence, and reisolation was achieved from cardiac tissue (34). At this point, ApoE-deficient mice seem to offer the most promise as a significant number of atheromas from which *C. pneumoniae* can be isolated have been seen after inoculation via the nasal route. Progression of disease has been identified after single or multiple inoculations, including macrophage adherence to the endothelium, foam cell accumulation within the subendothelium, and macroscopic appearance of fatty streaks and developed atheroma (44). The real value of data generated from mice may be that nasal inoculation of *C. pneumoniae* can result in a persistent infection of the arterial wall in areas that are associated with a developing atheromatous lesion. The limitation of this model, based on the available published data, remains the difficulty in defining the extent to which the presence of this organism contributes to the development of the fatty streak, given that under the experimental conditions, control mice will also develop disease. For now it appears that additional work in mice will need to be performed in order to create permissive conditions under which controls do not develop disease. These conditions, however, may have been achieved in the rabbit model.

Among rabbit models, it has been difficult to demonstrate disease after intranasal challenge in the Watanabe heritable hyperlipidemic rabbits (45). Better success has been seen by three groups using New Zealand White rabbits. One-month-old New Zealand White rabbits were given an intranasal challenge with *C. pneumoniae* and fed with standard chow (17). Controls were inoculated with buffer. Two of the eleven infected rabbits developed an atherosclerotic plaque with evidence of *C. pneumoniae* inclusions by immunocytochemistry, one of which was also found to have a lymphocytic infiltrate within the arterial wall. From one of these lesions, the organism was grown in culture. None of the five control animals was found to have atheroma. This experiment has been confirmed with a greater number of animals, all sacrificed at the same timepoint after infection (17a).

In another laboratory, using New Zealand White rabbits fed a diet enriched with a small amount of cholesterol (0.25%), two of nine infected rabbits were found to have evidence of *C. pneumoniae* in the arterial wall by immunofluorescence compared to none of controls (46). In addition, the infected animals were found to have a greater maximal intimal thickness, percentage of luminal circumference involved, and plaque area index compared to controls. In a third lab, 5 of 13 New Zealand rabbits fed standard chow developed atherosclerotic changes in the aorta including a cell proliferative response, slight intimal thickening, and a lymphocytic infiltration after inoculation with *C. pneumoniae* strain K7 at baseline and week 3, compared to no evidence of disease in 15 of 15 uninfected controls. All five infected animals with aortic pathology were found to have evidence of *C. pneumoniae* in the arterial wall by either immunocytochemistry or in situ hybridization (35).

The strength of these data rests on the reproducibility of the findings from different laboratories. In each case approximately 25% of infected animals develop arterial disease in which *C. pneumoniae* can be identified. The pathologic changes noted include a lymphocytic infiltration of the subendothelial space, intuitively suggesting an acute cell-mediated immunologic response to an intracellular pathogen. The distribution of early to late changes typically seen with atherogenesis also implies that the findings may be related to the disease in question. In comparison to the murine models, it also appears that in the rabbit model conditions can be set to minimize the development of atherosclerosis in the control population.

The limitations of these data include the variability in the experimental conditions, the differences in endpoint definitions (for example, intimal wall thickness versus lymphocytic infiltration), and the relatively small total number of animals studied thus far. Even given these limitations, there is a body of evidence accumulating which substantiates the claim that infection with this intracellular pathogen results in a response within the arterial wall which ultimately leads to cholesterol deposition and the generation of an atherosclerotic plaque.

## HOW COULD THE IMMUNE RESPONSE TO INFECTION WITH *C. PNEUMONIAE* INFLUENCE THE DYNAMICS OF ATHEROGENESIS?

While evidence is becoming available to support this association of chlamydial infection and the development of an atherosclerotic plaque, there remain significant questions as to how chlamydial cell biology and the human immune response to this infection are relevant to the pathogenesis of atherosclerosis. How is it possible that this organism can survive for prolonged periods of time in the vascular space, simultaneously evading eradication while invoking an inflammatory response? In order to explore this connection it may be useful to review some recent developments in our understanding of chlamydial cell biology.

Figure 1 outlines a possible scenario regarding the intracellular development of *Chlamydia trachomatis*, though there is a general belief that these findings also relate to *C. pneumoniae* (5). The chlamydial elemental body enters the cell and is localized within a phagosome. It then differentiates into a reticulate body, the metabolically active stage of the lifecycle, and begins to undergo cell division. However, if conditions become unfavorable, the organism appears to develop into what has been described as aberrant chlamydia, sometimes referred to as persistent bodies. One such trigger of the formation of persistent bodies is nutrient deprivation, specifically tryptophan depletion, which may be a consequence of the activity on the host cell of cytokines such as interferon gamma. These persistent bodies are

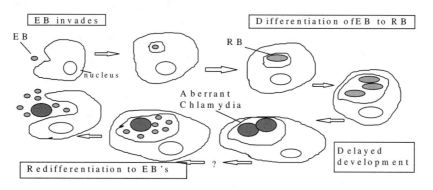

**Figure 1.** Altered intracellular development of *Chlamydia*. (Reprinted with permission from reference 35.)

known to survive in vitro for prolonged periods; they are metabolically relatively inactive and have an altered outer membrane constituency, expressing less major outer membrane protein, which is felt to be partially immunoprotective, (53) and more heat shock protein, which is felt to be highly immunopathogenic. When conditions become permissive, there is differentiation back into elemental bodies which are released or rupture from the host cell.

Evidence that *C. pneumoniae* may lie dormant in a cell may be found in a murine model of *C. pneumoniae* pneumonitis (37). Mice are inoculated intranansally with the organism. After 4 weeks one can find evidence of *C. pneumoniae* by PCR but not by culture. This PCR-positive result alone could represent residual nonviable organisms and not latent or persistent infection. To answer this question the animals are given either saline or cortisone. One can see in Table 3 that after two or four doses of therapy, all the cultures still remain sterile, though some portion of the animals are positive by PCR. Only after six courses of therapy do we see positive cultures in the steroid-treated group. Cultures from the saline-treated animals remain negative. These findings suggest two conclusions. First, a positive PCR in this setting may be a marker of latent disease. Second, though speculative, it is plausible that the administration of steroids (possibly through alterations in the immune response) induces a latent infection to become productive. There are data that suggest certain exposures of infected cell lines to interferon gamma can influence the balance between latency and active chlamydial replication (6). Along these same lines, there are also data demonstrating an increase in *C. pneumoniae* inclusion-forming units in two of three isolates when hydrocortisone is added to the culture media of infected HEp-2 cells (70).

In addition to these in vitro and animal model data supporting the possibility of a persistent state in the life cycle of chlamydiae, there are also clinical syndromes associated with latent, subclinical but chronic inflammatory disease. *C. trachomatis* is the cause of trachoma, one of the leading causes of blindness in certain areas of the developing world. It is a chronic inflammatory disease secondary to an unrelenting immune response to persistent *C. trachomatis* antigens, recognized clinically as elemental bodies in microscopic examinations of conjunctival scrapings. Of some concern has been the finding of these elemental bodies even after apparently adequate treatment, presumably a consequence of reexposure to the organism but also possibly due to incomplete eradication initially.

A well-described association between chronic pelvic inflammatory disease due to *C. trachomatis* and persistent inflammation in the fallopian tubes is seen even

**Table 3.** Impact of cortisone administration on recovery of *C. pneumoniae* from infected mice[a]

| Doses | Culture positive/total | | DNA positive/total | |
|---|---|---|---|---|
| | Saline | Cortisone | Saline | Cortisone |
| 2 | 0/10 | 0/10 | 5/10 | 3/10 |
| 4 | 0/10 | 0/10 | 3/10 | 2/10 |
| 6 | 0/10 | 6/13 | 2/10 | 6/13 |

[a]Mice were inoculated intranasally with *C. pneumoniae*; 4 weeks later, they were given either saline or cortisone. (Reprinted with permission from reference 37.)

after antibiotic therapy (35). Chronic infection of the cervical tract for as long as 1 year has also been documented (39). In addition to infection by *C. trachomatis*, pneumonia due to *C. psittaci* has been noted long after possible exposure to the organism. Latent infection due to *C. pneumoniae* is less well described; however, this pathogen has also been isolated from respiratory tract infections after clinical disease has subsided, and it has been associated with episodes of cough and bronchospasm that have persisted for months (12, 27). All of these examples describe how chlamydiae can be associated with a chronic infection, but how does this relate to atherogenesis? A brief overview of the role of inflammation in atherosclerosis may provide some insight.

An atherosclerotic plaque is a consequence of an interrelationship between cholesterol deposition in the subendothelial space and an inflammatory process composed of activated macrophages and lymphocytes all occurring under a collagenous fibrous cap. It has long been observed that the risk of occlusion of a coronary artery is only weakly correlated with the extent of luminal obstruction (3, 4, 16, 38, 49). In other words, the risk of a coronary artery occlusion is not much greater with an 80% stenosis when compared to the risk associated with a 20% stenosis. This seeming inconsistency is a consequence of the fact that the trigger of an acute obstruction is exposure of the subendothelial contents to the intravascular space, an event which occurs due to rupture of the fibrous cap. The likelihood of rupture of the cap is more closely correlated with the extent of inflammation within the plaque than to the size of the lipid deposit (71).

One of the hallmarks of a mature atheromatous plaque is the presence of foamy macrophages. An unstable plaque has many of these foamy macrophages distributed throughout it, producing a number of enzymes (such as metalloproteinases) capable of degrading collagen (14). Also throughout the plaque are T lymphocytes which can be seen distributed throughout the body of the plaque after staining of a carotid atheroma with anti-CD3 (66). While the antigen specificity of these cells is not thoroughly understood, there are early reports that they may be responding to heat shock proteins, (75) some fraction of which appear to be directed at antigens derived from *C. pneumoniae* (25, 26). This is a critical area of investigation in the evolution of our understanding of the role of *C. pneumoniae* in atherosclerosis. If a local immune response is directed at *C. pneumoniae* specifically, the possibility that the organism is merely an innocent bystander becomes far less plausible. Whatever the specificities, these T lymphocytes are presumably interacting with macrophages within the plaque, producing a cytokine response and driving the production of enzymes involved in the inflammatory response. To underscore the importance of this inflammatory response, pathologic examination of 20 atheromas taken from patients who had died of myocardial infarction revealed that activated macrophages and T lymphocytes were the dominant cell types at sites of plaque rupture associated with occlusive thrombi (71). Taken together, these data indicate that atherosclerosis is a local inflammatory disorder associated with activated macrophages and lymphocytes.

The lipid hypothesis of atherosclerosis asserts that oxidized low-density lipoprotein (LDL) cholesterol is responsible for activation of macrophages, and there is ample evidence to support this theory. Perhaps, however, this inflammation is also being driven by antigens derived from microorganisms and presented to T cells by tissue macrophages. Once these macrophages are activated, they secrete metallo-proteinases and collagenases which can weaken the fibrous cap, predisposing it to acute rupture. The subendothelial surface components are then exposed to circulating clotting factors leading to thrombosis of the vessel. A direct effect on endothelial cell function leading to procoagulant activity after infection with *C. pneumoniae* has also recently been demonstrated (18).

There is also mounting clinical evidence of the inflammatory nature of cardio-vascular disease related to atherogenesis. Four recent clinical papers found a correlation between circulating markers of inflammation and a future risk of cardiovascular events (28, 42, 60, 69). Measurements of C-reactive protein, using enzyme-linked immunosorbent assay (ELISA) techniques with sensitivities of 0.05 to 0.08 $\mu g/\mu l$ (more sensitive than is found in routine clinical applications) have been shown to predict one's future risk of cardiovascular events. In one paper, this risk was reduced by the use of aspirin (57). Whether aspirin is having its effect because of to its antithrombotic or its antiinflammatory activity is not clear, but these findings again underlie the belief that atherogenesis is an inflammatory process.

This line of evidence provides support for the role of a microorganism such as *C. pneumoniae* in the inflammatory component of the atherosclerotic plaque. But is there any potential association between *C. pneumoniae* infection and cholesterol deposition? Pending more conclusive evidence, there is a series of findings which indirectly suggests that a role in the process is plausible, summarized in Fig. 2, which represents a schematic representation of a foamy macrophage within an atherosclerotic plaque. The macrophage has internalized *C. pneumoniae*, either as an elemental or persistent body within the phagosome. Exogenous antigens derived

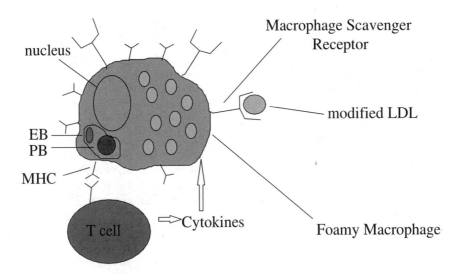

**Figure 2.** Model of an activated macrophage in an atheromatous plaque. EB, element body; PB, persistent body; MHC, major histocompatibility complex.

from *C. pneumoniae*, or host-derived heat shock proteins expressed as a consequence of infection, are then presented to T cells which in turn release cytokines into the local milieu that activate this and other macrophages. Activation of the macrophage enhances any number of functions, including surface expression of the macrophage scavenger receptor, as has been demonstrated with cytomegalovirus (CMV) infection (77). The scavenger receptor binds to chemically modified lipids. It binds to the lipotechoic acids of gram-positive organisms and lipopolysaccharides of certain gram-negative organisms (15). It also binds to oxidized LDL, which is then internalized. Microscopically, the cell takes on a foamy appearance as more lipid is internalized until at some point the cell ruptures, a process which serves to take up cholesterol from the circulation and concentrate it within the subendothelial space.

Whether this uptake and concentration of LDL are quantitatively contributing to the overall collection of subendothelial cholesterol was recently assessed in an animal model (65). A mouse in which the gene coding for the macrophage scavenger receptor had been deleted was crossed with an apolipoprotein E (apoE)-deficient mouse. The progeny of this cross were found to have a significant reduction in the size of their atherosclerotic plaques compared to the parent apoE deficient animals. The conclusion from this experiment is that the macrophage scavenger receptor may play a significant role in the accumulation of cholesterol within an atheroma. If infection of a macrophage with *C. pneumoniae* specifically results in an increase in the expression of this receptor, a clear connection can be made between the immune response to this pathogen and the deposition of fat within the arterial wall.

## ARE WE READY FOR CLINICAL TRIALS?

There is clearly much more work that needs to be done to consolidate the role of *C. pneumoniae* in the pathogenesis of atherosclerosis. From a strictly pragmatic approach to this area however, the available data may serve to justify the conduct of clinical trials assessing the merits of antibiotic intervention given the extraordinary morbidity and mortality associated with coronary artery disease. There have been two recently published antibiotic intervention trials. By admission of the authors, these studies are too small to provide anything other than provocative observations. Nonetheless, when viewed as pilot studies, they may offer some useful insights.

The first published study is a prospective, double-blind, randomized trial in which patients with a remote history of myocardial infarction (MI) and elevated IgG titers to *C. pneumoniae* were randomized to one or two courses of azithromycin or to placebo (23). Subjects with titers less than 1:64 were followed for clinical events, which included cardiovascular death, unstable angina, coronary revascularization, or myocardial infarction. Forty patients received azithromycin, 20 received placebo, 20 had elevated titers but were not randomized, 74 had intermediate titers, and 59 had negative titers (Table 4). The patients were all male and had a typical distribution of risk factors for coronary artery disease. Those with negative titers for chlamydia had a 7% event rate, during the mean 18 months of follow-up.

**Table 4.** Effect of azithromycin on incidence of cardiovascular events[a]

| C. pneumonia titer | Treatment | n | No. of cardiovascular events (%) | Odds ratio[b] |
|---|---|---|---|---|
| Negative | None | 55 | 4 (7) | |
| <1:64 | None | 74 | 11 (15) | 2.0 (0.6–6.8) |
| ≥1:64 | None/placebo | 40 | 11 (28) | 4.2 (1.2–15.5) |
| | | | | 5.0 (1.3–20)[c] |
| ≥1:64 | Azithromycin | 40 | 3 (8) | 0.9 (0.2–4.6) |

[a]Reprinted from reference 23 with permission from the publisher and author.
[b]Adjusted odds ratio (95% confidence interval), controlling for age, diabetes, hypertension, smoking, hypercholesterolemia, revascularization, and compared to subjects with negative titers to C. pneumoniae.
[c]Odds ratio compared to azithromycin-treated group.

Patients with intermediate titers had a 15% event rate, while those with titers greater than 1:64 had a 28% event rate, resulting in an odds ratio for this group of 4.2. Those subjects with elevated titers who received azithromycin had an incidence of cardiovascular events of 8%, similar to the negative titer subjects.

The criticisms of this study include the difficulty in assigning statistical significance to any individual finding, given that adjustments for multiple comparisons are not built into the overall alpha level. In addition, it is often difficult to ensure similar follow-up for subjects who are simply followed compared to those who are receiving study medication. Also, the sample population is based on a certain level of medical care provided solely to individuals within a catchment area surrounding London, England, so extrapolation to other communities may be difficult. Its strength can be seen in its confirmation of the fourfold increased risk of cardiovascular events with elevated titers to C. pneumoniae, as has been seen in the previous epidemiologic studies. Whether antibiotic intervention results in a reduction of risk will need to be studied in a larger cohort of subjects, given the small number of treated patients in this trial.

The second published study was a double-blind, randomized trial of roxithromycin (150 mg per day for 30 days) compared to placebo in patients with evidence of coronary artery disease manifest as unstable angina or an active non-Q wave infarction (24). The endpoints for this trial were the incidence of recurrent ischemia, acute myocardial infarction, or death due to ischemia within 30 days postrandomization. There were 102 patients randomized to roxithromycin and 100 to placebo. The groups were evenly matched at baseline, half of these patients had a previous myocardial infarction. In the composite endpoint of myocardial infarction, ischemic death, and recurrent angina, there were two events in the roxithromycin arm and nine on the placebo arm (Table 5). One of the two events among subjects given roxithromycin occurred within 72 hours of randomization.

In comparison to the first series, this cohort of patients included those who did not have a history of a previous MI, there were no inclusion criteria based on titers to C. pneumoniae, and the composite endpoint did not include a revascularization procedure. Given these differences, it is interesting to note that the treatment effect of antibiotic intervention was approximately 75% in each study. The limitation of this trial again rests on the small sample size and the statistical issues involved in

**Table 5.** Effect of roxithromycin on incidence of cardiovascular events[a]

| Event | No. of events in group treated with: | | P value |
| | Roxithromycin (n = 102) | Placebo (n = 100) | |
|---|---|---|---|
| Angina | 2 | 5 | 0.831 |
| Acute MI[b] | 0 | 2 | 0.732 |
| Death | 0 | 2 | 0.732 |
| MI + death | 0 | 4 | 0.116 |
| MI + death + angina | 2 | 9 | 0.064 |
| MI + death + angina | 1[c] | 9 | 0.036 |

[a]Reprinted from reference 24.
[b]MI, myocardial infarction.
[c]Excludes event occurring within first 72 h.

multiple comparisons. Also, the follow-up period was relatively brief, making assessments of the durability of the clinical response difficult to interpret. Of interest, however, is that the incidence of the individual components of the composite endpoint—angina, death, and acute MI—all trend in the same direction as the overall result, providing some level of internal consistency in the findings.

A number of trial design issues are raised within these two studies that may serve to guide the conduct of future clinical trials. The incidence of clinical events in patients with atherosclerosis is relatively low. Future trials may therefore require significant sample populations, in the range of thousands as opposed to hundreds of subjects, to provide meaningful results. The exact size of the trials will also hinge on the treatment effects. Of course, a 70% effect size, if confirmed, will help to reduce the sample size requirements. Interestingly, if effect sizes in this range are confirmed, one may be able to speculate as to the mechanism driving the response, an issue that needs to be considered given that some antibiotics have properties beyond their antimicrobial effects. Typical antibiotic treatment studies will demonstrate efficacy in the range of 75 to 95% compared to placebo whereas an effect size of 10 to 15% is considered robust when anticoagulant or antiinflammatory interventions are studied. The tetracyclines are known to have anticollagenase properties, making the mechanism behind any effect difficult to fully assess (21). Macrolides, and specifically erythromycin, have been associated with a small immune-modulating effect, though there are scant data with azithromycin or roxithromycin in this regard.

How long should therapy be continued? There is a concern that *C. pneumoniae* may not be readily eradicated by available agents. Reisolation of organisms after presumably adequate therapy, both in animal models and in clinical experience, has been reported. Although the reason for this finding is not well understood, it is possible that the immune response may create conditions that drive the organism into its latent state. As persistent bodies are felt to be relatively metabolically inactive, antibiotics which work by inhibition of protein synthesis may not be capable of inducing cell death. If any metabolic activity at all is needed, however, and antibiotic exposure to the organisms is maintained, it is conceivable that killing could ultimately occur. The two published studies used relatively brief courses of therapy, providing exposures of 2 to 4 weeks. The optimal duration of therapy, however, will remain a topic of debate until further evidence of efficacy becomes available.

The epidemiologic data suggest that higher titers may be associated with a greater risk of cardiovascular events. On a patient-specific basis, however, there are likely to be patients with low antibody titers that are harboring organisms (56). Better diagnostic criteria are necessary to define the population at risk. In addition to antibody titer, markers of inflammation such as C-reactive protein, measures of active *C. pneumoniae* infection such as circulating PCR positive monocytes, (47) or combinations of these may prove to be more useful for patient selection.

## Are We There Yet?

A number of lines of investigation have provided support for an association between infection with *C. pneumoniae* and atherogenesis. On their own, each has significant limitations, yet if they are taken as a whole, the link is tightened. Epidemiologic investigation can suggest an estimate of risk, and the geographic diversity of the studies published to date offer greater confidence in the results but epidemiologic associations cannot provide evidence of causality. The histopathologic studies provide evidence that the pathogen can be found at the site of disease; however, it cannot be determined from these studies that the disease is caused by the pathogen. While the innocent bystander hypothesis is a theoretically plausible consideration, *Chlamydia* is not known to be an innocent bystander in other settings and is in fact well known to be immunopathogenic. It would also be unusual to isolate a known pathogen from a sterile site at which a well-described disease is actively progressing and not strongly consider the organism to have a pathogenic role. Animal model data has providing tantalizing evidence that intranasal inoculation with *C. pneumoniae* results in the formation of an atherosclerotic plaque. Animal models are inherently limited in their applicability to human disease, especially in settings where a complex cell-mediated immune response may be central to underlying process. The genetic alterations in lipid metabolism in New Zealand White rabbits may also not be relevant to human atherosclerosis. Nonetheless, the fact that atherosclerosis has not been described with infection in these rabbits with other pathogens highlights the uniqueness of chlamydia in this regard. The overlap in the pathogenesis of *C. pneumoniae* and atherogenesis, specifically regarding activation of macrophages and the potential role of the macrophage scavenger receptor, also provides a plausible construct for this association. Still, the role of oxidized LDL cannot be minimized as the sole explanation for this inflammation, until it is demonstrated that *C. pneumoniae* infection results in a local increase in oxidized LDL. In addition, our understanding of the persistent state of the chlamydial life cycle is rudimentary, and its applicability to human disease has not been explored. While the clinical trials are providing suggestive results, the data are based on studies too underpowered to support firm conclusions.

## CONCLUSIONS

The association of *C. pneumoniae* and atherosclerosis is likely to evolve from additional pieces of supportive evidence. These will include additional investigations of chlamydial cell biology, specifically on the nature of the persistent body and its sensitivity to antibiotics; further studies on the antigen specificity of T cells in the atherosclerotic plaque; quantitative analyses of the extent to which macrophage scavenger receptor expression is modulated by *C. pneumoniae* infection; expanded assessments of the effect of infection with *C. pneumoniae* on endothelial function (including its effect on coagulability); and additional studies optimizing the timing and duration of antibiotic intervention, presumably in rabbit models initially, with the goal of mitigating the vascular response to this injury. Whether the investigation of this common respiratory pathogen and the most pervasive disease in Western society, linked by coincidence or as coconspirators, leads to tangible improvements in human health will depend on the results of large-scale clinical trials.

## REFERENCES

1. **Adamy, G.** 1930. Klinische Studie über die Psittakose. *Dtsch. Arch. Klin. Med. P.* **169**:301.

2. **Aldous, M. B., J. T. Grayston, S.-P. Wang, and H. M. Foy.** 1992. Seroepidemiology of *Chlamydia pneumoniae* TWAR infection in Seattle families, 1996–1979. *J. Infec. Dis.* **166**:646–649.

3. **Ambrose, J. A., and V. Fuster.** 1997. Can we predict future acute coronary events in patients with stable coronary artery disease? *JAMA* **277**:343–344.

3a. **American Heart Association.** 1995. *Heart and Stroke Facts: 1995 Statistical Supplement*, p. 1–4. American Heart Association, Dallas, Tex.

4. **Ambrose, J. A., M. A. Tannenbaum, D. Alexopoulus, C. E. Hjemdahl-Monsen, J. Leavy, M. Weiss, S. Borrico, R. Gorlin, and V. Fuster.** 1998. Angiographic progression of coronary artery disease and the development of myocardial infarction. *J. Am. Coll. Cardiol.* **12**:56–62.

5. **Beatty, W. L., R. P. Morrison, and G. I. Byrne.** 1994. Persistent chlamydiae: from cell culture to a paradigm for chlamydial pathogenesis. *Microbiol. Rev.* **58**:686–699.

6. **Beatty, W. L., G. I. Byrne, and R. P. Morrison.** 1993. Morphologic and antigenic characterization of interferon γ-mediated persistent *Chlamydia trachomatis* infection in vitro. *Proc. Natl. Acad. Sci. USA* **90**:3998–4002.

7. **Campbell, L. A., R. O'Brien, A. L. Cappuccio, C. C. Kuo, S. Wang, D. Stewart, D. L. Patton, P. K. Cummings, and J. T. Grayston.** 1995. Detection of *Chlamydia pneumoniae* TWAR in human coronary atherectomy tissues. *J. Infect. Dis.* **172**:585–588.

8. **Cappuccio, A., L. A. Jackson, R. A. Schmidt, and J. T. Grayston.** 1995. Detection of *Chlamydia pneumoniae* in coronary artery and other tissue specimens obtained at autopsy, abstr. D-174, p. 279. *In Abstracts of the 95th General Meeting of the American Society for Microbiology 1995*. American Society for Microbiology, Washington, D.C.

9. **Cappuccio, A. L., D. L. Patton, C. C. Kuo, and L. A. Campbell.** 1994. Detection of *Chlamydia trachomatis* deoxyribonucleic acid in monkey models (Macaca nemestrina) of salpingitis by in situ hybridization implications for pathogenesis. *Am. J. Obstet. Gynecol.* **171**:102–110.

10. **Cook, P. J., D. Honeybourne, G. Y. Lip, D. G. Beevers, and R. Wise.** 1995. Chlamydia pneumoniae and acute arterial thrombotic disease. *Circulation* **92**:3148–3149. (Letter.)

11. **Dahlen, G. T., J. Boman, L. S. Birgander, and B. Lindblom.** 1995. Lp(a) lipoprotein, IgG, IgA and IgM antibodies to *Chlamydia pneumoniae* and HLA class II genotype in early coronary artery disease. *Atherosclerosis* **114**:165–174.

12. **Dalhoff, K., V. Redecke, J. Braun, and M. Maass.** *Chlamydia (C) pneumoniae*: Immunopathologic symptoms and persistent infection, abstr. K-9, p. 330. *In Abstracts of the 37th Interscience Conference on Antimicrobial Agents and Chemotherapy*. American Society for Microbiology, Washington, D.C.

13. **Danesh, J., R. Collins, and R. Peto.** 1997. Chronic infections and coronary heart disease: Is there a link? *Lancet* **350**:430–436.

14. **Davies, M. J.** 1997. The composition of coronary artery plaques. *N. Engl. J. Med.* **336**:1312–1314.

15. **Dunne, D., D. Resnick, J. Greenberg, M. Krieger, and R. A. Joiner.** 1994. The type 1 macrophage scavenger receptor binds to gram-positive bacteria and recognizes lipotechoic acid. *Proc. Natl. Acad. Sci. USA* **91:**1863–1867.

16. **Falk, E., P. K. Shah, and V. Fuster.** 1995. Coronary plaque disruption. *Circulation* **92:**657–671.

17. **Fong, I. W., B. Chiu, E. Viira, M. W. Fong, D. Jang, and J. Mahony.** 1997. Rabbit model for *Chlamydia pneumoniae* infection. *J. Clin. Microbiol.* **35:**48–52.

17a.**Fong, I. W.** 1997. Personal communication.

18. **Fryer, R. H., E. P. Schwobe, M. L. Woods, and G. M. Rodgers.** 1997. Chlamydia species infect human vascular endothelial cells and induce procoagulant activity. *J. Invest. Med.* **45:**168–174.

19. **Gieffers, J., and M. Maass.** 1995. Serological response to *C. pneumoniae* in coronary heart disease, abstr. 495, p. 95. *In Abstracts of the 7th European Congress of Clinical Microbiology and Infectious Diseases,* Vienna, Austria, 1995.

20. **Godzik, K. L., E. R. O'Brien, S. Wang, and C. Kuo.** 1995. In vitro susceptibility of human vascular wall cells to infection with *Chlamydia pneumoniae. J. Clin. Microbiol.* **33:**2411–2414.

21. **Golub, L., N. Ramanurthy, T. McNamara, B. Gomes, M. Wolff, A. Casino, A. Kapoor, J. Zambon, S. Ciancio, M. Schneir, et al.** 1984. Tetracyclines inhibit tissues collagenase activity. A new mechanism in the treatment of periodontal disease. *J. Periodontal Res.* **19:**651–655.

22. **Grayston, J. T., C. C. Kuo, A. S. Coulson, L. A. Campbell, R. D. Lawrence, M. J. Lee, E. D. Strandness, and S. Wang.** 1995. *Chlamydia pneumoniae* (TWAR) in atherosclerosis of the carotid artery. *Circulation* **92:**3397–3400.

23. **Gupta, S., E. W. Leatham, D. Carrington, M. A. Mendall, J. C. Kaski, and A. J. Camm.** 1997. Elevated Chlamydia pneumoniae antibodies, cardiovascular events, and azithromycin in male survivors of myocardial infarction. *Circulation* **96:**404–407.

24. **Gurfinkel, E., G. Bozovich, A. Daroca, E. Beck, and B. Mautner for the ROXIS Study Group.** 1997. Randomized trial of roxithromycin in non-Q wave coronary syndromes: ROXIS pilot study. *Lancet* **350:**404–407.

25. **Halme, S., P. Saikku, and H. M. Surcel.** 1997. Characterization of *Chlamydia pneumoniae* antigens using human T cell clones. *Scand. J. Immunol.* **45:**378–384.

26. **Halme, S., H. Syrjala, A. Bloigu, P. Saikku, M. Leinonen, J. Airaksinen, and H. M. Surcel.** 1997. Lymphocyte responses to chlamydia antigens in patients with coronary heart disease. *Eur. Heart J.* **18:**1095–1101.

27. **Hammerschlag, M. R., K. Chirgwin, P. M. Roblin, M. Gelling, W. Dumornay, L. Mandel, P. Smith, and J. Schacter.** 1992. Persistent infection with *Chlamydia pneumoniae* following acute respiratory illness. *Clin. Infect. Dis.* **14:**178–182.

28. **Haverkäte, F., S. G. Thompson, S. D. Pyke, J. R. Gallimore, and M. B. Pepys for the ECAT Study Group.** 1997. Production of C-reactive protein and risk of coronary events in stable and unstable angina. *Lancet* **349:**462–466.

29. **Jackson, L. A., L. A. Campbell, C. Kuo, D. I. Rodriguez, A. Lee, and J. T. Grayston.** 1997. Isolation of *Chlamydia pneumoniae* from a carotid endarterectomy specimen. *J. Infect. Dis.* **176:**292–295.

30. **Kaukoranta-Tolvanen, S., K. Laitinen, P. Saikku, and M. Leinonen.** 1994. *Chlamydia pneumoniae* multiples in human endothelial cells in vitro. *Microb. Pathog.* **16:**313–319.

31. **Kuo, C. C., A. Shor, L. A. Campbell, H. Fukushi, D. L. Patton, and J. T. Grayston.** 1993. Demonstration of *Chlamydia pneumoniae* in atherosclerotic lesions of coronary arteries. JID **167:**841–849.

32. **Kuo, C. C., A. M. Gown, E. P. Benditt, and J. T. Grayston.** 1993. Detection of *Chlamydia pneumoniae* in aortic lesions of atherosclerosis by immunocytochemical stain. *Arterioscler. Thromb.* **13:**1501–1504.

33. **Kuo, C. C., J. T. Grayston, L. A. Campbell, Y. A. Goo, R. W. Wissler, and E. P. Benditt.** 1995. *Chlamydia pneumoniae* (TWAR) in coronary arteries of young adults (15–34 years old). *Proc. Natl. Acad. Sci. USA* **92:**6911–6914.

34. **Laitinen, K., H. Alakarppa, A. Laurila, and M. Leinonen.** 1997. Animal models for *Chlamydia pneumonia* infection. *Scand. J. Infect. Dis.* **104**(Suppl.):15–17.

35. **Laitinen, K., A. Laurila, M. Leinonen, and P. Saikku.** 1997. Atherosclerotic changes in normocholesterolemic rabbits after *Chlamydia pneumoniae* infection, abstr. B-83. *In Abstracts of the 37th*

*Interscience Conference on Antimicrobial Agents and Chemotherapy.* American Society for Microbiology, Washington, D.C.

36. **Maass, M., P. M. Engel, and S. Kruger.** 1996. Presence of *Chlamydia pneumoniae* in atheromatous lesions of the carotid arteries, abstr. C-158, p. 29. *In Abstracts of the 96th General Meeting of the American Society for Microbiology 1996.* American Society for Microbiology, Washington, D.C.

37. **Malinverni, R., C-C. Kuo, and J. T. Grayston.** 1995. Experimental *Chlamydia pneumoniae* (Cpn) pneumonitis in mice: evidence of persistent infection. *In Abstracts of the 95th American Society for Microbiology General Meeting 1995,* American Society for Microbiology, Washington, D.C.

38. **Mann, J. M., and M. J. Davies.** 1996. Vulnerable plaque: relation of characteristics to degree of stenosis in human coronary arteries. *Circulation* **94:**928–931.

39. **McCormack, W. M., S. Alpert, D. E. McComb, R. L. Nichols, D. Z. Semine, and S. H. Zinner.** 1979. Fifteen-month follow-up study of women infected with *Chlamydia tachomatis.* **300:**123–125.

40. **Melnick, S. L., E. Shahar, A. R. Folsom, J. T. Grayston, P. D. Sorlie, S. P. Wang, and M. Szklo.** 1993. Past infection by *Chlamydia pneumoniae* strain TWAR and asymptomatic carotid atherosclerosis. *Am. J. Med.* **95:**499–504.

41. **Mendall, M. A., D. Carrington, D. Strachan, et al.** 1995. *Chlamydia pneumoniae*: risk factors for seropositivity and association with coronary heart disease. *J. Infect.* **30:**121–128.

42. **Mendall, M. A., P. Patel, L. Ballam, D. Strachan, and T. C. Northfield.** 1996. C reactive protein and its relation to cardiovascular risk factors: a population based cross sectional study. *Br. Med. J.* **312:**1061–1065.

43. **Minick, C. R., C. G. Fabricant, J. Fabricant, and M. M. Latrena.** 1979. Atheroarteriosclerosis induced by infection with a herpesvirus. *Am. J. Pathol.* **96:**673–706.

44. **Moazed, T. C., C. Kuo, J. T. Grayston, and L. A. Campbell.** 1997. Murine models of *Chlamydia pneumoniae* infection and atherosclerosis. *J. Infect. Dis.* **175:**883–890.

45. **Moazed, T. C., C. Kuo, D. L. Patton, J. T. Grayston, and L. A. Campbell.** 1996. Experimental rabbit models of *Chlamydia pneumoniae* infection. *Am. J. Pathol.* **148:**667–676.

46. **Muhlstein, J. B., J. L. Anderson, E. H. Hammond, L. Zhao, S. Trehan, E. P. Schwobe, and J. F. Carlquist.** 1998. Infection with *Chlamydia pneumoniae* accelerates the development of atherosclerosis and treatment with azithromycin prevents it in a rabbit model, p. 43, abstr. 4.14. *In Program and Abstracts of the Fourth International Conference on the Macrolides, Azalides, Streptogramins and Ketolides.*

47. **Muhlstein, J. B., J. F. Carlquist, E. H. Hammond, E. Radicke, M. J. Thompson, S. Trehan, and J. L. Anderson.** 1998. Detection of *Chlamydia pneumoniae* bacteremia in patients with symptomatic coronary atherosclerosis, p. 43, abstr. 4.13. *In Program and Abstracts of the Fourth International Conference on the Macrolides, Azalides, Streptogramins and Ketolides.*

48. **Muhlstein, J. B., E. H. Hammond, J. F. Carlquist, E. Radicke, M. J. Thomson, L. A. Karagounis, M. L. Woods, and J. L. Anderson.** 1996. Increased incidence of *Chlamydia pneumoniae* species within the coronary arteries of patients with symptomatic atherosclerotic versus other forms of cardiovascular disease. *J. Am. Coll. Cardiol.* **27:**1555–1561.

49. **Mulcahy, D., S. Husain, G. Zalos, A. Rehman, N. P. Andrews, W. H. Scheneke, N. L. Geller, and A. A. Quyyumi.** 1997. Ischemia during ambulatory monitoring as a prognostic indicator in patients with stable coronary artery disease. *JAMA* **277:**318–324.

50. **Ong, G., B. J. Thomas, A. O. Mansfield, B. R. Davidson, and D. Taylor-Robinson.** 1996. Detection and widespread distribution of *Chlamydia pneumoniae* in the vascular system and its possible implications. *J. Clin. Pathol.* **49:**102–106.

51. **Ossewaarde, J. M., C. Vallinga, E. J. M. Feskens, and D. Kromhout.** 1995. Infection with *C. pneumoniae* as a risk factor for coronary heart disease. *Atherosclerosis* **115**(Suppl.):S13. (Abstract 41.)

52. **Ouchi, K., B. Fujii, Y. Kanamoto, H. Miyazaki, and T. Nakazawa.** Detection of *Chlamydia pneumoniae* in atherosclerotic lesions of coronary arteries and large arteries, abstr. K-37, p. 294. *In Abstracts of the 35th Interscience Conference on Antimicrobial Agents and Chemotherapy.* American Society for Microbiology, Washington, D.C.

53. **Pal, S., I. Theodor, E. M. Peterson, and L. M. de la Maza.** 1997. Immunization with an acellular vaccine consisting of the outer membrane complex of *Chlamydia trachomatis* induces protection against a genital challenge. *Infect. Immun.* **65:**3361–3369.

54. Patel, P., M. A. Mendall, D. Carrington, D. P. Strachan, E. Leatham, N. Molineaux, J. Levy, C. Blakeston, C. A. Seymour, A. J. Camm, and T. C. Northfield. 1995. Association of *Helicobacter pylori* and *Chlamydia pneumoniae* infections with coronary heart disease and cardiovascular risk factors. *Br. Med. J.* **311**:711–714.

55. Patton, D. L., M. Askienazy-Elbhar, J. Henry-Suchet, L. A. Campbell, A. Cappussio, W. Tannous, S. P. Wang, and C. C. Kuo. 1994. Detection of *Chlamydia trachomatis* in fallopian tube tissue in women with postinfectious tubal infertility. *Am. J. Obst. Gyn.* **17**:95–101.

56. Puolakkainen, M., C. Kuo, A. Shor, S. Wang, J. T. Grayston, and L. A. Campbell. 1993. Serological response to *Chlamydia pneumoniae* in adults with coronary arterial fatty streaks and fibrolipid plaques. *J. Clin. Microbiol.* **31**:2212–2214.

57. Pyorala, K. 1996. CHD prevention in clinical practice. *Lancet* **348**(Suppl. I):s26–s28.

58. Saikku, P., M. Leinonen, K. Mattila, M.-R. Ekman, M. S. Nieminen, R. H. Makela, J. K. Huttunen, and V. Valtonen. 1988. Serological evidence of an association of a novel chlamydia, TWAR, with chronic coronary heart disease and acute myocardial infarction. *Lancet* **ii**:983–985.

59. Ramirez, J. A., and the *Chlamydia pneumoniae*/Atherosclerosis Study Group. 1996. Isolation of *Chlamydia pneumoniae* from the coronary artery of a patient with coronary atherosclerosis. *Ann. Intern. Med.* **125**:979–982.

60. Ridker, P. M., M. Cushman, M. J. Stampfer, R. P. Tracey, and C. H. Hennekens. 1997. Inflammation, aspirin, and the risk of cardiovascular disease in apparently healthy men. *N. Engl. J. Med.* **336**:973–979.

61. Saikku, P., M. Leinonen, L. Tonkanen, E. Linnanmakel, M. Ekman, V. Manninen, M. Mänttäri, M. H. Frick, and J. K. Huttunen. 1992. Chronic *Chlamydia pneumonia* infection as a risk factor for coronary heart disease in the Helsinki Heart Study. *Ann. Intern. Med.* **116**:273–278.

62. Shor, A., C. C. Kuo, and D. L. Patton. 1992. Detection of *Chlamydia pneumoniae* in coronary arterial fatty streaks and atheromatous plaques. *S. Afr. Med. J.* **82**:158–161.

63. Sutton, G. C., J. A. Denmakis, T. O. Anderson, and R. A. Morrissey, with the Idiopathic Myocardial Disease Study Group of the Cook County Hospital. 1971. Serologic evidence of a sporadic outbreak in Illinois of infection by Chlamydia (psittacosis-LGV agent) in patients with primary myocardial disease and respiratory disease. *Am. Heart J.* **81**:597–607.

64. Sutton, G. C., R. A. Morrissey, J. R. Tobin, and T. O. Anderson. 1967. Pericardial and myocardial disease associated with serologic evidence of infection by agents of the psittacosis-lymphogranuloma venereum group (Chlamydiaceae). *Circulation* **26**:830–838.

65. Suzuki, H., Y. Kurihara, M. Takeya, N. Kamada, M. Kataoka, K. Jishage, O. Ueda, H. Sakaguchi, T. Higashi, T. Suzuki, Y. Takashima, Y. Kawabe, O. Cynshi, Y. Wada, M. Honda, H. Kurihara, H. Aburatani, T. Doi, A. Matsumoto, S. Azuma, T. Noda, Y. Toyoda, H. Itakura, Y. Yazaki, T. Kodoma, et al. 1997. A role for macrophage scavenger receptors in atherosclerosis and susceptibility to infection. *Nature* **386**:292–295.

66. Swanson, S. J., A. Rosenzweig, J. G. Seidman, and P. Libby. 1994. Diversity of T cell antigen receptor V beta gene utilization in advanced human atheroma. *Arterioscler. Thromb.* **14**:1210–1214.

67. Thom, D. H., J. T. Grayston, D. S. Siscovick, S. Wang, N. S. Weiss, and J. R. Daling. 1992. Association of prior infection with *Chlamydia pneumoniae* and angiographically demonstrated coronary artery disease. *JAMA* **268**:68–72.

68. Thom, D. M., S. P. Wang, J. T. Grayston, D. S. Siscovik, D. K. Stewart, R. A. Kronmal, and N. S. Weiss. 1991. *Chlamydia pneumoniae* strain TWAR antibody and angiographically demonstrated coronary artery disease. *Arterioscler. Thromb.* **11**:547–551.

69. Tracy, R. P., R. N. Lemaitre, B. M. Psaty, D. G. Ives, R. W. Evans, M. Cushman, E. N. Meilahn, and L. H. Kuller. 1997. Relationship of C-reactive protein to risk of cardiovascular disease in the elderly. *Arterioscler. Thromb. Vasc. Biol.* **17**:1121–1127.

70. Tsumura, N., U. Emre, P. Roblin, and M. R. Hammerschlag. 1996. Effect of hydrocortisone succinate on growth of *Chlamydia pneumoniae* in vitro. *J. Clin. Microbiol.* **34**:2379–2381.

71. Van de Wal, A. C., A. E. Becker, C. M. Van der Loos, and P. K. Das. 1994. Site of intimal rupture or erosion of thrombosed coronary atherosclerotic plaques is characterized by an inflammatory process irrespective of the dominant plaque morphology. *Circulation* **89**:36–44.

72. Varghese, P. J., C. A. Gaydos, S. B. Arumugham, D. G. Pham, T. C. Quinn, and C. U. Tuazon. 1995. Demonstration of *Chlamydia pneumoniae* in coronary atheromas specimens from young pa-

tients with normal cholesterol from the southern part of India, abstr. 53, p. 30. *In Abstracts of the 33rd Annual Meeting of the Infectious Diseases Society of America 1995.* Infectious Diseases Society of America, Washington, D.C.

73. **Weiss, S. M., P. M. Roblin, C. A. Gaydos, D. Cummings, D. L. Patton, N. Schulhoff, J. Shani, R. Frankel, K. Penney, T. C. Quinn, M. R. Hammerschlag, and J. Schachter.** 1996. Failure to detect *Chlamydia pneumoniae* in coronary atheromas of patients undergoing atherectomy. *J. Infect. Dis.* **173:**957–962.

74. **Weiss, S., P. Roblin, A. Kutlin, B. Paigen, and M. Hammerschlag.** 1997. *Chlamydia pneumoniae* (Cp) does not promote atherosclerosis in a mouse model, abstr. B-82. *In Abstracts of the 37th Interscience Conference on Antimicrobial Agents and Chemotherapy.* American Society for Microbiology, Washington, D.C.

75. **Wick, G., G. Schett, A. Amberger, R. Kleindienst, and Q. Xu.** 1995. Is atherosclerosis an immunologically mediated disease? *Immunol. Today* **16:**27–33.

76. **Workowski, K. A., M. F. Lampe, K. G. Wong, M. B. Watts, and W. E. Stamm.** 1993. Long-term eradication of *Chlamydia trachomatis* genital infection after antimicrobial therapy. Evidence against persistent infection. *JAMA* **270:**2071–2075.

77. **Zhou, Y. F., E. Guetta, Z. X. Yu, T. Finkel, and S. E. Epstein.** 1996. Human cytomegalovirus increases modified LDL uptake and scavenger receptor mRNA expression in vascular smooth muscle cells. *J. Clin. Invest.* **98:**2129–2138.

78. **Zhou, Y. F., M. B. Leon, M. A. Waclawiw, J. J. Popma, Z. X. Yu, T. Finkel, and S. E. Epstein.** 1996. Association between prior cytomegalovirus infection and the risk of restenosis after coronary atherectomy. *N. Engl. J. Med.* **335:**624–630.

*Emerging Infections 2*
Edited by W. M. Scheld, W. A. Craig, and J. M. Hughes
© 1998 ASM Press, Washington, D.C.

*Chapter 6*

# Cholera and *Vibrio cholerae*: New Challenges from a Once and Future Pathogen

## *Robert V. Tauxe and Timothy J. Barrett*

Cholera is a severe diarrheal illness caused by several strains of *Vibrio cholerae* that produce a powerful enterotoxin. Although other organisms occasionally cause similar illness, the term "cholera" is reserved for illness caused by infection with toxigenic strains of *V. cholerae* O1 or O139. This distinctive epidemic disease emerged on the global stage early in the 19th century and subsequently swept throughout the world in successive pandemic waves, seven by the most accepted historical account (64) (Table 1). Cholera arrived in Europe and North America at the height of the industrial revolution; the subsequent epidemics in the crowded cities had a profound impact on the development of institutions of public health. Fear of cholera led to the establishment of permanent municipal health departments and disease surveillance well before the microbe that caused it was known (71). The discovery that cholera was associated with contaminated water supplies spurred the "sanitary revolution," leading to municipal water and sewage treatment systems and the control of many diseases in the developed world. Then, early in the 20th century, epidemic cholera almost disappeared except for a persistent focus around the Bay of Bengal.

This lull broke dramatically in 1961, when the seventh and ongoing pandemic began in Indonesia (Fig. 1). This pandemic was caused by a different biotype of *Vibrio cholerae* O1, called the El Tor biotype, after the Egyptian quarantine station where it had been isolated early in the 1900s. The new pandemic spread rapidly across Asia and within a decade reached Africa with catastrophic consequences (38, 42). In the 1970s enhanced worldwide surveillance led to the surprising discovery of cases of cholera in southern United States and in northeastern Australia. These cases were caused by distinctive strains of toxigenic *Vibrio cholerae* O1 of biotype El Tor, apparently unrelated to the pandemic (9, 10, 14). Identification of these cases led to the new appreciation that *V. cholerae* O1 has a natural reservoir in coastal areas and rivers; patients were infected after consuming undercooked

---

***Robert V. Tauxe and Timothy J. Barrett*** • Division of Bacterial and Mycotic Diseases, National Center for Infectious Diseases, Centers for Disease Control and Prevention, Atlanta, GA 30333.

**Table 1.** Cholera pandemics since 1817[a]

| No. | Yrs | Origin | Pandemic organism |
| --- | --- | --- | --- |
| 1 | 1817–1823 | India | Unknown |
| 2 | 1829–1851 | India | Unknown |
| 3 | 1852–1859 | India | Unknown |
| 4 | 1863–1879 | India | Unknown |
| 5 | 1881–1896 | India | *V. cholerae* O1, classical biotype |
| 6 | 1899–1923 | India | *V. cholerae* O1, classical biotype |
| 7 | 1961–present | Sulawesi, Indonesia | *V. cholerae* O1, El Tor |
| 8? | 1992–present | Madras, India | *V. cholerae* O139 |

[a]Data for pandemics 1 to 6 are from reference 64.

crustacea or drinking untreated water in the absence of human sewage contamination. In contrast to the static focus on the Gulf of Mexico, the seventh pandemic itself arrived on the west coast of South America in 1991 and spread with phenomenal speed and intensity through that continent and Central America (82).

Cholera is not a historical curiosity but a major and continuing public health challenge. The seventh and current pandemic continues in many countries, where the infrastructure that guarantees clean water and safe food is missing or unmaintained. It is a particular challenge in slums that circle the growing cities of the developing world, in makeshift refugee camps, and in Central Asian republics that were formerly part of the Soviet Union. Unlike previous cholera pandemics, which tended to pass through a region and disappear, the current pandemic has now persisted more than three decades and may continue indefinitely. In 1996, 78 countries reported cases of cholera, and the pandemic persists in Asia, Africa, and Latin

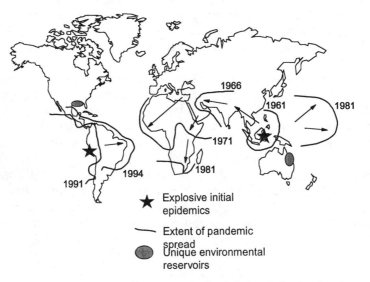

**Figure 1.** Spread of the seventh global pandemic of cholera, indicating the advancing edge of the epidemic at successive points in time.

America (Fig. 2) (4). Seven countries, all in Africa, reported incidence of more than 100 cases per 100,000 persons in 1996 (Fig. 3). This successful re-emerging pathogen is well adapted to the modern developing world.

Fortunately, effective treatment for cholera is now well established and inexpensive. Rapid replacement of lost electrolytes and fluids with oral and intravenous solutions reduces the case-fatality rate from more than 25 to less than 1% (79). Indeed, the development of oral rehydration therapy for cholera and other dehydrating diarrheal illnesses ranks as one of the critical medical discoveries of the 20th century. Unfortunately, this effective and inexpensive treatment is still not universally available. In 1996, the reported death rate for cholera was over 10% in five African countries with epidemic cholera, and there were substantial continentwide differences in the fatality rate (Table 2) (4).

## RECENT MICROBIOLOGIC OBSERVATIONS ON DIVERSITY IN *VIBRIO CHOLERAE*

The causative bacterium was described by Robert Koch in 1886, following its isolation and characterization during an epidemic in Egypt in the fifth pandemic (45). *Vibrio cholerae* is a comma-shaped gram-negative halophilic rod that swims with rapid darting movements, propelled by a single polar flagellum. It grows best in slightly saline watery environments and is exquisitely sensitive to sunlight, desiccation, and acidity. A large number of different serogroups have been described for *Vibrio cholerae* on the basis of their O antigens; however, all strains associated with epidemic disease were toxigenic members of serogroup O1 or most recently O139 (72). Within the O1 serogroup, two common serotypes (called Inaba and Ogawa) are recognized and represent antigenic variations of the O1 antigen. It has been clear for decades that a variety of different strains could cause epidemics. The

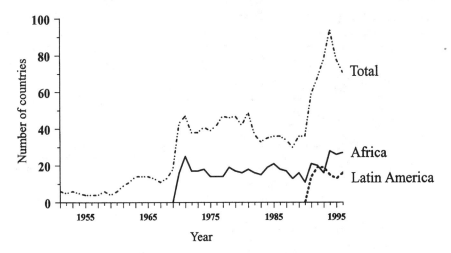

**Figure 2.** Number of countries reporting cholera to the World Health Organization, 1951 to 1996. Data are from the World Health Organization.

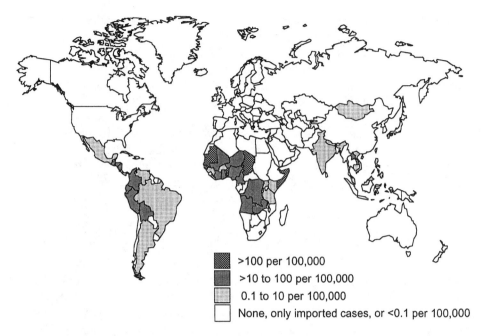

**Figure 3.** Reported incidence of cholera, by country, 1996. Data are from the World Health Organization.

*V. cholerae* O1 strains isolated by Koch and those described early in the 20th century in the sixth pandemic are now known as classical biotype strains to distinguish them from the El Tor biotype strains, which cause the current global pandemic. El Tor biotype is now worldwide in its distribution, while classical biotype strains are found only in coastal Bangladesh (75). The differentiation of the two biotypes has traditionally been based on phenotypic characterization including hemolysis of sheep red blood cells, bacteriophage susceptibility, Voges-Proskauer reaction, polymyxin B susceptibility, and hemagglutination of chicken red blood cells (13). Early isolates of the El Tor biotype were strongly hemolytic, but most recent isolates are not, greatly diminishing the value of this simple test (5). However, nonhemolytic El Tor strains still carry a hemolysin gene that is not present

**Table 2.** Reported cases and case fatality ratios by continent in 1996[a]

| Continent | Cases | Deaths | Case fatality ratio (%) |
| --- | --- | --- | --- |
| Africa | 108,535 | 6,216 | 5.7 |
| Asia | 10,142 | 122 | 1.2 |
| Australia and Oceania | 4 | 0 | 0 |
| Europe | 25 | 0 | 0 |
| North and Central America | 6,383 | 143 | 2.2 |
| South America | 18,260 | 208 | 1.1 |

[a]Data are from the World Health Organization.

in classical strains, and an oligonucleotide probe for this gene seems to be biotype specific (3).

Strains of *V. cholerae* of many serotypes are common in brackish and freshwater environments around the world. The organism is well adapted to life in warm water environments, where it may have invertebrate hosts. It produces chitinase, an enzyme that dissolves the crustacean exoskeleton, and may have a natural association with copepods or other microcrustacea (41, 62). The properties that confer pathogenic and epidemic potential are incompletely defined. The most obvious is the ability to produce cholera toxin, a protein exotoxin composed of one active A subunit and five binding B subunits, which resembles the heat labile toxin of enterotoxigenic *Escherichia coli*. The genes for this toxin are part of a linked cluster of genes that code for cholera toxin subunits A and B (and other less well understood accessory genes) as part of a "virulence cassette." Simple toxigenicity is necessary but probably not sufficient to achieve epidemic potential, as toxigenic strains of other serotypes that have not caused epidemics have been described (59). A second important virulence factor is the attachment factor known as the toxin-coregulated pilus (TCP) (53). This pilus appears to mediate colonization in the gut, perhaps by attachment to gut mucosal cells. A modified toxigenic strain lacking TCP did not colonize, cause disease, or evoke an immune response when given to human volunteers (39). The expression of both cholera toxin and TCP is controlled by the ToxR regulon and is switched on and off in response to environmental stimuli; this regulatory ability could also be considered a virulence factor. The virulence cassette has recently been shown to be transferred by a filamentous phage that can transfer toxigenicity to other strains that already possess TCP (90). This means that cholera toxin, the primary virulence factor of *V. cholerae*, was acquired through horizontal gene transfer from another unknown microbial source (49, 56).

The emergence of epidemic *V. cholerae* O139 infections in 1992 proves that the O1 lipopolysaccharide surface antigen itself is not necessary for the organism to cause epidemic cholera. This singular event provides an instructive example of pathogen evolution. Outbreaks of severe cholera-like illness in Madras, India, in 1992 were caused by strains of *V. cholerae* that did not agglutinate in antisera to 138 defined serogroups and were thus designated group 139 (22). The strains resemble typical El Tor strains phenotypically and produce cholera toxin and typical cholera illness. Epidemiologic investigations indicate that they are transmitted through contaminated water and food, just as is *V. cholerae* O1 (40). Indeed, by many molecular and phenotypic measures, these organisms are extremely similar to El Tor strains of serogroup O1. The principal difference lies in the genes that produce the O antigen. In O139 strains, a major portion of these genes is missing, so that O-antigen synthesis and the O antigen itself is truncated (27). The dominant surface antigen of O139 is a polysaccharide capsule, rather than a typical O antigen, and the genes that code for synthesis of the capsule have largely replaced the genes that code for enzymes that synthesized the O antigen (27, 77). This documented evolutionary switch from lipopolysaccharide antigen to polysaccharide capsule is unique among bacteria. Although the mechanism for this block deletion/replacement mutation has not been defined, modification by phage is one possible explanation.

The epidemiologic consequences of antigenic conversion were dramatic. A cholera epidemic spread rapidly in populations already immunized by natural infection with *V. cholerae* O1, through India, into Bangladesh and southeast Asia, reaching Thailand by 1993 (15, 21, 40). Though cholera in Bengal has been largely a disease of childhood and adults are usually protected by earlier and recurrent exposures, this epidemic affected many adults, indicating that natural immunity provided by preceding O1 infections had little protective effect against O139 infection. Because the O139 strains produce the same cholera toxin as El Tor strains, this lack of protection suggests that the dominant protective immunogen is the O antigen itself, rather than antibodies to cholera toxin, which would have been evoked by preceding infection with O1 strains. The appearance of this new virulent serogroup in India appears to be a unique bacterial example of an "antigenic escape" mutation, an evolutionary event occurring in the setting of high levels of immunity that is analogous to antigenic shift in the influenza virus. For unclear reasons, O139 has gone into decline since 1994, persisting around the Bay of Bengal but not spreading further in Asia or into Africa (2). It would be premature to call this the 8th pandemic. In most areas where O139 has declined, it has been replaced by new clones of *V. cholerae* O1 that are different from those originally displaced by O139 (74).

Less dramatic antigenic conversion within serogroup O1 of *V. cholerae* has long been recognized. The ability to switch between Ogawa and Inaba serotypes may provide some ability to evade the host immune response, but vibriocidal antibody titers to both serotypes are typically equivalent in patients recovering from cholera (7). The mechanism for the switch from Ogawa to Inaba serotype has been shown to be a deletion in the *rfbT* gene (54). Inaba-to-Ogawa shifts can occur if this deletion is precisely corrected. Such an event was observed during the epidemic in Latin America where all early isolates were serotype Inaba, but later isolates, indistinguishable by other subtyping methods, were serotype Ogawa (4a, 87).

As a pathogen, toxigenic *V. cholerae* has remarkable host specificity. The organism does not cause disease in animals other than humans, and no role for the toxin or TCP has yet been identified in the aquatic environment. This host specificity is not explained by the biologic activity of cholera toxin, which can induce intestinal secretions in many mammalian tissue systems. Perhaps the utility of the toxin to the organism lies in the intense diarrhea it causes in the human gut, which contaminates the environment and transmits the organism to other human hosts. If so, the evolutionary events that led to cholera must have occurred relatively recently, after humans were numerous enough to sustain transmission. Cholera may have had a substantial local effect on the human population. For unclear reasons, persons of blood group O are more likely to have severe disease after infection (37, 78). Blood group O is relatively rare in the population living on the Bay of Bengal, which may reflect the evolutionary selection of cholera in this human population (37).

A curious phenotypic variation has been recently observed. Some "sticky" strains of toxigenic *V. cholerae* O1 autoagglutinate, forming rough-surfaced colonies on agar and polybacterial particles in solution (60). These so called "rugose" strains are infectious and can withstand environmental stress, including chlorine disinfectants, better than solitary bacteria. Their public health significance is unclear.

## NEW INSIGHTS FROM MOLECULAR SUBTYPING

Molecular subtyping has expanded our understanding of this persistent pathogen in recent years. Three major methods used have included multilocus enzyme electrophoresis (MEE), which depends on allelic variation in "housekeeping" enzymes, ribotyping (RT), which depends on variation in the number and location on the chromosome of the conserved genes for 16s rRNA, and pulsed-field gel electrophoresis (PFGE), which depends on the presence and location of target sites for restriction endonuclease enzymes on the bacterial chromosome (6). Though they differ in the degree of differentiation they provide and in ease of application, these three methods have yielded complementary results. Each method easily distinguishes the 7th pandemic El Tor strains from earlier classical strains, indicating that a substantial evolutionary gulf separates the two biotypes. Similarly, each method separates the U.S. Gulf Coast and Australian strains as distinct subgroups unto themselves. This means that these two environmental foci are not directly related to the 7th epidemic and may represent either the residua of earlier epidemics or toxigenic El Tor strains that lack capacity or opportunity to cause an epidemic. Finally, these methods indicate that surprising diversity exists within the 7th pandemic and among the various O139 strains.

Among toxigenic El Tor strains characterized at the Centers for Disease Control and Prevention, we have identified 4 MEE profiles (33), 11 ribotype subtypes (65), and 39 PFGE patterns (16). Some of these appear to be geographically restricted, and some are cosmopolitan (Fig. 4). The distribution of strains is not static and rapid shifts can occur. The seventh pandemic is not a single event but is a mosaic of separate and overlapping epidemics that can spread quickly. For example, in the summer of 1991, shortly after the South American epidemic began, a second unique dissemination of a different subtype of *V. cholerae* serogroup O1, biotype El Tor occurred (33, 47). Easily recognized by its multiple antimicrobial resistance (MAR) to sulfisoxazole, streptomycin, and furazolidone, and characterized as ribotype 6a and PFGE type cluster 15,64,65, this strain was detected virtually simultaneously in Mexico, in several parts of Asia, and in Romania. The MAR strains have subsequently spread throughout Central America and have become the dominant strain there, despite the simultaneous presence of the South American epidemic strain (31, 47). Between 1992 and 1994, the proportion of *V. cholerae* O1 infections in the United States caused by MAR strains increased from 3 to 94%, virtually all of which were associated with foreign travel (52). The geographic origin of the MAR strain is unknown. Its sudden global appearance on three continents in the summer of 1991 is difficult to explain by any mechanism other than air transport, though no links were recognized at the time. The MAR variant illustrates how the current pandemic is sustained by the appearance and rapid global dissemination of new strains.

Molecular diversity can also help clarify cryptogenic outbreaks. For example, in 1991 simultaneous cases of cholera occurred in two unrelated persons at opposite

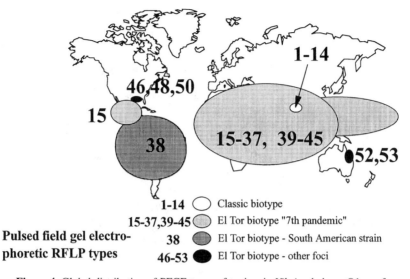

**Figure 4.** Global distribution of PFGE types of toxigenic *Vibrio cholerae* O1 as of 1992 (from reference 16). Nontoxigenic types are not shown.

ends of the Hawaiian island of Oahu on the same day (57). Despite intensive investigation, only one other infection was diagnosed serologically in a relative, and the source was not identified although both patients reported consuming different raw seafoods. The two strains were indistinguishable by ribotype (type 6b) and PFGE (pattern 34) and closely resembled other strains previously related to the Philippines, a primary source of Hawaiian seafoods. The ability to assign these strains a probable source and to distinguish them from the Latin American epidemic focused control measures and reassured public health authorities. Similarly, a small outbreak of cholera in the state of Maryland was traced to imported fresh coconut milk from Thailand, and the strains from the ill persons matched by ribotype (types 5 and 3) and PGFE (pattern 25) with strains previously identified in Southeast Asia (16, 65, 84).

Molecular characterization also sheds some light on the South American epidemic itself. The source of the strain of toxigenic *V. cholerae* O1 El Tor that arrived in Peru in 1991 has been unclear. It is a typical El Tor in nearly all respects and resembles other strains of the seventh pandemic by ribotyping, a member of the widely distributed ribotype 5 (65). It has a single and consistent PFGE profile distinct from strains isolated elsewhere and representing just one more pattern among many in the pandemic (16). The Peruvian strains can also be distinguished by MEE on the basis of a single variant enzyme; the genetic basis for this convenient difference rests on a 16-kb insertion in the *pepN* gene, probably representing a single genetic event (CDC unpublished data). Since 1991, strains from the epidemic in South America continue to exhibit a remarkable homogeneity, retaining a dominant PFGE profile and pansusceptibility to antimicrobials in most areas. As that combination of PFGE profile and MEE type has not been identified elsewhere, except in direct relation to travelers from Latin America, the source of the epidemic cannot be assigned with confidence. Characterization of nontoxigenic *V. cholerae* O1 strains previously isolated from Latin America indicates that these strains are very divergent from the current epidemic strains, suggesting that it is unlikely that the epidemic arose when a previously nontoxigenic local strain acquired the toxin (33). The general similarity of Latin American epidemic strains to others in the seventh pandemic cluster strongly suggests that a single importation event from an unidentified reservoir in the Old World occurred, with subsequent rapid spread of that strain.

Molecular characterization of *V. cholerae* O139 strains also reveals a surprising diversity, even among strains collected near the beginning of the epidemic. One such survey identified 4 similar PFGE patterns and 2 ribotypes among 23 strains (66). This suggests that the conversion event that led to O139 either happened simultaneously to several different strains of toxigenic O1 biotype El Tor or happened several times in slightly different manners; both are consistent with the hypothesis of phage-mediated conversion (66). This diversity has persisted and even expanded as the epidemic evolved, even as the infections became less frequent (34). The characteristic multiple resistance pattern of the O139 strains proved to be conferred by a novel self-transmissible genetic element that integrates into the chromosome and can transfer resistance for three antimicrobial agents between *V. cholerae* and *E. coli* (91). Curiously, the prevalence of this resistance is reported to be waning in the most recent O139 strains (2).

Studies of the molecular taxonomy of epidemic *V. cholerae* suggest that the sixth and seventh pandemics were caused by independently derived clones. DNA sequencing of the *asd* gene in sixth and seventh pandemic strains, along with nontoxigenic, non-O1 environmental isolates, revealed no differences within each pandemic but showed each pandemic to be more closely related to certain non-O1 isolates than to the other pandemic (44). *V. cholerae* O139 genes were identical to those of the seventh pandemic strains. This study confirmed earlier work by the same authors in which ribotyping showed major differences between the sixth and seventh pandemic isolates and found O139 isolates to be most similar to O1 isolates of the early seventh pandemic (43). Such data strongly suggest that new strains capable of causing epidemic cholera have arisen on several occasions in the past. We can anticipate that more are likely to arise in the future.

Sequencing the cholera toxin gene itself yields a taxonomy different from that of the organism. At least three variant gene sequences of the B subunit gene have been described. One is common to both the classical biotype and the U.S. Gulf Coast El Tor strains, one is found in Australian El Tor strains, and one in other El Tor strains of the seventh pandemic, including those from Latin America (63). The presence of similar toxin genes in both the classical biotype and one lineage of El Tor biotype is further evidence of the horizontal mobility of the toxin genes.

## EMERGENCE AND GEOGRAPHIC SPREAD

The episodic history of cholera pandemics and the genetic diversity of *V. cholerae* suggest that previous global waves may have reflected similar emergence of other pandemic strains. However, neither the time of the transfer of cholera toxin to *V. cholerae* O1 nor the nature of those strains has been clearly defined. Epidemic cholera is not clearly described in early Mediterranean or Arabic medical texts, though a compatible disease appears in medieval Indian manuscripts (64). Toxigenic *V. cholerae* O1 could have been established for many years in the brackish waters of the Bay of Bengal, infecting those who drank or consumed raw shellfish from those waters, in an ecologic pattern common to many other vibrios.

Epidemic cholera was easily recognized by 1817, when it affected European troops and local residents in India. The epidemic rapidly spread to Southeast Asia, China, Arabia, and Persia, reaching the Mediterranean coast of Syria by 1822. From there, the epidemic spread rapidly throughout the rest of the inhabited world (64). The global spread of cholera was probably hastened by the establishment of global European empires and the resulting increase in international trade. Later in the 19th century, steamships, riverboats, and trains increased the speed and decreased the cost of travel, making spread even more rapid. The annual Muslim pilgrimage to Mecca (Hajj) played a role in cholera pandemics 4 through 6 (64).

In the current pandemic, several mechanisms have been documented by which *V. cholerae* can be introduced into new geographic areas. The first and perhaps the most important is via a person who travels while harboring an incubating infection. History is replete with anecdotes of cholera outbreaks following the arrival of ill travelers. Transient asymptomatic carriage is frequent in *V. cholerae* infection, so the transportation event can be difficult to identify. In recent years, travel-associated cases identified in the United States introduced the organism repeatedly from other continents, though rarely with evidence of further transmission (52). In one remarkable event, a dish of local fresh fruit prepared in the United States by a recently returned and asymptomatically infected traveler transmitted the infection (1). Epidemic *V. cholerae* can also be transported in foods themselves. This is almost never the result of commercial food transport but rather the informal transport of "suitcase foods" to relatives. Several well-documented outbreaks have followed the consumption of foods purchased in a developing world market and brought informally in suitcases to relatives in the U.S. (18, 20, 35, 88). International transfer via commercial food has been documented only once, following the importation of fresh frozen coconut milk produced by an unlicensed factory in Thailand (84).

A third mode of transfer, via the ballast water of freighter ships, may be important in some circumstances. This mode was discovered after toxigenic *V. cholerae* O1 of the Latin American epidemic subtype were detected in a Gulf Coast oyster bed in 1992 (19). Thorough investigation did not identify a land-based sewage contamination source. The oyster beds were near a ship channel leading into an inner harbor, and the same Latin American epidemic strain of *V. cholerae* O1 was identified repeatedly in samples of ballast water being discharged from freighters arriving from Latin America (55). The double-hulled freighter ship, a post World War II innovation, routinely takes on and discharges ballast water in harbors to maintain a constant displacement with different cargoes. In the process, hundreds of thousands of gallons of harbor water and attendant flora and fauna are transported around the world. This mechanism can explain the introduction of cholera into harbor cities, a phenomenon that has been repeatedly observed when cases of cholera arise in persons eating raw shellfish from the harbor. In 1991, a specific freighter from China was suspected as a possible source of introduction of cholera into Peru, as the epidemic began in a harbor town visited by that freighter and early cases seemed anecdotally to be associated with raw seafoods processed in harbor water (82).

## The Genesis of Epidemics

Once the pathogen is introduced, an outbreak or epidemic will not occur unless there are special permissive circumstances. The feces of a returning traveler are quickly rendered harmless by standard sewage treatment or even by a well-maintained outhouse. *V. cholerae* has not been documented to spread directly from one person to another without intermediary contamination of food or water. An epidemic will occur only if the organisms are able to reach an open channel of waterborne or food-borne transmission. This was readily achieved in many 19th century cities, where gross sewage contamination of water systems and the absence of sewage or water treatment made large epidemics possible. Seminal epidemiologic observations in London and Hamburg identified the catastrophic efficiency with which contaminated municipal water systems could spread the disease (64, 76).

Today similar conditions prevail in many parts of the developing world. In Latin America, epidemiologic investigations identified several specific mechanisms for epidemic transmission (81). In rural areas, streams and rivers that are communal laundry and bathing facilities as well as the source of drinking water serve to spread the organism. In urban areas, poorly maintained water systems where water flow is intermittent often have pressure drops that pull sewage from adjacent sewage pipes into the drinking water. Even if the water was clean when it was first drawn from a deep well, it can be heavily contaminated by the time it reaches the unsuspecting recipient. The mistaken belief that water need not be chlorinated as long as it is clean at the well head has allowed many epidemics to flourish. Where water supplies are distant or intermittent, water is fetched and stored in the home. The design of the water storage container is critical, as clean water can easily become contaminated if it is scooped out by hand (58).

Food-borne transmission is an important component of many epidemics and has been the predominant mode of transmission in some (32). Moist grains eaten without reheating or acidification are a common vehicle as *Vibrio cholerae* can grow rapidly on rice, lentils, or other cooked grains (46). Condiments that acidify the grain, such as tomatoes or yogurt, can prevent this growth. In many parts of the world, street-vended foods and beverages are a recurrent source of cholera (47, 51, 69). Street vendors are a regular feature of urban life and often prepare food under nonhygienic circumstances. Raw or undercooked seafoods are also a recurrent food vehicle, either because they are naturally contaminated or because they are harvested from or processed with contaminated water. In the United States, the few cases of nontravel associated cholera that occur are almost entirely associated with eating undercooked local shellfish from the Gulf of Mexico (92).

Preventing cholera transmission means knowing which of these routes of transmission dominate and taking effective action to block them. Epidemiologic investigation may be necessary to target control measures correctly. For example, in an epidemic in Portugal in 1974, initial cases were associated with raw shellfish, but the epidemic worsened after widespread concern greatly increased the consumption of bottled water. An epidemiologic investigation showed that the bottled water itself was the source of much of the cholera, as the water source that was used had become contaminated (11, 12). More recently, a large urban outbreak occurred in Guatemala in the presence of a chlorinated and safe water supply, due to contamination of street-vended beverages (47). In the 1991 cholera epidemic in Ecuador, simultaneous transmission occurred via several mechanisms, indicating that control measures were needed at several levels (93).

## Persistence of the Seventh Pandemic

*Vibrio cholerae* O1, and perhaps O139, has a natural habitat in brackish bodies of water. The recurrence of cholera caused by the El Tor biotype strains of *V. cholerae* O1 along the U.S. coast of the Gulf of Mexico since at least 1973 and in Australian rivers since at least 1977 indicates that these organisms can persist long term in the environment, even in the absence of human fecal contamination. This environmental reservoir means that wherever the current pandemic strains are introduced around the world, they may find natural ecosystems permitting their long-term persistence and hence become endemic diseases. Such foci can serve to reintroduce the organism to other areas where it may be only intermittent. We can expect the current pandemic to persist indefinitely.

This prospect is distinctly different from earlier pandemics. Despite repeated global introductions, the classical strains did not persist anywhere outside of the Indian subcontinent. Biologic differences between the El Tor biotype and the classical biotype may help to explain the persistence of the current pandemic. Compared to classical strains, El Tor strains are more likely to produce inapparent infections (36), to persist longer in the environment (8), to multiply more rapidly following inoculation into foods (46), and to evoke less complete immunity (26). The degree to which these characteristics are shared by all strains of El Tor is not clear. The possibility of intraspecies competition is raised by recent observations from India and Bangladesh, where classical biotype strains are confined to a few rural coastal areas and where first El Tor, then O139, and then again El Tor strains have dominated further inland and in the urban areas (2, 75). How these organisms might compete with each other in the environment, in some as yet unidentified invertebrate host, or even in human populations remains to be defined.

Other environmental variables may influence the likelihood of persistent epidemics. Many serotypes of *V. cholerae* exhibit strong seasonal changes in environmental prevalence, reaching high counts in association with warm water and zooplankton counts (41, 86). Changes in rainfall and temperature may affect the prevalence; in colonial India cholera epidemics were noted to be particularly likely to occur during the year after a drought, through mechanisms that remain obscure (70). Some may speculate that the environmental changes related to El Niño could alter an underlying ecology, but there are also much more direct and obvious effects. Floods and washouts wrought havoc with sewers and water mains in Peru during the El Niño episode of 1982. The sewers and mains had not been completely repaired by 1991, contributing substantially to the severity of the epidemic there. In the early 1980s in the Sahel, droughts, crop failure, and famine turned people into eco-refugees, deprived of their usual foods and cooking fuels. Those droughts may also have been related to El Niño and were a time of resurgent cholera in Africa (80).

## NEW STRATEGIES FOR CONTROL

The introduction of *V. cholerae* via travelers and ships is difficult to prevent, as border checks and "cordons sanitaires" have been uniformly unsuccessful in limiting the spread of cholera epidemics. Even universal vaccination would have little impact, as the vaccines do not prevent asymptomatic carriage. Recent International Maritime Organization regulations requiring freighter captains to exchange ballast water at sea before entering the next port may decrease the volumes of harbor water transferred, but this transfer mechanism is likely to persist until a new generation of freighters is built with continuous flow ballast tanks (19).

Epidemic cholera can be controlled by reducing the risk of sustained transmission following introduction. In the developed world, this control was achieved by the engineered separation of the human fecal stream from our water and food streams. In the developing world, similar measures are slowly taking place but will take substantial investment over decades to complete. Simple interim strategies exist, however. In an emergency, people can be encouraged to boil their water and to avoid particularly dangerous foods, though these measures often are difficult to sustain. Other more sustainable interventions have been shown to be protective at the household level. These include storing drinking water in narrow-mouthed containers, into which hands are not easily introduced, and chlorinating or acidifying the water in the home (58). Cooking seafoods, reheating leftover grains before eating them, and using acidifying condiments are other protective habits that can be useful control strategies in cholera epidemics. Providing safe water storage vessels and chlorine solutions for routine water treatment in the home can institutionalize many of these habits if a simple commercial infrastructure for making and distributing vessels and chlorine can be put in place (67). Such an intervention was easily sustained for a year in a village trial in Bolivia and lowered the overall incidence of diarrheal illness by 44% in participating families (68). The system has also been adapted for use by street vendors to prepare beverages and to provide clean water for washing. In a field trial of this system, street vendors were able to produce clean water for these uses, and the contamination of served beverages was significantly less than from street vendors using traditional implements (21a).

Can the population be immunized against cholera? Natural infection with toxigenic El Tor *V. cholerae* O1 produces partial, temporary, and serogroup-specific protection. To date, vaccines have given similar results. An inexpensive cholera vaccine that provided long-term protection against cholera would be a major advance. The search for better cholera vaccines has yielded a substantially improved understanding of virulence mechanisms and of the nature of a protective immune response. Vaccine research is hampered by the lack of a good animal model, making volunteer trials and extensive field trials necessary. Three vaccines are now commercially available in some countries, but only the parenteral killed vaccine tested extensively in the early 1970s is licensed in the United States (17). This vaccine provides 50% protection for 6 months. Two oral vaccines are marketed in Europe: a whole-cell killed vaccine that includes a B-subunit toxin moiety (WC-BS) (23–25, 73) and a live attenuated vaccine from the Center for Vaccine Development, CVD 103-HgR (48, 50). When WC-BS vaccine was tested extensively in a field trial in Bangladesh in a location where both El Tor and classical strains were present, it had a protective efficacy in the first year of the trial of 62% (23). Efficacy waned after 2 years and was substantially lower among persons of blood group O (24), among children, and against infection with El Tor biotype as opposed to classical biotype (25). In a recent open trial of a killed WC vaccine without the B subunit, similar results were obtained, indicating that the B subunit itself may confer little specific benefit (85). In a trial among Peruvian military recruits, short-term efficacy in protecting against El Tor cholera in the first 2 months after vaccination was 86% (73). The efficacy of the CVD 103-HgR vaccine has been measured in volunteer challenge studies conducted in North America. Efficacy is 62 to 64% against any diarrhea when challenged with El Tor strains and 100% when challenged with classical strains (50). Duration of protection has been documented for as long as 6 months but has not been tested beyond that. The appearance of the O139 serogroup has complicated the search for effective vaccines, which may now need to be polyvalent. Several other live attenuated vaccines are under development, including vaccines against O139 strains (29, 83).

Although the newer vaccines are a substantial improvement over the parenteral vaccine, they are not yet ready for general public health use. Among travelers, cholera is an exceedingly rare event, and routine vaccination is not recommended (17). The cost of delivery, incomplete protection, and the requirement for regular booster doses make vaccination unattractive for populationwide use. Cost-benefit analyses indicate that in an optimal setting of high incidence and low delivery cost, the savings are not substantial and depend critically on the incidence of cholera (28). In many settings, vaccine is not as cost effective as other strategies for reducing morbidity and mortality (30, 61). In the epidemic setting, use of vaccines is particularly problematic (89). The first priority is to prevent death by ensuring access to adequate treatment. The second is to provide safe water to threatened households, with adequate residual disinfectant levels to prevent recontamination. A vaccination campaign launched at the height of the epidemic could easily draw scarce public health resources away from these life-saving activities without providing immediate benefit, as immune protection would take several weeks to establish. The ideal moment to vaccinate would be shortly before the epidemic begins and after other preventive measures have been taken. Epidemics are unpredictable events. The strategy of vaccinating the entire population in advance would be expensive and could engender a false sense of security.

The presence of an environmental reservoir, the relative frequency of inapparent infections and asymptomatic carriers, the appearance of more than one serogroup, and the lack of a vaccine that provides lifelong protection mean that eradication of the disease is very unlikely. Prevention measures that are independent of serogroup are attractive as they are likely to remain effective regardless of current or future antigenic diversity. The control of cholera in the developed world through 19th century sanitary engineering is a crowning public health achievement. Protecting the rapidly growing populations of the developing world today is an achievable goal. Appropriate technologies and training for water treatment and storage, for sanitation, and for safer food handling are likely to have a direct impact on cholera and on a variety of other diseases transmitted through contaminated water and food. Sustainable and locally controlled means of water treatment, such as better water storage vessels and water disinfection by the consumer, may be an interim solution that can help communities gain experience in providing necessary services for themselves.

Epidemic cholera remains a marker of severe underdevelopment, a sign that the basic sanitary infrastructure of a society is below a critical threshold that separates the human fecal stream from the water and food supply. This is not a natural phenomenon but rather a consequence of the way people live. We can hope that, just as it did in Europe and North America a century ago, cholera will spur sanitary reform and modern public health in the growing democracies of today's developing world.

## REFERENCES

1. **Ackers, M., R. Pagaduan, G. Hart, K. D. Greene, S. Abbott, E. Mintz, and R. V. Tauxe.** 1997. Cholera and sliced fruit: Probable transmission from an asymptomatic carrier in the United States. *Int. J. Infect. Dis.* **1:**212–214.

2. **Albert, M. J., N. A. Bhuiyan, K. A. Talkuder, A. S. G. Faruque, S. Nahar, S. M. Faruque, M. Ansaruzzaman, and M. Rahman.** 1997. Phenotypic and genotypic changes in *Vibrio cholerae* O139 Bengal. *J. Clin. Microbiol.* **35:**2588–2592.

3. **Alm, R. A., and P. A. Manning.** 1990. Biotype specific probe for *Vibrio cholerae* serogroup O1. *J. Clin. Microbiol.* **28:**823–824.

4. **Anonymous.** 1997. Cholera in 1996. *Weekly Epidemiol. Rec.* **31:**229–235.

4a. **Barrett, T. J.** Unpublished data.

5. **Barrett, T. J., and P. A. Blake.** 1981. Epidemiologic usefulness of changes in hemolytic activty of *Vibrio cholerae* biotype El Tor during the seventh pandemic. *J. Clin. Microbiol.* **13:**126–129.

6. **Barrett, T. J., and D. N. Cameron.** 1998. Cholera, p. 1–17. *In* J. M. Rhodes, and J. D. Milton (ed.), Methods in molecular medicine. Humana Press, Totowa, N.J.

7. **Barrett, T. J., and J. C. Feeley.** 1994. Serologic diagnosis of *Vibrio cholerae* infections, p. 135–141. *In* I. K. Wachsmuth, P. A. Blake, and Ø. Olsvik (ed.), Vibrio cholerae *and Cholera: Molecular to Global Perspectives.* American Society for Microbiology, Washington, D.C.

8. **Benenson, A. S., S. Z. Ahmad, and R. O. Oseasohn.** 1965. Person-to-person transmission of cholera, p. 332–336. *In* O. A. Bushnell and C. S. Brookhyser (ed.), *Proceedings of the Cholera Research Symposium; Honolulu, Hawaii, 24–29 January 1965.* Public Health Service, Bethesda, Md.

9. **Blake, P. A.** 1994. Endemic cholera in Australia and the United States, p. 309–319. *In* I. K. Wachsmuth, P. A. Blake, and Ø. Olsvik (ed.), Vibrio cholerae *and Cholera: Molecular to Global Perspectives.* American Society for Microbiology, Washington, D.C.

10. **Blake, P. A., D. T. Allegra, J. D. Snyder, T. J. Barrett, L. McFarland, C. T. Caraway, J. C. Feeley, J. P. Craig, J. V. Lee, N. D. Puhr, and R. A. Feldman.** 1980. Cholera—a possible endemic focus in the United States. *N. Engl. J. Med.* **302:**305–309.

11. **Blake, P. A., M. L. Rosenberg, J. B. Costa, P. S. Ferreira, C. L. Guimaraes, and E. J. Gangarosa.** 1977. Cholera in Portugal, 1974. I. Modes of transmission. *Am. J. Epidemiol.* **105:**337–343.

12. **Blake, P. A., M. L. Rosenberg, J. Florencia, J. B. Costa, L. D. P. Quinino, and E. J. Gangarosa.** 1977. Cholera in Portugal, 1974. II. Transmission by bottled mineral water. *Am. J. Epidemiol.* **105:** 344–348.

13. **Bopp, C. A., B. A. Kay, and J. G. Wells.** 1994. Laboratory methods for the diagnosis of *Vibrio cholerae*. Centers for Disease Control and Prevention, Atlanta, Ga.

14. **Bourke, A. T. C., Y. N. Cossins, B. R. W. Gray, T. J. Lunney, N. A. Rostron, R. V. Holmes, E. R. Griggs, D. J. Larsen, and V. R. Kelk.** 1986. Investigation of cholera acquired from the riverine environment in Queensland. *Med. J. Aust.* **144:**229–234.

15. **Boyce, T. G., E. D. Mintz, K. D. Greene, J. G. Wells, J. C. Hockin, D. Morgan, and R. V. Tauxe.** 1995. *Vibrio cholerae* O139 Bengal infections among tourists to Southeast Asia: An intercontinental foodborne outbreak. *J. Infect. Dis.* **172:**1401–1404.

16. **Cameron, D. N., F. M. Khambaty, I. K. Wachsmuth, R. V. Tauxe, and T. J. Barrett.** 1994. Molecular characterization of *Vibrio cholerae* O1 strains by pulsed-field electrophoresis. *J. Clin. Microbiol.* **32:**1685–1690.

17. **Centers for Disease Control.** 1988. Cholera vaccine: Recommendations of the Immunization Practices Advisory Committee. *Morbid. Mortal. Weekly Rep.* **37:**617–624.

18. **Centers for Disease Control.** 1991. Cholera—New York, 1991. *Morbid. Mortal. Weekly Rep.* **40:** 516–518.

19. **Centers for Disease Control.** 1992. Isolation of *Vibrio cholerae* O1 from oysters—Mobile Bay, 1991–1992. *Morbid. Mortal. Weekly Rep.* **42:**91–93.

20. **Centers for Disease Control.** 1995. Cholera associated with food transported from El Salvador—Indiana, 1994. *Morbid. Mortal. Weekly Rep.* **44:**385–386.

21. **Centers for Disease Control.** 1995. Update: *Vibrio cholerae* O1—Western hemisphere, 1991–1994; and *V. cholerae* O139—Asia, 1994. *Morbid. Mortal. Weekly Rep.* **44:**215–219.

21a.**Centers for Disease Control and Prevention.** Unpublished data.

22. **Cholera Working Group.** 1993. Large epidemic of cholera-like disease in Bangladesh caused by *Vibrio cholerae* O139 synonym Bengal. *Lancet* **342:**387–390.

23. **Clemens, J. D., J. R. Harris, D. A. Sack, J. Chakraborty, F. Ahmed, B. F. Stanton, M. U. Khan, B. A. Kay, N. Huda, M. R. Khan, M. Yunus, M. R. Rao, A.-M. Svennerholm, and J. Holmgren.** 1988. Field trial of oral cholera vaccines in Bangladesh: Results of one year of follow-up. *J. Infect. Dis.* **158:**60–69.

24. **Clemens, J. D., D. A. Sack, J. R. Harris, J. Chakraborty, M. R. Khan, S. Huda, F. Ahmed, J. Gomes, M. R. Rao, A.-M. Svennerholm, and J. Holmgren.** 1989. ABO Blood groups and cholera: New observations on specificity of risk and modification of vaccine efficacy. *J. Infect. Dis.* **159:** 770–773.

25. **Clemens, J. D., D. A. Sack, J. R. Harris, F. van Loon, J. Chakraborty, F. Ahmed, M. R. Rao, M. R. Khan, M. Yunus, N. Huda, B. F. Stanton, B. F. Kay, S. Walter, R. Eeckels, A.-M. Svennerholm, and J. Holmgren.** 1990. Field trial of oral cholera vaccines in Bangladesh: Results from three-year follow-up. *Lancet* **335:**270–273.

26. **Clemens, J. D., F. van Loon, D. A. Sack, M. R. Rao, F. Ahmed, J. Chakraborty, B. A. Kay, M. R. Khan, M. D. Yunus, J. R. Harris, and A.-M. Svennerholm.** 1991. Biotype as determinant of natural immunizing effect of cholera. *Lancet* **337:**883–884.

27. **Comstock, L. E., J. A. Johnson, J. M. Michalski, J. G. Morris Jr., and J. B. Kaper.** 1996. Cloning and sequence of a region encoding a surface polysaccharide of *Vibrio cholerae* O139 and characterization of the insertion site in the chromosome of *Vibrio cholerae* O1. *Mol. Microbiol.* **19:** 815–826.

28. **Cookson, S. T., D. Stamboulian, J. Demonte, J. Quero, C. M. De Arquiza, A. Aleman, A. Lepetic, and M. M. Levine.** 1997. A cost-benefit analysis of programmatic use of CVD 103 HgR live oral cholera vaccine in a high-risk population. *Int. J. Epidemiol.* **26:**212–219.

29. **Coster, T. S., K. P. Killeen, M. K. Waldor, D. T. Beattie, D. R. Spriggs, J. R. Kenner, A. Trofa, J. C. Sadoff, J. J. Mekalanos, and D. N. Taylor.** 1995. Safety, immunogenicity, and efficacy of live attenuated *Vibrio cholerae* O139 vaccine prototype. *Lancet* **345:**949–952.

30. **Cvjetanovic, B.** 1974. Economic considerations in cholera control, p. 435–445. *In* D. Barua, and W. Burroughs (ed.), *Cholera.* The W.B. Saunders Co., Philadelphia, Pa.

31. **Dubon, J. M., C. J. Palmer, A. L. Ager, G. Shor-Posner, and M. K. Baum.** 1997. Emergence of multiple drug-resistant *Vibrio cholerae* in San Pedro Sula, Honduras. *Lancet* **349:**924.

32. **Estrada-Garcia, T., and E. D. Mintz.** 1996. Cholera: Foodborne transmission and its prevention. *Eur. J. Epidemiol.* **12:**461–469.

33. **Evins, G. M., D. N. Cameron, J. G. Wells, K. D. Greene, T. Popovic, S. Giono-Cerezo, I. K. Wachsmuth, and R. V. Tauxe.** 1995. The emerging diversity of the electrophoretic types of *Vibrio cholerae* in the Western Hemisphere. *J. Infect. Dis.* **172:**173–179.

34. **Faruque, S. M., K. M. Ahmed, A. K. Siddique, K. Zaman, A. R. M. Alim, and M. J. Albert.** 1997. Molecular analysis of toxigenic *Vibrio cholerae* O139 Bengal strains isolated in Bangladesh between 1993 and 1996: Evidence for emergence of a new clone of the Bengal Vibrios. *J. Clin. Microbiol.* **35:**2299–2306.

35. **Finelli, L., D. Swerdlow, K. Mertz, H. Ragazonni, and K. Spitalny.** 1992. Outbreak of cholera associated with crab brought from an area with epidemic disease. *J. Infect. Dis.* **166:**1433–1435.

36. **Gangarosa, E. J., and W. H. Mosley.** 1974. Epidemiology and control of cholera, p. 381–403. *In* D. Barua and W. Burrows (ed.), *Cholera.* The W. B. Saunders Co., Philadelphia, Pa.

37. **Glass, R. I., J. Holmgren, C. E. Haley, M. R. Khan, A.-M. Svennerholm, B. J. Stoll, K. M. B. Hossain, R. E. Black, M. Yunus, and D. Barua.** 1985. Predisposition for cholera of individuals with O blood group: possible evolutionary significance. *Am. J. Epidemiol.* **121:**791–796.

38. **Goodgame, R. W., and W. B. G. Greenough III.** 1975. Cholera in Africa: A message for the West. *Ann. Intern. Med.* **82:**101–106.

39. **Herrington, D. A., R. H. Hall, G. Losonsky, J. J. Mekalanos, R. K. Taylor, and M. M. Levine.** 1988. Toxin, toxin-coregulated pili, and the toxR regulon are essential for *Vibrio cholerae* pathogenesis in humans. *J. Exp. Med.* **168:**1487–1492.

40. **Hoge, C. W., L. Bodhidatta, P. Echeverria, M. Deesuwan, and P. Kitporka.** 1996. Epidemiologic study of *Vibrio cholerae* O1 and O139 in Thailand: At the advancing edge of the eighth pandemic. *Am. J. Epidemiol.* **143:**263–268.

41. **Huq, A., P. A. West, B. Small, M. I. Huq, and R. R. Colwell.** 1984. Influence of water temperature, salinity, and pH on survival and growth of toxigenic *Vibrio cholerae* serovar O1 associated with live copepods in laboratory microcosms. *Appl. Environ. Microbiol.* **48:**420–424.

42. **Kamal, A. M.** 1974. The seventh pandemic of cholera, p. 1–14. *In* D. Barua and W. Burrows (ed.), *Cholera.* The W. B. Saunders Co., Philadelphia, Pa.

43. **Karaolis, D. K. R., R. Lan, and P. R. Reeves.** 1994. Molecular evolution of the seventh-pandemic clone of *Vibrio cholerae* and its relationship to other pandemic and epidemic *V. cholerae* isolates. *J. Bacteriol.* **176:**6199–6206.

44. **Karaolis, D. K. R., R. Lan, and P. R. Reeves.** 1995. The sixth and seventh cholera pandemics are due to independent clones derived from environmental, nontoxigenic, non-O1 *Vibrio cholerae. J. Bacteriol.* **177:**3191–3198.

45. **Koch, R.** 1884. An address on cholera and its bacillus. *Br. Med. J.* **2:**403–407.

46. **Kolvin, J. L., and D. Roberts.** 1982. Studies on the growth of *Vibrio cholerae* biotype eltor and biotype classical in foods. *J. Hyg. Camb.* **89:**243–252.

47. **Koo, D., A. Aragon, V. Moscoso, M. Gudiel, L. Bietti, N. Carillo, J. Chojoj, B. Gordillo, F. Cano, D. N. Cameron, J. G. Wells, N. H. Bean, and R. V. Tauxe.** 1996. Epidemic cholera in Guatemala, 1993: Transmission of a newly introduced epidemic strain by street vendors. *Epidemiol. Infect.* **116:**121–126.

48. **Lagos, R., A. Avendano, V. Prado, I. Horwitz, S. Wasserman, G. Losonsky, S. Cryz, J. B. Kaper, and M. M. Levine.** 1995. Attenuated live cholera vaccine strain CVD 103-HgR elicits significantly higher serum vibriocidal antibody titers in persons of blood group O. *Infect. Immun.* **63:**707–709.

49. **Levin, B. R., and R. V. Tauxe.** 1996. Cholera: nice bacteria and bad viruses. *Curr. Biol.* **6:**1389–1391.

50. **Levine, M. M., and C. O. Tacket.** 1994. Recombinant live oral vaccines, p. 395–413. *In* I. K. Wachsmuth, P. A. Blake, and Ø. Olsvik (ed.), *Vibrio cholerae and cholera: Molecular to Global Perspectives.* American Society for Microbiology, Washington, D.C.

51. **Lim-Quizon, M. C., R. M. Benabaye, F. M. White, M. M. Dayrit, and M. E. White.** 1994. Cholera in metropolitan Manila: Foodborne transmission via street vendors. *Bull. W. H. O.* **72:**745–749.

52. **Mahon, B. E., E. D. Mintz, K. D. Greene, J. G. Wells, and R. V. Tauxe.** 1996. Reported cholera in the United States, 1992–1994: A reflection of global changes in cholera epidemiology. *JAMA* **276:**307–312.

53. **Manning, P. A.** 1997. The *tcp* gene cluster of *Vibrio cholerae*. *Gene* **192:**63–70.

54. **Manning, P. A., U. H. Stroeher, and R. Morona.** 1994. Molecular basis for O-antigen biosynthesis in *Vibrio cholerae* O1: Ogawa-Inaba switching, p. 77–94. *In* I. K. Wachsmuth, P. A. Blake, and Ø. Olsvik (ed.), Vibrio cholerae *and cholera: Molecular to Global Perspectives.* American Society for Microbiology, Washington, D.C.

55. **McCarthy, S. A., R. M. McPherson, and A. M. Guarino.** 1992. Toxigenic *Vibrio cholerae* O1 and cargo ships entering Gulf of Mexico. *Lancet* **339:**624.

56. **Mekalanos, J. J., E. J. Rubin, and M. K. Waldor.** 1997. Cholera: molecular basis for emergence and pathogenesis. *FEMS Immunol. Med. Microbiol.* **18:**241–248.

57. **Mintz, E. D., P. V. Effler, L. Maslankowski, V. Ansdell, E. Pon, T. J. Barrett, and R. V. Tauxe.** 1994. A rapid public health response to a cryptic outbreak of cholera in Hawaii. *Am. J. Public Health* **84:**1988–1991.

58. **Mintz, E. D., F. M. Reiff, and R. V. Tauxe.** 1995. Safe water treatment and storage in the home; A practical new strategy to prevent waterborne disease. *JAMA* **273:**948–953.

59. **Morris, J. G., Jr.** 1994. Non-O Group 1 *Vibrio cholerae* strains not associated with epidemic disease, p. 103–115. *In* I. K. Wachsmuth, P. A. Blake, and Ø. Olsvik (ed.), Vibrio cholerae *and Cholera: Molecular to Global Perspectives.* American Society for Microbiology, Washington, D.C.

60. **Morris, J. G., Jr., M. B. Sztein, E. W. Rice, J. P. Nataro, G. A. Losonsky, P. Panigrahi, C. O. Tacket, and J. A. Johnson.** 1996. *Vibrio cholerae* O1 can assume a chlorine-resistant rugose survival form that is virulent for humans. *J. Infect. Dis.* **174:**1364–1368.

61. **Naficy, A., M. R. Rao, C. Paquet, D. Antona, A. Sorkin, and J. D. Clemens.** 1998. Treatment and vaccination strategies to control cholera in sub-Saharan refugee settings: a cost-effectiveness analysis. *JAMA* **279:**521–525.

62. **Nalin, D. R.** 1976. Cholera, copepods and chitinase. *Lancet* **ii:**958.

63. **Olsvik, O., J. Wahlberg, B. Petterson, M. Uhlen, T. Popovic, I. K. Wachsmuth, and P. I. Fields.** 1993. Use of automated sequencing of polymerase chain-reaction-generated amplicons to identify three types of cholera toxin subunit B in *Vibrio cholerae* O1 strains. *J. Clin. Microbiol.* **31:**22–25.

64. **Pollitzer, R.** 1959. *Cholera.* WHO Monograph Series no. 43. World Health Organization, Geneva, Switzerland.

65. **Popovic, T., C. Bopp, O. Olsvik, and K. Wachsmuth.** 1993. Epidemiologic application of a standardized ribotype scheme for *Vibrio cholerae* O1. *J. Clin. Microbiol.* **31:**2474–2482.

66. **Popovic, T., P. I. Fields, O. Olsvik, J. G. Wells, G. M. Evins, D. N. Cameron, J. J. Farmer III, C. A. Bopp, I. K. Wachsmuth, R. B. Sach, M. J. Albert, G. B. Nair, T. Shimada, and J. C. Feeley.** 1995. Molecular subtyping of toxigenic *Vibrio cholerae* O139 causing epidemic cholera in India and Bangladesh, 1992–1993. *J. Infect. Dis.* **171:**122–127.

67. **Quick, R. E., L. V. Venczel, O. Gonzalez, E. D. Mintz, A. K. Highsmith, A. Espada, E. Damiani, N. H. Bean, E. H. De Hannover, and R. V. Tauxe.** 1996. Narrow-mouthed water storage vessels and in situ chlorination in a Bolivian community: A simple method to improve drinking water quality. *Am. J. Trop. Med. Hyg.* **54:**511–516.

68. **Quick, R., L. Venczel, E. Mintz, C. Bopp, L. Soleto, N. Bean, and R. Tauxe.** 1995. Diarrhea prevention in Bolivia through safe water storage vessels and locally produced mixed oxidant disinfectant, abstr. K142, p. 313. Program Abstr. 35th Intersci. Conf. Antimicrob. Agents Chemother. American Society for Microbiology, Washington, D.C.

69. **Ries, A. A., D. J. Vugia, L. Beingolea, A. M. Palacios, E. Vasquez, J. G. Wells, N. G. Baca, D. L. Swerdlow, M. Pollack, N. H. Bean, L. Seminario, and R. V. Tauxe.** 1992. Cholera in Piura, Peru: A modern urban epidemic. *J. Infect. Dis.* **166:**1429–1433.

70. **Rogers, L.** 1957. Thirty years' research on the control of cholera epidemics. *Br. Med. J.* **2:**1193–1197.

71. **Rosenberg, C. E.** 1987. The cholera years—tthe United States in 1832, 1849, and 1866. University of Chicago Press, Chicago, Il.

72. **Sakazaki, R.** 1992. Bacteriology of Vibrio and related organisms, p. 37–56. *In* D. Barua and W. B. Greenough III (ed.), *Cholera*, 2nd ed. Plenum Publishing, New York, N.Y.

73. **Sanchez, J. L., B. Vasquez, R. E. Begue, R. Meza, G. Castellares, C. Cabezas, D. M. Watts, A.-M. Svennerholm, J. C. Sadoff, and D. N. Taylor.** 1994. Protective efficacy of oral whole-cell/recombinant-B-subunit cholera vaccine in Peruvian military recruits. *Lancet* **344:**1273–1276.

74. **Sharma, C., G. B. Nair, A. K. Mukhopadhyay, S. K. Bhattacharya, R. K. Ghosh, and A. Ghosh.** 1997. Molecular characterization of *Vibrio cholerae* O1 biotype El Tor strains isolated between 1992 and 1995 in Calcutta, India—Evidence for the emergence of a new clone of the El Tor biotype. *J. Infect. Dis.* **175:**1134–1141.

75. **Siddique, A. K., A. H. Baqui, A. Eusof, K. Haider, M. A. Hossain, I. Bashir, and K. Zaman.** 1991. Survival of classic cholera in Bangladesh. *Lancet* **337:**1125–1127.

76. **Snow, J.** 1936. *Snow on Cholera, Being a Reprint of Two Papers.* The Commonwealth Fund, Oxford University Press, London, England.

77. **Stroeher, U. H., G. Parasivam, B. K. Dredge, and P. A. Manning.** 1997. Novel *Vibrio cholerae* O139 genes involved in lipopolysaccharide biosynthesis. *J. Bacteriol.* **179:**2740–2747.

78. **Swerdlow, D. L., E. D. Mintz, M. Rodriguez, E. Tejada, C. Ocampo, L. Espejo, T. J. Barrett, J. Petzelt, N. H. Bean, L. Seminario, and R. V. Tauxe.** 1994. Severe life-threatening cholera associated with blood group O in Peru: Implications for the Latin American epidemic. *J. Infect. Dis.* **170:**468–472.

79. **Swerdlow, D. L., and A. A. Ries.** 1992. Cholera in the Americas: Guidelines for the clinician. *JAMA* **267:**1495–1499.

80. **Tauxe, R. V., S. D. Holmberg, A. Dodin, J. G. Wells, and P. A. Blake.** 1988. Epidemic cholera in Mali: high mortality and multiple routes of transmission in a famine area. *Epidemiol. Infect.* **100:** 279–289.

81. **Tauxe, R. V., E. D. Mintz, and R. E. Quick.** 1995. Epidemic cholera in the New World: translating field epidemiology into new prevention strategies. *Emerg. Infect. Dis.* **1:**141–146.

82. **Tauxe, R., L. Seminario, R. Tapia, and M. Libel.** 1994. The Latin American epidemic, p. 321–350. *In* I. K. Wachsmuth, P. A. Blake, and Ø. Olsvik (ed.), Vibrio cholerae *and Cholera: Molecular to Global Perspective.* American Society for Microbiology, Washington, D.C.

83. **Taylor, D. N., C. O. Tacket, G. Losonsky, O. Castro, J. Gutierrez, R. Meza, J. P. Nataro, J. B. Kaper, S. S. Wasserman, R. Edelman, M. M. Levine, and S. J. Cryz.** 1997. Evaluation of a bivalent(CVD 103-HgR/CVD 111) live oral cholera vaccine in adult volunteers from the United States and Peru. *Infect. Immun.* **65:**3852–3856.

84. **Taylor, J. L., J. Tuttle, T. Pramukul, K. O'Brien, T. J. Barrett, B. Jolbaito, Y. L. Lim, D. J. Vugia, J. G. Morris, R. V. Tauxe, and D. M. Dwyer.** 1993. An outbreak of cholera in Maryland associated with imported commercial frozen fresh coconut milk. *J. Infect. Dis.* **167:**1330–1335.

85. **Trach, D. D., J. D. Clemens, N. T. Ke, H. T. Thuy, N. D. Son, D. G. Canh, P. V. D. Hang, and M. R. Rao.** 1997. Field trial of a locally produced, killed, oral cholera vaccine in Vietnam. *Lancet* **349:**231–235.

86. **Ventura, G., L. Roberts, and R. Gilman.** 1992. *Vibrio cholerae* non-O1 in sewage lagoons and seasonality in Peru cholera epidemic. *Lancet* **339:**937–938.

87. **Vugia, D. J., M. Rodriquez, R. Vargas, C. Ricse, C. Ocampo, R. Llaque, J. L. Seminario, K. G. Greene, R. V. Tauxe, and R. V. Blake.** 1994. Epidemic cholera in Trujillo, Peru 1992: utility of a clinical case definition and shift in *Vibrio cholerae* O1 serotype. *Am. J. Trop. Med. Hyg.* **50:** 566–569.

88. **Vugia, D., A. Shefer, J. Douglas, K. Greene, R. Bryant, and S. Werner.** 1997. Cholera from raw seaweed transported from the Philippines to California. *J. Clin. Microbiol.* **35:**284–285.

89. **Waldman, R. J.** 1998. Cholera vaccination in refugee settings. *JAMA* **279:**552–553.

90. **Waldor, M. K., and J. J. Mekalanos.** 1996. Lysogenic conversion by a filamentous phage encoding cholera toxin. *Science* **272:**1910–1914.

91. **Waldor, M. K., H. Tschape, and J. J. Mekalanos.** 1996. A new type of conjugative transposon encodes resistance to sulfamethoxazole, trimethoprim, and streptomycin in *Vibrio cholerae* O139. *J. Bacteriol.* **178:**4157–4165.

92. **Weber, J. T., W. C. Levine, D. P. Hopkins, and R. V. Tauxe.** 1994. Cholera in the United States, 1965–1991; risks at home and abroad. *Arch. Intern. Med.* **154:**551–556.

93. **Weber, J. T., E. D. Mintz, R. Canizares, A. Semiglia, I. Gomez, R. Sempertegui, A. Davila, K. G. Greene, N. D. Puhr, D. N. Cameron, F. C. Tenover, T. J. Barrett, N. H. Bean, C. Ivey, R. V. Tauxe, and P. A. Blake.** 1994. Epidemic cholera in Ecuador: multidrug resistance and transmission by water and seafood. *Epidemiol. Infect.* **112:**1–11.

*Emerging Infections 2*
Edited by W. M. Scheld, W. A. Craig, and J. M. Hughes
© 1998 ASM Press, Washington, D.C.

*Chapter 7*

# Reemerging Infections: Recent Developments in Pertussis

## *Erik L. Hewlett*

Although pertussis (whooping cough) technically qualifies as a reemerging infection by virtue of its increase in reported cases over the last 15 years, there is no doom and gloom about the future of this fascinating illness. In fact, this is a very exciting time in pertussis research with the recent development, testing, and licensure of less reactive acellular pertussis vaccines for use in routine childhood immunization (7, 49, 65). Despite the important recent progress summarized in this chapter, there are substantial barriers to overcome in the long-term mission of controlling or eliminating this disease.

It is not uncommon to encounter the question of why one still is concerned about pertussis in 1998, as the general perception persists that this is a pediatric illness well controlled with the present immunization program. This view became even more prevalent with the recent licensure of acellular vaccines, which addressed in large part public concern about reactogenicity of the whole-cell pertussis vaccine and its postulated role in neurologic sequelae (2, 5, 23, 45, 51). As discussed below, pertussis is much more complicated than represented by this perception.

## EPIDEMIOLOGY

Pertussis is a cyclic disease with peaks of incidence at 3- to 4-year intervals (14, 20, 23, 51). There was a nadir in reported cases in the United States in 1976, and the number has increased in a cyclic manner since then (4). Concurrently, there has been an increase in the proportion of cases in age groups older than 10 years. This latter observation is certainly due to the facts that pertussis immunization ends with the preschool booster at age 4 to 6 years and that there is no routine immunization of adolescents and adults against pertussis. This public health policy has resulted in a shift in age-specific incidence of pertussis from the prevaccine era to the present (14, 20, 22, 23, 75). Prior to the mid-1950s, pertussis was most common

---

*Erik L. Hewlett* • Departments of Medicine and Pharmacology, University of Virginia School of Medicine, Box 419, Health Sciences Center, Charlottesville, VA 22908.

in children from ages 2 to 10, and virtually everyone had this illness as a child. Adults had immunity maintained from their childhood disease by repeated exposure. Currently, the highest incidence is in infants less than 6 months of age who have not yet received a full course of primary immunization. In addition, there has been a progressive increase in pertussis in the group whose vaccine immunity is fading, namely those individuals more than 10 years of age (14).

This epidemiologic pattern is dramatically illustrated by an epidemic in Vermont in 1996 (8). From January to June of that year, there were only 10 cases of pertussis reported in the state. From June to December, however, there were 270 cases. Victims ranged in age from 27 days to 87 years, but only 4% were <1 year old. There was a striking bimodal distribution with the main peak in the 10 to 14 year age group and a smaller peak in the 40 to 49 year group. The mean duration of symptoms was 33 days. While extreme in the extent of adolescent and adult involvement, this example highlights the potential for disease in an immunized population and raises questions about the manifestations and recognition of this illness in the adult age group.

There is a growing body of literature dealing with the presentation and severity of pertussis in adults (10, 22, 43, 74, 81). For example, in a study of university students visiting student health facilities with cough 6 days or longer in duration, 26% were found to have serologic evidence of recent infection with *B. pertussis* (72). Other reports support the concept that one-third to one-quarter of adolescent or adult patients with cough of greater than a week may have pertussis (27, 74, 75, 105). Beyond the statistics, however, the following vignette provides a graphic illustration of the epidemiology and clinical features of this disease.

> A 3-year-old girl, up-to-date on her immunizations, developed a hacking cough without wheezing after returning from a summer vacation in Colorado. Over the next 2 weeks, her cough became paroxysmal, worse at night and with one period when she experienced episodes every 15 minutes. She was seen by several physicians and diagnosed as having asthma and/or a viral upper respiratory infection. Approximately 4 weeks into her illness, her father, a physician and administrator at an academic medical center, began to experience a cough which quickly became spasmodic in nature and worse in the daytime. When his cough episodes reached the point of causing cough syncope and near loss of consciousness, he sought medical attention. An otolaryngologist could not visualize his vocal cords without local anesthetic because on repeated attempts the examination precipitated cough paroxysms. The father was diagnosed as having mycoplasma infection and was treated with erythromycin, without relief. At 3 weeks into his illness (7 weeks into his daughter's course), he was given beclomethasone by inhaler, resulting in a dramatic reduction in cough frequency and severity. Similar therapy also provided symptomatic relief for his daughter. Neither father nor daughter was ever cultured for pertussis, but both were strikingly seropositive when

studied more than 4 and 8 weeks, respectively, after onset of symptoms.

It is frequently stated that the primary reason to be concerned about pertussis in adults is the potential for spread of the infection to susceptible infants in whom the disease can be severe and even life threatening. But the clinical situation described above documents that there are other issues involved. Pertussis is often not a trivial illness in adults. Reported complications include myocardial infarction, pneumothorax, herniated lumbar disc, encephalopathy, and (as in this case) syncopal episodes (10, 22, 40, 81, 92, 94, 105). Interestingly, in some ways the aging adult can be considered comparable to the infant in vulnerability to sequelae of pertussis, at least in part by virtue of the presence of other underlying health problems. Clearly, the diagnosis of pertussis should be considered in the setting of adults' experiencing cough greater than 1 week in duration. Furthermore, when the diagnosis is made, it should not be taken lightly in the adult population.

## DIAGNOSIS

Without detailing the limitations of previously used methods of diagnosis for identification of *B. pertussis* in clinical specimens, it is fair to say that PCR assays for pertussis have come of age (13, 24, 28, 34, 37, 41, 48, 53, 60, 61, 66, 76, 85, 86, 102). The major advantage of this approach is that the organisms do not need to be viable and able to grow on artificial medium. This point is illustrated in a recent publication by Edelman et al., in which PCR and culture were compared in pertussis patients receiving erythromycin treatment (29). After 4 days of therapy, 56% of patients were culture positive and 89% were PCR positive. After 7 days, no patients were culture positive, but 56% were still PCR positive.

A variety of primers have been used for pertussis PCR assays, and this technology is available in an increasing number of centers (48, 66). Serology is also being used increasingly to identify patients with pertussis, although this approach is more effective for epidemiologic purposes than in acute diagnosis (67). It is important to note, however, that there is still the need for recovery of the causative organism, whenever possible, to track serotypes in the population and (when clinically indicated) to monitor antibiotic susceptibility. At least one erythromycin-resistant isolate of *B. pertussis* has been reported (59). Despite this observation, erythromycin remains the drug of choice for pertussis, with trimethoprim-sulfamethoxazole as an alternative for patients allergic to or unable to tolerate erythromycin. *B. pertussis* and *B. parapertussis* exhibit good in vitro sensitivity to fluoroquinolones (52), but clinical testing is necessary to determine if these agents will be effective for treatment of adults.

## PATHOPHYSIOLOGY

Despite a great deal of interest in and investigation of the subject, much remains to be learned about the pathogenesis of pertussis (44, 46, 78, 82). This infection is localized to the respiratory tract. Almost certainly, *B. pertussis* reaches that site via aerosol droplets produced by the cough of an actively infected individual. Elegant studies by a number of scientists have established that the armamentarium of virulence factors produced by *B. pertussis* (listed in Table 1) is not expressed constitutively. Rather, their production is carefully controlled by the *bvg* (bordetella virulence genes) system, which senses the environment and determines when the organism has encountered appropriate conditions to cause a change from its avirulent form (38, 68, 90, 103). Not surprisingly, this regulatory system allows for the attachment factors, such as filamentous hemagglutinin and pertactin, to be produced first, followed later by the toxins which cause disease by altering host physiology and protecting the bacterium against clearance by the immune system (90).

*Bordetella pertussis* produces a collection of surface molecules which appear to serve as adhesins for the bacterial interactions with host cells. These include filamentous hemagglutinin (FHA), pertactin (PRN), and several serologically distinct fimbriae (FIM) (98). In addition, there is evidence that pertussis toxin located on the surface of the bacterium can function as an attachment factor (99), and there is another *bvg*-regulated molecule, tracheal colonization factor, which may be involved in adhesion (32). While most of these have been studied in vitro for their ability to contribute to the binding of *B. pertussis* to cultured cells, little is known about the role for each in the complex sequence of events which is required for this organism to cause disease. The existence of multiple adhesins suggests that there is significant redundancy in the attachment of this organism. Nevertheless, attachment factors have been targeted in the development of acellular vaccines with the objective of preventing establishment of infection, rather than just the manifestations of disease (15, 83).

Recently, *B. pertussis* has been found to share with other respiratory pathogens (mostly gram positive organisms) the ability to bind to the human complement regulatory protein, C4BP (12). This interaction between bacterium and host factor is dependent on expression of FHA, and its role in establishment of infection is currently being investigated.

Tracheal cytotoxin (TCT) is an intriguing disaccharide, tetrapeptide molecule which appears to be important pathophysiologically but is not produced in a *bvg*-regulated manner (26, 63). This toxin is generated during processing of the bacterial

**Table 1.** Virulence factors of *B. pertussis*

| Factor | Putative function(s) | Component in licensed acellular vaccine(s) |
|---|---|---|
| *bvg*[a] regulated | | |
| Filamentous hemagglutinin (FHA) | Adhesin | Yes |
| Pertactin (PRN) | Adhesin | Yes |
| Fimbriae (FIM) | Adhesin | Yes |
| Tracheal colonization factor | Possible adhesin | No |
| Pertussis toxin (PT) | Toxin, possible adhesin | Yes |
| Adenylate cyclase toxin (ACT) | Inhibition of phagocytes | No |
| *bvg*[a] independent | | |
| Tracheal cytotoxin (TCT) | Ciliostasis and respiratory cell death | No |

[a]*bvg*, bordetella virulence genes.

peptidoglycan layer into monomeric subunits that would normally be recycled by the bacterium. *B. pertussis*, however, is defective in transporting the monomers back into the cytoplasm, resulting in their release at levels sufficient to cause epithelial cytopathology (34a). TCT has been demonstrated to cause ciliostasis and ultimately death of respiratory epithelial cells in vitro by a mechanism involving induction of interleukin-1 (IL-1) and nitric oxide synthase in the target cells (42, 63, 64). Examination of specimens from patients dying of pertussis has revealed histopathological changes consistent with those elicited by TCT in vitro, suggesting that this molecule may be an important factor in development of the clinical manifestations of pertussis (104).

Although striking in their biological effects in vitro (adenylate cyclase toxin and pertussis toxin) and in vivo (pertussis toxin), the exact role for these other toxins in development and progression of clinical disease remains a matter for speculation (46, 80, 82, 100). Adenylate cyclase toxin (AC toxin) is a bacterial adenylate cyclase which can be delivered to the interior of host cells to raise cAMP levels (25, 50). Its known effects in vitro are inhibition of phagocyte function, prevention of bacterial killing, and induction of apoptosis (25, 56, 79). In animal models, it is critical for establishment of infection and elicitation of pulmonary inflammation and causes apoptosis of pulmonary cells (35, 55). It is possible (but heretofore untested) that this toxin also elicits mucous and fluid secretion from the respiratory mucosa by a cAMP-dependent mechanism during the course of infection.

Although a related species, *B. parapertussis*, does not produce pertussis toxin (PT) because of mutations in the promotor region (11), and does cause a pertussis-like illness, PT appears to be an important molecule in determining the extent and severity of clinical disease associated with *Bordetella pertussis* infection (46, 80, 82). This member of the family of ADP-ribosylating toxins modifies several regulatory G-proteins (101). There is not an established target cell/tissue through which its actions are linked to the manifestations of pertussis, but speculation ranges from local effects in the respiratory tract to actions at systemic sites including the central nervous system. The role of PT as a protective antigen is described below.

## PREVENTION OF DISEASE

Immunization with whole cell pertussis vaccine has been the mainstay of public health measures against this illness since the mid-1950s. There is no doubt that this type of vaccine has been effective in reducing the incidence of pertussis, but it has had its controversial aspect—its reactogenicity and hypothesized role in severe neurological injury (2, 5, 23, 45, 51, 75). For these reasons, there has been a major international effort to develop nonwhole cell pertussis vaccines over the past 20 to 25 years, which culminated in the testing and licensure of several products in the United States and elsewhere within the last two years (9, 21, 30, 49). These so-called "acellular" pertussis vaccines consist of one, two, three, or four (counting two serotypes of fimbriae as one antigen) components, namely the virulence factors of *B. pertussis* which have been shown to elicit protection in animal studies (see Table 1). These products have been extensively studied and characterized; the results of that work have been published and will not be discussed in detail here (6, 23, 49, 57, 89).

The components in each vaccine are listed in Table 2. The only single-component vaccine is made from PT alone, prepared with hydrogen peroxide treatment for toxoiding (9, 58, 97). The two-component products from three different manufacturers contain PT and FHA but differ in the methods of preparation and detoxification, as well as in quantity of antigens and selection of adjuvant (6, 9, 36, 39, 47, 62, 93). There are two vaccines which contain three components—PT, FHA, and PRN (6, 9, 36, 39, 47, 91). One of those contains the only genetically toxoided PT (36, 77). Finally, two manufacturers produce four-component vaccines, which vary significantly in their composition and preparation processes (6, 9, 39, 47, 95).

The results of field trials in which these vaccines were evaluated for clinical efficacy are listed in Table 2. Many of the trials were different in design, and the data from each should be considered individually. There are, however, important conclusions about these data taken as a group—acellular pertussis vaccines are less reactogenic than whole-cell vaccine and provide some level of protection against the World Health Organization (WHO) definition of pertussis (paroxysmal cough for 3 weeks or longer and laboratory confirmation) (3). There was, in addition, a general trend toward greater protection by the vaccines which contained more antigens. The whole-cell pertussis vaccine used as a control in the Sweden (Stockholm) and Italy trials had an unexpectedly low efficacy which did not appear to be representative of whole-cell vaccine performance in general (9, 36, 39).

With licensure of several acellular products for routine childhood immunization and increasing recognition of this illness in adolescents and adults, consideration of disease control must include extending the target population for vaccination. Present immunization policy in the U.S. dictates that the last dose of DTP or DTaP be given at age 4 to 6 years, prior to entry into school. The reason for this cut-off is not clear but must have involved lack of appreciation of the potential seriousness of pertussis in adults, as well as concern about possible adverse consequences of immunization in that population. This public health issue is currently being addressed with a field trial in which acellular pertussis vaccine is being evaluated for safety and efficacy in subjects aged 18 to 65 years. Results from this study, which is supported by the National Institute of Allergy and Infectious Diseases, are likely to influence adult immunization protocols in the U.S. and elsewhere.

In field trials conducted in Sweden in 1986 to 1987, two acellular products were found to have lower-than-expected efficacy and (importantly) there was no direct correlation between antibody level against one or the other or both antigen and protection (1,96). Those data led to an expanded investigation to find potential markers of immunity during the multiple trials required in the testing of the current acellular vaccines. The outcome, however, was the same—there is no single level of antibody against one pertussis antigen which is reflective of protection. This situation is difficult for the regulatory authorities charged with testing and licensing pertussis vaccines, but it has prompted a debate and exploration of the mechanism(s) by which these vaccines protect. The latest developments in that endeavor are presented below.

**Table 2.** Results from seven acellular pertussis vaccine trials

| Trial location | Design[a] | Manufacturer[d] | Vaccine components[e] | Doses | Efficacy[b] (95% CI) | Reference |
|---|---|---|---|---|---|---|
| Sweden (Goteborg) | DBP | AM | PT | 3 | 71 (63–78) | 97 |
| Sweden (Stockholm) | DBP | SKB | PT, FHA | 3 | 59 (51–66) | 39 |
| | | C-C | PT, FHA, PRN, FIM | 3 | 85 (81–89) | 39 |
| | | C-US | Whole cell | 3 | 48 (37–58) | 39 |
| Italy (Rome) | DBP | SKB | PT, FHA, PRN | 3 | 84 (76–90) | 36 |
| | | CB | PT, FHA, PRN | 3 | 84 (76–90) | 36 |
| | | C-US | Whole cell | 3 | 36 (14–52) | 36 |
| Germany (Erlangen) | DB for DTaP/DTP, unblinded for DT placebo | WL | PT, FHA, PRN, FIM | 4 | 83 (76–88)[c] | 95 |
| Germany (Mainz) | PHC | L | Whole cell | 4 | 93 (89–96)[c] | 95 |
| | | SKB | PT, FHA, PRN | 3 | 89 (77–95) | 91 |
| | | B | Whole cell | 3 | 97 (83–100) | 91 |
| Germany (Munich) | CC | C-US | PT, FHA | 4 | 96 (87–99) | 62 |
| | | B | Whole cell | 4 | 97 (79–100) | 62 |
| Senegal | DB for DTaP/DTP, unblinded PHC for unvaccinated individuals | PM | PT, FHA | 3 | 85 (66–93) | 93 |
| | | PM | Whole cell | 3 | 96 (86–99) | 93 |

[a]Trial design notations/abbreviations: DBP, double blind placebo; DB, double blind; PHC, prospective household contact; CC, case-control.
[b]Efficacy using WHO case definition.
[c]Efficacy using modified WHO case definition, including whoop and/or vomiting.
[d]Manufacturers: AM, North American Vaccine-AmVax; B, Behring; CB, Chiron Biocine; C-C, Connaught-Canada; C-US, Connaught-US; L, Lederle; PM, Pasteur Merieux; SKB, SmithKline Beecham; WL, Wyeth-Lederle.
[e]Components: FHA, filamentous hemagglutinin; FIM, fimbriae; PRN, pertactin; PT, pertussis toxin.

## MECHANISMS OF IMMUNITY

Despite the fact that whole-cell pertussis vaccine has been used successfully for more than 40 years, the mechanism by which it elicits protection remains a matter of speculation. The only variable shown to correlate with immunity is a high serum agglutinin titer (69, 88). These observations from the 1940s were clarified by Mink et al., who showed that agglutinin titers correlated best with IgG antifimbrial antibodies (73). Nevertheless, the presence of pertussis agglutinating antibodies does not appear adequate to explain the efficacy of pertussis vaccines, especially for vaccines containing only two or three components not including fimbriae.

In the 1940s, whole-cell pertussis vaccines were shown to protect mice against intracerebral challenge with strain 18323 of *B. pertussis*, a procedure which became known as the Kendrick test, in recognition of its developer, Pearl Kendrick (54). Development of the various acellular vaccines was predicated on the hypothesis that individual antigens, such as PT, FHA, PRN, and fimbriae (alone or in combination) can stimulate an immune response which will prevent disease and/or infection (83). In contrast to the whole-cell vaccine, not all of these products routinely pass the Kendrick test, despite the fact that their protective effects have been demonstrated in human trials. This set of circumstances provides a difficult situation for regulatory authorities who are responsible for testing of acellular pertussis vaccines for licensure and lot release. It also raises further questions about the mechanisms by which vaccines protect in the Kendrick test and the relevance of that procedure to human disease. Together, these observations have prompted an enhanced level of investigation of the possible mechanisms of vaccine-elicited protection against and natural clearance of *B. pertussis*.

Hints that cell-mediated immunity might play a role in protection against pertussis began with the work of Cheers and Gray (19). These include the demonstration that *B. pertussis* can enter and survive within eukaryotic cells, such as HeLa cells, macrophages, and neutrophils (31, 33). The potential relevance of this information from in vitro studies was enhanced by the detection of organisms within alveolar macrophages of HIV-infected patients, who may experience chronic infection with *B. pertussis* (16, 17). Mills et al. have found that passive transfer of $CD4^+$ Th1 cells to immunodeficient mice can confer protection against challenge with *B. pertussis* (70) and that effective immunization in mice required development of cell-mediated immune response (84).

Several investigators have observed cell-mediated immunity against components of the organism in individuals convalescent from pertussis and in vaccine recipients (18). Mills and associates have studied lymphocytes obtained from Swedish children during and after acute pertussis, using the release of cytokines as an indication of the type of cells responding to various stimuli (87). The results revealed that the Th1 subtype of $CD4^+$ T cells is involved in the immune response to infection with *B. pertussis*. While not yet conclusive about the mechanism of immunity, these discoveries will serve as the basis for further investigation of cell-mediated immunity in recovery from this disease and its prevention by immunization. Most recently, Mills et al. have described a respiratory challenge model of pertussis in mice in which a combined contribution of humoral and cellular responses against an assortment of bacterial antigens appears to be responsible for clearance and protection (71).

## CONCLUSIONS

In summary, it is important to recognize that pertussis is a relevant diagnostic consideration in patients of all ages who present with cough of >1 week in duration, especially if that cough is paroxysmal. The diagnosis of pertussis is moving toward increasing use of PCR and (for patients later in their course) serology. Although there remains a great deal more to learn about the pathophysiology of pertussis, it appears that the illness results from the contribution of multiple virulence factors, including several adhesins and toxins.

Although not directly comparable, acellular pertussis vaccines are, in general, effective in preventing moderately severe disease (paroxysmal cough of >21 days in duration). The mechanisms of host clearance and vaccine immunity remain unclear, but there is increasing evidence of a role for some combination of humoral and cell-mediated immune responses in these processes. Future clinical investigation will focus on potential benefit of additional antigens for the acellular vaccines, their duration of protection, and whether they might be used for protection of the adult population which is now recognized as experiencing an increasing incidence of pertussis. Combination of acellular pertussis vaccine with antigens from other organisms to yield multicomponent products of adequate efficacy is an additional challenge already facing manufacturers and regulatory authorities.

## REFERENCES

1. **Anonymous.** 1988. Placebo-controlled trial of two acellular pertussis vaccines in Sweden—protective efficacy and adverse events. *Lancet* i:955–960.
2. **Anonymous.** 1991. *In* C. P. Howson, C. J. Howe, and H. V. Fineberg (ed.), *Adverse Effects of Pertussis and Rubella Vaccines.* National Academy Press, Washington, D.C.
3. **Anonymous.** 1991. WHO meeting on case definition of pertussis. World Health Organization, Geneva, Switzerland.
4. **Anonymous.** 1993. Resurgence of pertussis—United States, 1993. *Morbid. Mortal. Weekly Rep.* **42:**952–960.
5. **Anonymous.** 1994. *In* K. R. Stratton, C. J. Howe, and R. B. Johnston (ed.), *DPT Vaccine and Chronic Nervous System Dysfunction: a new Analysis.* National Academy Press, Washington, D.C.
6. **Anonymous.** 1997. Proceedings of International Symposium on Pertussis Vaccine Trials. October 30–November 1, 1995; Rome, Italy. *Dev. Biol. Stand.* **89:**1–410.
7. **Anonymous.** 1996. Food and Drug Administration approval of an acellular pertussis vaccine for the initial four doses of the diphtheria, tetanus, and pertussis vaccination series. *Morbid. Mortal. Weekly Rep.* **45:**676–677.
8. **Anonymous.** 1997. Pertussis outbreak—Vermont, 1996. *Morbid. Mortal. Weekly Rep.* **46:**822–826.
9. **Anonymous.** 1997. Pertussis vaccination: use of acellular pertussis vaccines among infants and young children. Recommendations of the Advisory Committee on Immunization Practices (ACIP). *Morbid. Mortal. Weekly Rep.* **46:**1–25.
10. **Aoyama, T., Y. Takeuchi, A. Goto, H. Iwai, Y. Murase, and T. Iwata.** 1992. Pertussis in adults. *Am. J. Dis. Child.* **146:**163–166.
11. **Arico, B., and R. Rappuoli.** 1987. *Bordetella parapertussis* and *Bordetella bronchiseptica* contain transcriptionally silent pertussis toxin genes. *J. Bacteriol.* **169:**2847–2853.

12. **Berggard, K., E. Johnsson, F. R. Mooi, and G. Lindahl.** 1997. *Bordetella pertussis* binds the human complement regulator C4BP: role of filamentous hemagglutinin. *Infect. Immun.* **65:**3638–3643.

13. **Birkebaek, N. H., I. Heron, and K. Skjodt.** 1994. *Bordetella pertussis* diagnosed by polymerase chain reaction. *APMIS* **102:**291–294.

14. **Black, S.** 1997. Epidemiology of pertussis. *Pediatr. Infect. Dis. J.* **16:**S85–89.

15. **Brennan, M. J., and R. D. Shahin.** 1996. Pertussis antigens that abrogate bacterial adherence and elicit immunity. *Am. J. Respir. Crit. Care Med.* **154:**S145–149.

16. **Bromberg, K., H. Mendez, and E. Handelsman.** 1995. Chronic infection with *B. pertussis* (BP) in HIV-infected children. *Pediatr. Res.* **37:**107A. (Abstract 1008.)

17. **Bromberg, K., G. Tannis, and P. Steiner.** 1991. Detection of *Bordetella pertussis* associated with the alveolar macrophages of children with human immunodeficiency virus infection. *Infect. Immun.* **59:**4715–4719.

18. **Cassone, A., C. M. Ausiello, F. Urbani, R. Lande, M. Giuliano, A. La Sala, A. Piscitelli, and S. Salmaso.** 1997. Cell-mediated and antibody responses to *Bordetella pertussis* antigens in children vaccinated with acellular or whole-cell pertussis vaccines. *Arch. Pediatr. Adolesc. Med.* **151:**283–289.

19. **Cheers, C., and D. F. Gray.** 1969. Macrophage behaviour during the complaisant phase of murine pertussis. *Immunology* **17:**875–887.

20. **Cherry, J. D.** 1984. The epidemiology of pertussis and pertussis immunization in the United Kingdom and the United States: a comparative study. *Curr. Probl. Pediatr.* **14:**1–78.

21. **Cherry, J. D.** 1997. Comparative efficacy of acellular pertussis vaccines: an analysis of recent trials. *Pediatr. Infect. Dis. J.* **16:**S90–96.

22. **Cherry, J. D., L. J. Baraff, and E. Hewlett.** 1989. The past, present, and future of pertussis. The role of adults in epidemiology and future control. *West. J. Med.* **150:**319–328.

23. **Cherry, J. D., P. A. Brunell, G. S. Golden, and D. Karzon.** 1988. Report of the task force on pertussis and pertussis vaccine. *Pediatrics* **81:**939–984.

24. **Cimolai, N., C. Trombley, and D. O'Neill.** 1996. Diagnosis of whooping cough: a new era with rapid molecular diagnostics. *Pediatr. Emerg. Care* **12:**91–93.

25. **Confer, D. L., and J. W. Eaton.** 1982. Phagocyte impotence caused by an invasive bacterial adenylkate cyclase. *Science* **217:**948–950.

26. **Cookson, B. T., A. N. Tyler, and W. E. Goldman.** 1989. Primary structure of the peptidoglycan-derived tracheal cytotoxin of *Bordetella pertussis*. *Biochemistry* **28:**1744–1749.

27. **Deville, J. G., J. D. Cherry, P. D. Christenson, E. Pineda, C. T. Leach, T. L. Kuhls, and S. Viker.** 1995. Frequency of unrecognized *Bordetella pertussis* infections in adults. *Clin. Infect. Dis.* **21:**639–642.

28. **Douglas, E., J. G. Coote, R. Parton, and W. McPheat.** 1993. Identification of *Bordetella pertussis* in nasopharyngeal swabs by PCR amplification of a region of the adenylate cyclase gene. *J. Med. Microbiol.* **38:**140–144.

29. **Edelman, K., S. Nikkari, O. Ruuskanen, Q. He, M. Viljanen, and J. Mertsola.** 1996. Detection of *Bordetella pertussis* by polymerase chain reaction and culture in the nasopharynx of erythromycin-treated infants with pertussis. *Pediatr. Infect. Dis. J.* **15:**54–57.

30. **Edwards, K. M.** 1993. Acellular pertussis vaccines—a solution to the pertussis problem? *J. Infect. Dis.* **168:**15–20.

31. **Ewanowich, C. A., A. R. Melton, A. A. Weiss, R. K. Sherburne, and M. S. Peppler.** 1989. Invasion of HeLa 229 cells by virulent *Bordetella pertussis*. *Infect. Immun.* **57:**2698–2704.

32. **Finn, T. M., and L. A. Stevens.** 1995. Tracheal colonization factor: a *Bordetella pertussis* secreted virulence determinant. *Mol. Microbiol.* **16:**625–634.

33. **Friedman, R. L., K. Nordensson, L. Wilson, E. T. Akporiaye, and D. E. Yocum.** 1992. Uptake and intracellular survival of *Bordetella pertussis* in human macrophages. *Infect. Immun.* **60:**4578–4585.

34. **Glare, E. M., J. C. Paton, R. R. Premier, A. J. Lawrence, and I. T. Nisbet.** 1990. Analysis of a repetitive DNA sequence from *Bordetella pertussis* and its application to the diagnosis of pertussis using the polymerase chain reaction. *J. Clin. Microbiol.* **28:**1982–1987.

34a. **Goldman, W. E.** Personal communication.

35. **Goodwin, M. S., and A. A. Weiss.** 1990. Adenylate cyclase toxin is critical for colonization and pertussis toxin is critical for lethal infection by *Bordetella pertussis* in infant mice. *Infect. Immun.* **58:**3445–3447.

36. **Greco, D., S. Salmaso, P. Mastrantonio, M. Giuliano, A. E. Tozzi, A. Anemona, M. L. Ciofi degli Atti, A. Giammanco, P. Panei, W. C. Blackwelder, D. L. Klein, and S. G. F. Wassilak.** 1996. A controlled trial of two acellular vaccines and one whole-cell vaccine against pertussis. *N. Engl. J. Med.* **334:**341–348.

37. **Grimprel, E., P. Begue, I. Anjak, F. Betsou, and N. Guiso.** 1993. Comparison of polymerase chain reaction, culture, and western immunoblot serology for diagnosis of *Bordetella pertussis* infection. *J. Clin. Microbiol.* **31:**2745–2750.

38. **Gross, R., and N. H. Carbonetti.** 1993. Differential regulation of *Bordetella pertussis* virulence factors. *Zentralbl Bakteriol.* **278:**177–186.

39. **Gustafsson, L., H. O. Hallander, P. Olin, E. Reizenstein, and J. Storsaeter.** 1996. A controlled trial of a two-component acellular, a five-component acellular, and a whole-cell pertussis vaccine. *N. Engl. J. Med.* **334:**349–355.

40. **Halperin, S. A., and T. J. Marrie.** 1991. Pertussis encephalopathy in an adult: case report and review. *Rev. Infect. Dis.* **13:**1043–1047.

41. **He, Q., J. Mertsola, H. Soini, and M. K. Viljanen.** 1994. Sensitive and specific polymerase chain reaction assays for detection of *Bordetella pertussis* in nasopharyngeal specimens. *J. Pediatr.* **124:**421–426.

42. **Heiss, L. N., J. R. Lancaster, Jr., J. A. Corbett, and W. E. Goldman.** 1994. Epithelial autotoxicity of nitric oxide: role in the respiratory cytopathology of pertussis. *Proc. Natl. Acad. Sci. USA* **91:**267–270.

43. **Herwaldt, L. A.** 1993. Pertussis and pertussis vaccines in adults. *JAMA* **269:**93–94.

44. **Hewlett, E. L.** 1995. Bordetella species, p. 2078–2084. *In* G. L. Mandell, J. E. Bennett, and R. Dolin (ed.), *Principles and Practices of Infectious Diseases*, 4th ed. Churchill Livingstone, New York, N.Y.

45. **Hewlett, E. L.** 1996. *Bordetella pertussis* and the central nervous system, p. 655–666. *In* W. M. Scheld, R. J. Whitley, and D. T. Durack (ed.), *Infections of the Central Nervous System,* 2nd ed. Raven Press, New York, N.Y.

46. **Hewlett, E. L.** 1997. Pertussis: current concepts of pathogenesis and prevention. *Pediatr. Infect. Dis. J.* **16:**S78–84.

47. **Hewlett, E. L.** 1997. Preparation and composition of acellular pertussis vaccines. Consideration of potential effects on vaccine efficacy. *Dev. Biol. Stand.* **89:**143–151.

48. **Hewlett, E. L.** New developments in pertussis, p. 1–12. *In* G. L. Mandell, J. E. Bennett, and R. Dolin (ed.), *Principles and Practice of Infectious Diseases Update,* vol. 5, no. 2. Churchill Livingstone, New York, N.Y.

49. **Hewlett, E. L., and J. D. Cherry.** 1997. New and improved vaccines against pertussis, p. 387–416. *In* G. S. Cobon, J. B. Kaper, G. C. Woodrow, and M. M. Levine (ed.), *New Generation Vaccines,* 2nd ed. Marcel Dekker, Inc., New York, N.Y.

50. **Hewlett, E. L. and V. M. Gordon.** 1988. Adenylate cyclase toxin of *Bordetella pertussis,* p. 193–209. *In* A. C. Wardlaw and R. Parton (ed.), *Pathogenesis and Immunity in Pertussis.* John Wiley and Sons, New York, N.Y.

51. **Hodder, S. L. and E. A. Mortimer, Jr.** 1992. Epidemiology of pertussis and reactions to pertussis vaccine. *Epidemiol. Rev.* **14:**243–267.

52. **Hoppe, J. E., and C. G. Simon.** 1990. In vitro susceptibilities of *Bordetella pertussis* and *Bordetella parapertussis* to seven fluoroquinolones. *Antimicrob. Agents Chemother.* **34:**2287–2288.

53. **Houard, S., C. Hackel, A. Herzog, and A. Bollen.** 1989. Specific identification of *Bordetella pertussis* by the polymerase chain reaction. *Res. Microbiol.* **140:**477–487.

54. **Kendrick, P. L., G. Eldering, M. K. Dixon, and J. Misner.** 1947. Mouse protection tests in the study of pertussis vaccine: a comparative series using the intracerebral route of challenge. *Am. J. Public Health* **37:**803–810.

55. **Khelef, N., C.-M. Bachelet, B. B. Vargaftig, and N. Guiso.** 1994. Characterization of murine lung inflammation after infection with parental *Bordetella pertussis* and mutants deficient in adhesins or toxins. *Infect. Immun.* **62:**2893–2900.

56. **Khelef, N., and N. Guiso.** 1995. Induction of macrophage apoptosis by *Bordetella pertussis* adenylate cyclase-hemolysis. *FEMS Microbiol. Lett.* **134:**27–32.

57. **Klein, D. L.** 1995. Report of the nationwide multicenter acellular pertussis trial. *Pediatrics* **96:** 547–603.

58. **Krantz, I., R. Sekura, B. Trollfors, J. Taranger, G. Zackrisson, T. Lagergard, R. Schneerson, and J. Robbins.** 1990. Immunogenicity and safety of a pertussis vaccine composed of pertussis toxin inactivated by hydrogen peroxide, in 18- to 23-month-old children. *J. Pediatr.* **116:**539–543.

59. **Lewis, K., M. A. Saubolle, F. C. Tenover, M. F. Rudinsky, S. D. Barbour, and J. D. Cherry.** 1995. Pertussis caused by an erythromycin-resistant strain of *Bordetella pertussis*. *Pediatr. Infect. Dis. J.* **14:**388–391.

60. **Li, Z., D. L. Jansen, T. M. Finn, S. A. Halperin, A. Kasina, S. P. O'Connor, T. Aoyama, C. R. Manclark, and M. J. Brennan.** 1994. Identification of *Bordetella pertussis* infection by shared-primer PCR. *J. Clin. Microbiol.* **32:**783–789.

61. **Lichtinghagen, R., R. Diedrich-Glaubitz, and B. von Horsten.** 1994. Identification of *Bordetella pertussis* in nasopharyngeal swabs using the polymerase chain reaction: evaluation of detection methods. *Eur. J. Clin. Chem. Clin. Biochem.* **32:**161–167.

62. **Liese, J. G., C. K. Meschievitz, E. Harzer, J. Froeschle, P. Hosbach, J. E. Hoppe, F. Porter, S. Stojanov, K. Niinivaara, A. M. Walker, and B. H. Belohradsky.** 1997. Efficacy of a two-component acellular pertussis vaccine in infants. *Pediatr. Infect. Dis. J.* **16:**1038–1044.

63. **Luker, K. E., J. L. Collier, E. W. Kolodziej, G. R. Marshall, and W. E. Goldman.** 1993. *Bordetella pertussis* tracheal cytotoxin and other muramyl peptides: distinct structure-activity relationships for respiratory epithelial cytopathology. *Proc. Natl. Acad. Sci. USA.* **90:**2365–2369.

64. **Luker, K. E., A. N. Tyler, G. R. Marshall, and W. E. Goldman.** 1995. Tracheal cytotoxin structural requirements for respiratory epithelial damage in pertussis. *Mol. Microbiol.* **16:**733–743.

65. **Marwick, C.** 1996. Acellular pertussis vaccine is licensed for infants. *JAMA* **276:**516–518.

66. **Meade, B. D., and A. Bollen.** 1994. Recommendations for use of the polymerase chain reaction in the diagnosis of *Bordetella pertussis* infections. *J. Med. Microbiol.* **41:**51–55.

67. **Meade, B. D., A. Deforest, K. M. Edwards, T. A. Romani, F. Lynn, C. H. O'Brien, C. B. Swartz, G. F. Reed, and M. A. Deloria.** 1995. Description and evaluation of serologic assays used in a multicenter trial of acellular pertussis vaccines. *Pediatrics* **96:**570–575.

68. **Miller, J. F., J. J. Mekalanos, and S. Falkow.** 1989. Coordinate regulation and sensory transduction in the control of bacterial virulence. *Science* **243:**916–922.

69. **Miller, J. J., Jr., R. J. Silverberg, T. M. Saito, and J. B. Humber.** 1943. An agglutinative reaction for *Hemophilus pertussis*. II. Its relation to clinical immunity. *J. Pediatr.* **22:**644–651.

70. **Mills, K. H., A. Barnard, J. Watkins, and K. Redhead.** 1993. Cell-mediated immunity to *Bordetella pertussis:* role of Th1 cells in bacterial clearance in a murine respiratory infection model. *Infect. Immun.* **61:**399–410.

71. **Mills, K. H. G., M. Ryan, E. Ryan, and B. P. Mahon.** 1998. A murine model in which protection correlates with pertussis vaccine efficacy in children reveals complementary roles for humoral and cell-mediated immunity in protection against *Bordetella pertussis*. *Infect. Immun.* **66:**594–602.

72. **Mink, C. M., J. D. Cherry, P. Christenson, K. Lewis, E. Pineda, D. Shlian, J. A. Dawson, and D. A. Blumberg.** 1992. A search for *Bordetella pertussis* infection in university students. *Clin. Infect. Dis.* **14:**464–471.

73. **Mink, C. M., C. H. O'Brien, S. Wassilak, A. Deforest, and B. D. Meade.** 1994. Isotype and antigen specificity of pertussis agglutinins following whole-cell pertussis vaccination and infection with *Bordetella pertussis*. *Infect. Immun.* **62:**1118–1120.

74. **Mink, C. M., N. M. Sirota, and S. Nugent.** 1994. Outbreak of pertussis in a fully immunized adolescent and adult population. *Arch. Pediatr. Adolesc. Med.* **148:**153–157.

75. **Mortimer, E. A., Jr.** 1990. Pertussis and its prevention: a family affair. *J. Infect. Dis.* **161:**473–479.

76. **Nelson, S., A. Matlow, C. McDowell, M. Roscoe, M. Karmali, L. Penn, and L. Dyster.** 1997. Detection of *Bordetella pertussis* in clinical specimens by PCR and a microtiter plate-based DNA hybridization assay. *J. Clin. Microbiol.* **35:**117–120.

77. **Nencioni, L., G. Volpini, S. Peppoloni, M. Bugnoli, T. DeMagistris, I. Marsili, and R. Rappuoli.** 1991. Properties of pertussis toxin mutant PT-9K/129G after formaldehyde treatment. *Infect. Immun.* **59**:625–630.

78. **Parton, R.** 1996. New perspectives on *Bordetella* pathogenicity. *J. Med. Microbiol.* **44**:233–235.

79. **Pearson, R. D., P. Symes, M. Conboy, A. A. Weiss, and E. L. Hewlett.** 1987. Inhibition of monocyte oxidative responses by *Bordetella pertussis* adenylate cyclase toxin. *J. Immunol.* **139**: 2749–2754.

80. **Pittman, M.** 1984. The concept of pertussis as a toxin-mediated disease. *Pediatr. Infect. Dis.* **3**: 467–486.

81. **Postels-Multani, S., H. J. Schmitt, C. H. Wirsing von König, H. L. Bock, and H. Bogaerts.** 1995. Symptoms and complications of pertussis in adults. *Infection* **23**:139–142.

82. **Rappuoli, R.** 1994. Pathogenicity mechanisms of *Bordetella*. *Curr. Top. Microbiol. Immunol.* **192**: 319–336.

83. **Rappuoli, R.** 1997. Rational design of vaccines. *Nat. Med.* **3**:374–376.

84. **Redhead, K., J. Watkins, A. Barnard, and K. H. G. Mills.** 1993. Effective immunization against *Bordetella pertussis* respiratory infection in mice is dependent on induction of cell-mediated immunity. *Infect. Immun.* **61**:3190–3198.

85. **Reizenstein, E., B. Johansson, L. Mardin, J. Abens, R. Möllby, and H. O. Hallander.** 1993. Diagnostic evaluation of polymerase chain reaction discriminative for *Bordetella pertussis, B. parapertussis,* and *B. bronchiseptica. Diagn. Microbiol. Infect. Dis.* **17**:185–191.

86. **Reizenstein, E., L. Lindberg, R. Möllby, and H. O. Hallander.** 1996. Validation of nested *Bordetella* PCR in pertussis vaccine trial. *J. Clin. Microbiol.* **34**:810–815.

87. **Ryan, M., G. Murphy, L. Gothefors, L. Nilsson, J. Storsaeter, and K. H. G. Mills.** 1997. *Bordetella pertussis* respiratory infection in children is associated with preferential activation of type 1 T helper cells. *J. Infect. Dis.* **175**:1246–1250.

88. **Sako, W.** 1947. Studies on pertussis immunization. *J. Pediatr.* **30**:29–40.

89. **Sato, Y., M. Kimura, and H. Fukumi.** 1984. Development of a pertussis component vaccine in Japan. *Lancet* **1**:122–126.

90. **Scarlato, V., B. Arico, A. Prugnola, and R. Rappuoli.** 1991. Sequential activation and environmental regulation of virulence genes in *Bordetella pertussis. EMBO J.* **10**:3971–3975.

91. **Schmitt, H. J., C. H. W. von Konig, A. Neiss, H. Bogaerts, H. L. Bock, H. Schulte-Wissermann, M. Gahr, R. Schult, J. U. Folkens, W. Rauh, and R. Clemens.** 1996. Efficacy of acellular pertussis vaccine in early childhood after household exposure. *JAMA* **275**:37–41.

92. **Shvartzman, P., R. Mader, and T. Stopler.** 1989. Herniated lumbar disc associated with pertussis. *J. Fam. Pract.* **28**:224–225.

93. **Simondon, F., M. P. Preziosi, A. Yam, C. T. Kane, L. Chabirand, I. Iteman, G. Sanden, S. Mboup, A. Hoffenbach, K. Knudsen, N. Guiso, S. Wassilak, and M. Cadoz.** 1997. A randomized double-blind trial comparing a two-component acellular to a whole-cell pertussis vaccine in Senegal. *Vaccine* **15**:1606–1612.

94. **Smith, S., and R. C. Tilton.** 1996. Acute *Bordetella pertussis* infection in an adult. *J. Clin. Microbiol.* **34**:429–430.

95. **Stehr, K., J. D. Cherry, U. Heininger, S. Schmitt-Grohe, M. Uberall, S. Laussucq, T. Eckhardt, M. Meyer, R. Engelhardt, and P. Christenson.** 1998. A comparative efficacy trial in Germany in infants who received either the Lederle/Takeda acellular pertussis component DTP (DTaP) vaccine, the Lederle whole-cell component DTP vaccine, or DT vaccine. *Pediatrics* **101**:1–11.

96. **Storsaeter, J., H. Hallander, C. P. Farrington, P. Olin, R. Möllby, and E. Miller.** 1990. Secondary analyses of the efficacy of two acellular pertussis vaccines evaluated in a Swedish phase III trial. *Vaccine* **8**:457–461.

97. **Trollfors, B., J. Taranger, T. Lagergard, L. Lind, V. Sundh, G. Zackrisson, C. Lowe, W. Blackwelder, and J. B. Robbins.** 1995. A placebo-controlled trial of a pertussis-toxoid vaccine. *N. Engl. J. Med.* **333**:1045–1050.

98. **Tuomanen, E.** 1988. *Bordetella pertussis* adhesins, p. 75–94. *In* A. C. Wardlaw and R. Parton (ed.), *Pathogenesis and Immunity in Pertussis.* John Wiley and Sons, Inc., New York, N.Y.

99. **Tuomanen, E., and A. Weiss.** 1985. Characterization of two adhesins of *Bordetella pertussis* for human ciliated respiratory-epithelial cells. *J. Infect. Dis.* **152**:118–125.

100. **Ui, M.** 1988. The multiple biological activities of pertussis toxin, p. 121–146. *In* A. C. Wardlaw and R. Parton (ed.), *Pathogenesis and Immunity in Pertussis.* John Wiley and Sons, Inc. New York, N.Y.

101. **Ui, M.** 1990. Pertussis toxin as a valuable probe for G-protein involvement in signal transduction, p. 45–78. *In* J. Moss and M. Vaughan (ed.), *ADP-Ribosylating Toxins and G Proteins.* American Society for Microbiology, Washington, D.C.

102. **Wadowsky, R. M., R. H. Michaels, T. Libert, L. A. Kingsley, and G. D. Ehrlich.** 1996. Multiplex PCR-based assay for detection of *Bordetella pertussis* in nasopharyngeal swab specimens. *J. Clin. Microbiol.* **34:**2645–2649.

103. **Weiss, A. A., E. L. Hewlett, G. A. Myers, and S. Falkow.** 1983. Tn5-induced mutations affecting virulence factors of *Bordetella pertussis. Infect. Immun.* **42:**33–41.

104. **Wilson, R., R. Read, M. Thomas, A. Rutman, K. Harrison, V. Lund, B. Cookson, W. Goldman, H. Lambert, and P. Cole.** 1991. Effects of *Bordetella pertussis* infection on human respiratory epithelium in vivo and in vitro. *Infect. Immun.* **59:**337–345.

105. **Wright, S. W., K. M. Edwards, M. D. Decker, and M. H. Zeldin.** 1995. Pertussis infection in adults with persistent cough. *JAMA* **273:**1044–1046.

*Emerging Infections 2*
Edited by W. M. Scheld, W. A. Craig, and J. M. Hughes
© 1998 ASM Press, Washington, D.C.

*Chapter 8*

# Epidemic Leptospirosis Associated with Pulmonary Hemorrhage in Nicaragua, Other Recent Outbreaks, and Diagnostic Testing: Issues and Opportunities

## *Bradley A. Perkins*

Leptospires have been recognized as a cause of human disease since 1915, when Inada described the etiology and transmission of what was then known as "Weil's disease," but today is more often called leptospirosis (10). Since that time there has been good progress in our understanding of its microbiology, animal reservoirs, transmission to humans, occupational and recreational risk factors, pathogenesis, pathology, clinical manifestations, and diagnosis (6, 8). However, the lack of simple, widely applicable diagnostic tests and the similarity of leptospirosis to other febrile diseases have hampered public health efforts to improve its control and prevention. Recently, there have been encouraging advances in diagnostic technology that may offer important opportunities in these areas (7). Much of this activity is stimulated by the recognition that leptospirosis may be an important under-recognized cause of febrile illness in the tropics (18). This chapter reviews the investigation of a large epidemic of leptospirosis in Nicaragua, two other recent smaller outbreaks, and the current status of diagnostic testing.

## NICARAGUA

In late 1995, following exceptionally heavy rainfall that resulted in local flooding in a rural area north of Lake Managua in Nicaragua, three persons died after presenting to the Achuapa Health Center with an acute febrile illness (4, 22). During the next 2 weeks, 400 persons from the neighboring towns of Achuapa and El Sauce (combined population of 37,030) were evaluated for acute onset of fevers, chills, headaches, and myalgias. By 7 November 1995, 150 persons had been hos-

*Bradley A. Perkins* • Division of Bacterial and Mycotic Diseases, National Center for Infectious Diseases, Centers for Disease Control and Prevention, Atlanta, GA 30333.

pitalized with more severe manifestations of disease including abdominal pain, hypotension, and respiratory distress. At least 13 died from respiratory distress associated with pulmonary hemorrhage.

Initial clinical speculation on the cause of this epidemic focused on dengue and dengue hemorrhagic fever, as well as a number of other arthropod- and rodent-borne rickettsial and viral pathogens. These diseases were ruled out by a battery of serologic, PCR-based, and histopathologic studies at the Centers for Disease Control and Prevention (CDC) in Atlanta, Ga. (4). Based on the histopathologic findings and reports of outbreaks of pulmonary hemorrhage resulting from leptospiral infection in China, Korea, and Brazil, Sherif Zaki and colleagues at CDC evaluated tissues from these patients using newly developed immunohistochemical stains for detection of leptospiral antigens in human tissues (14, 16, 23, 26). Figure 1 shows both intact leptospiral forms as well as granular leptospiral antigens staining in lung tissue of a patient who died of pulmonary hemorrhage. Liver and kidney tissues from these same patients revealed similar findings.

Leptospirosis is a zoonotic infection with a wide range of wild and domestic animal reservoirs that is caused by the spirochete *Leptospira interrogans* (8). *L. interrogans* is frequently further classified into serogroups and serovars, and the taxonomy of this species is being revised based on DNA relatedness (25). Transmission to humans usually occurs via skin or mucous membrane contact with urine from infected animals. The typical clinical manifestations of the disease include

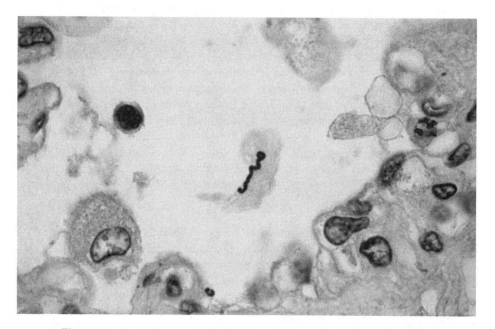

**Figure 1.** Leptospirosis associated with pulmonary hemorrhage. A single leptospire in alveolar space is seen by immunostaining in a lung sample from a patient who died of a pulmonary hemorrhage. Naphthol-fast red with hematoxylin counterstain was used. Original magnification, ×250. (Courtesy of Sherif R. Zaki.)

fever, headache, myalgias, and conjunctival suffusion; hemorrhage, meningitis, jaundice, and renal failure occur less frequently. Leptospires can be cultured from blood and urine but require special media and prolonged incubation for growth. The standard serologic reference assay is the microscopic agglutination test (MAT) in which patients' sera are reacted with a panel of leptospiral serovars (usually in the range of 20) and observed for agglutination with the patient sera. Penicillin or ampicillin is recommended for treatment of severe disease; doxycycline can be used for treatment of mild disease and chemoprophylaxis (21, 24).

Based on Zaki's observations, CDC initiated a collaborative investigation with the Nicaraguan Ministry of Health to describe the epidemic and identify the risk factors for invasive disease, identify the most important animal reservoirs for infection, and isolate and characterize leptospiral strains responsible for the epidemic. Figure 2 shows the epidemic curve of suspect leptospirosis cases among Achuapa and El Sauce town residents. For this analysis, a suspected leptospirosis case was defined as any person with a nonmalarial febrile illness. The peak of the epidemic occurred on 29 October when 250 cases were evaluated in the two health clinics serving these towns. A total of 2,259 cases occurred, resulting in a population-based attack rate of 6%. There were 15 deaths identified, resulting in a minimum mortality rate of 0.17%. The distribution of cases by sex was even, and the peak age-specific attack rates occurred in children 1 to 14 years of age.

A case-control study was undertaken in which cases were defined as residents of Achuapa and El Sauce who had been hospitalized with: (i) fever; (ii) headache, musculoskeletal pain, or chills; (iii) abdominal pain, respiratory distress, hemorrhagic manifestations, or hypotension; (iv) a negative blood smear for malaria. One control, matched by age and area of residence, was identified for each case, and a questionnaire that focused on both individual and household risk factors was administered. Sera were obtained from both cases and controls as well as from case and control household animals. The field conditions were extremely difficult, and

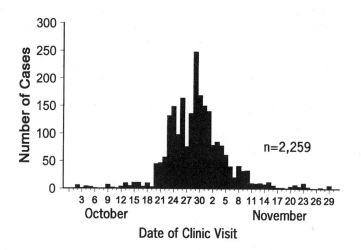

**Figure 2.** Epidemic curve of suspected leptospirosis cases from Achuapa and El Sauce, Nicaragua, for October and November 1995.

**Table 1.** Selected risk factors evaluated in the case-control study

| Risk factor | No. positive/no. evaluated (% positive) | | Univariate matched odds ratio (95% CI) |
| --- | --- | --- | --- |
| | Cases ($n = 51$) | Controls ($n = 51$) | |
| Walking in creeks | 28/49 (57.1) | 16/49 (32.6) | 7.0 (1.6–30.8) |
| Rodents in food preparation area | 13/38 (34.2) | 6/38 (15.6) | 4.5 (0.9–20.8) |
| Swimming in river/ creek | 23/50 (46) | 13/50 (26) | 3.0 (1.1–8.2) |
| Flooded residence | 26/48 (54) | 17/48 (35) | 2.8 (1.0–7.8) |
| Cook mainly in house | 11/50 (22) | 20/50 (40) | 0.3 (0.1–0.9) |
| Female sex | 23/51 (45.1) | 36/51 (70.6) | 0.1 (0.03–0.6) |

a number of the individuals enrolled in the case-control study could be reached only by horseback.

Table 1 shows univariate analyses of selected risk factors evaluated in the case-control study. Walking in the creeks, presence of rodents in the food preparation area, swimming in rivers or creeks during the month preceding illness, and having one's residence flooded were significantly associated with illness, whereas cooking mainly in the home and being female were associated with significant protection. When these factors were modeled with multivariate analysis, the only one that remained significant while controlling for sex was walking through creeks (estimated odds ratio of 12).

Microscopic agglutination test seropositivity by serovar, and overall, among persons enrolled in the case-control study is shown in Table 2. The canicola serovar is highly adapted to dogs as its major reservoir, whereas balum and mancarso tend to be associated with rodents. The animal reservoir for pyrogenes has not been well delineated. Table 3 shows a conservative analytic approach to the case-control household animal seropositivity data. These are matched data restricted to sets in which at least one of the animal types in question was present and which were tested against the case and control household sets. We found that there was a significant association with dog seropositivity in the case households that was not found when testing cattle, pigs, and rodents. This is the first study we are aware of that uses quantitative epidemiologic methods to link human leptospirosis to the most important animal reservoir during a large epidemic. It suggests, in light of the descriptive epidemiology showing an even sex distribution and highest attack

**Table 2.** MAT seropositivity by serovar among persons enrolled in the case-control study

| Serovar | No. (%) positive | | Odds ratio (95% CI) |
| --- | --- | --- | --- |
| | Cases ($n = 33$) | Controls ($n = 47$) | |
| Canicola | 18 (55) | 7 (15) | 7 (1–31) |
| Ballum | 12 (41) | 2 (4) | 10 (1–78) |
| Mankarso | 11 (33) | 0 (0) | Undefined (2–infinity) |
| Pyrogenes | 12 (36) | 5 (11) | 3 (0.9–12) |
| Overall | 19 (58) | 11 (23) | 4 (2–12) |

**Table 3.** MAT seropositivity by animal type at case and control households where at least one of the animal type was present and tested at matched case and control household sets

| Animal type | No. positive/no. evaluated (% positive) | | P value[a] |
|---|---|---|---|
| | Case houses | Control houses | |
| Dogs | 10/12 (83) | 3/12 (25) | 0.015 |
| Cattle | 3/5 (60) | 3/5 (60) | 0.48 |
| Pigs | 4/9 (44) | 7/9 (78) | 0.25 |
| Rodents | 2/8 (25) | 2/8 (25) | 0.48 |

[a]P values are for matched analyses.

rates in children, that dogs probably played a critical role in peridomestic amplification of human risk for exposure to leptospirosis.

There were 12 *L. interrogans* isolates collected during the investigation. Of the four isolates from humans, two were serovar canicola and two were serogroup pyrogenes with serovar identification pending. These last two isolates will probably represent a new serovar and are currently being evaluated in several reference laboratories. Six serovar canicola strains were isolated from dogs (from urine in 6 of 10 case household dogs tested). A serovar pomona strain was isolated from a pig, and a serovar canicola strain was isolated from a household mouse.

In summary, while it may be tempting to speculate that cases of pulmonary hemorrhage resulted from particular virulence factors associated with an as-yet-unidentified new leptospiral serovar, we think that the large number of cases allowed us to glimpse, in relatively large numbers, some well described but rare pulmonary manifestations of leptospirosis (12). The human serology and culture results suggest that there were multiple serovars involved. This is consistent with the importance of flooding in causing this epidemic as well as identifying walking through creeks as an independent risk factor. And lastly, there is reasonably strong evidence for the general importance of dogs in transmission of disease to humans during the epidemic. This is based on the particular leptospiral serovars identified (i.e., canicola), serology from persons enrolled in the case-control study, and the proportion of seropositive dogs in case households compared to control households.

## PUERTO RICO AND COSTA RICA

Two other recent observations illustrate the importance of flooding in transmission of leptospires to humans. In Puerto Rico, there was widespread flooding after a hurricane struck the island in September 1996. Following recognition of several severe leptospirosis cases after the hurricane, Sanders et al. did a systematic comparison of leptospirosis seropositivity among dengue-negative sera from suspected dengue patients in the prehurricane and posthurricane periods (17). Seven (10%) of 72 patient sera tested from the prehurricane period had evidence of acute leptospiral infection (using a newly developed IgM dipstick test with confirmation by MAT), and 19 (27%) of 70 posthurricane period sera were positive (relative risk [RR] = 2.8, 95% confidence interval [CI], 1.2 to 6.2; $P < 0.01$). These data suggest that there is significant endemic leptospirosis in Puerto Rico, but that flooding appeared to substantially increase risk for disease.

Also in 1996, the Illinois Department of Health was notified of five patients with an unknown febrile illness who had returned from a white-water rafting trip on flooded rivers in Costa Rica on 27 and 28 September 1996 (5). During an investigation, nine (35%) of 26 rafters on the trip were found to have had fever associated with rigors, headache, and myalgia. Two were hospitalized; both recovered. Acute and convalescent sera were collected from seven of the nine cases; all were negative for dengue, but five were positive for leptospirosis by either MAT or IgM ELISA or both. In univariate analyses, risk for illness was associated with reported ingestion of water (RR = 8.7, lower 95% CI = 1.5) and being submerged in water after falling into the river while rafting (RR = 6.0, lower 95% CI = 1.1). This investigation emphasizes the possible risks to U.S. travelers pursuing fresh-water-related recreational opportunities, and it again highlights the possible importance of flooding in increasing risk for disease.

## DIAGNOSTIC TESTING

Isolation of *L. interrogans* from human clinical specimens is the gold standard for diagnosis of leptospirosis and should be used to validate indirect means for diagnosis (e.g., serology- and PCR-based tests). Leptospires can be cultured from blood (early days of illness), cerebrospinal fluid (by end of first week of illness), and urine (second week of illness) (6). Unfortunately, isolation of *L. interrogans* is a slow process, usually requiring 1–2 weeks of incubation in specialized media, making culture impractical for routine clinical diagnosis. To be useful, a test must allow identification of infection early enough to initiate meaningful therapy, and it must be appropriate for use in developing as well as developed countries.

Serologic tests developed for diagnosis of leptospirosis run the gambit of formats including: agglutination (microscopic and macroscopic), complement fixation, immune (indirect) hemagglutination, immune hemolysis, immunofluorescence, and ELISA (6). As previously mentioned, the reference standard serologic test is the MAT (microscopic agglutination test), but similar to culture it is not appropriate for clinical diagnosis because it is only available in highly specialized reference laboratories due to its complexity (e.g., the World Health Organization [WHO], Collaborating Centers for Leptospirosis at CDC in Atlanta, and several other countries including Australia, the United Kingdom, and The Netherlands). In the United States, the tests most frequently available for leptospirosis are the indirect hemagglutination test, macroscopic (slide) agglutination, and ELISA. The indirect hemagglutination test was developed in the early 1970s at CDC, but its performance in some reference laboratories may lack adequate sensitivity and specificity (5a, 19).

Several new ELISA format tests have been recently evaluated with encouraging results (1, 13, 15). Some of these tests are designed to detect IgM antibodies, offering possible diagnostic utility early in illness using single acute serum specimens. Perhaps the most exciting recent developments have come with testing of dipstick format assays for detection of leptospiral IgM antibodies (9). These tests may be appropriate for use in developing countries where most leptospirosis cases occur. They offer the possibility of aiding physicians in distinguishing leptospirosis from diseases like dengue or malaria in which clinical presentations may be similar but appropriate therapy is quite different.

A number of pathologic methods involving microscopic evaluation of human tissues have been shown to be useful in diagnosis of leptospirosis. These include dark-field microscopy, special stains (e.g., Dieterle's, Steiner's, and Warthin-Starry silver impregnation stains), immunohistochemical (IHC) staining, and in situ hybridization (ISH) methods (6, 26). Interpretation of dark-field microscopy and special staining require specialized expertise in distinguishing leptospires from other normal human tissues. Immunohistochemical (IHC) staining (using immuno-alkaline phosphatase or immunoperoxidase) and in situ hybridization (ISH) (using biotin-labelled leptospiral DNA) methods are excellent techniques for rapid identification of leptospires in human tissues. If performed correctly, they should have high sensitivity and specificity (26).

Another area of recent progress is in design and testing of DNA probes for use in the polymerase chain reaction (PCR) to detect leptospires (3, 11, 20, 27). This technology has been applied for detection of infection as well as for more rapid subtyping of leptospires. Some evaluations have suggested that PCR detection of leptospiral DNA in the urine may be more sensitive than culture (2). While this technology may be useful for diagnosis in some developed countries and in specific research studies, it does not appear to address (at least at the present time) the major public health challenge of providing physicians in developing countries with useful diagnostic technology for leptospirosis.

## CONCLUSIONS

The epidemic in Nicaragua and the smaller outbreaks in Puerto Rico and Costa Rica demonstrate the difficulties associated with recognition of leptospirosis, both because of its similarity to other febrile diseases and the lack of simple, widely applicable diagnostic tests. In all three examples, there was a clear association with flooding. This raises the possibility of being able to predict periods when the risk for human transmission may be increased so that surveillance can be enhanced and preventive measures can be implemented (e.g., decreasing exposure or chemoprophylaxis). Case-control studies, like that done in Nicaragua that linked human cases to household animals through animal serosurveys, are a powerful epidemiologic approach to identify the most important animal reservoirs during epidemics. This kind of information is critical if control of leptospirosis in animals is to be part of efforts to prevent human disease.

In areas like Puerto Rico where there is evidence of substantial leptospirosis even in the absence of flooding, population-based surveillance is needed so that public health efforts to improve its control and prevention can be prioritized. In less developed tropical countries, systematic efforts are needed to determine the endemic burden of leptospirosis. To do this, better diagnostic tests for leptospirosis are desperately needed to allow physicians to make the diagnosis of leptospirosis and provide appropriate antibiotic therapy and also to provide estimates of burden of disease.

Development of new diagnostic tests including ELISA and dipstick format tests to detect IgM antibodies on acute serum specimens, immunohistochemistry, and PCR-based detection of leptospiral DNA, provide opportunities for developed and developing countries to improve or implement diagnostic testing for leptospirosis. To facilitate this, several WHO Collaborating Centers for Leptospirosis are conducting a multilaboratory evaluation of newly developed diagnostic tests. The purpose of these efforts is to validate the sensitivity and specificity of these tests compared to gold standards including culture and MAT (acute and convalescent sera with fourfold rise in titer). If early observations with these tests are substantiated, this information will be widely disseminated, and pilot projects to demonstrate their utility will be conducted in several countries. Improving the ability of physicians to diagnose leptospirosis is a critical step in understanding the public health importance of the disease and developing more effective means for its control and prevention.

**Acknowledgments.** I gratefully acknowledge the contributions of the Nicaraguan Epidemic Working Group at the Ministry of Health in Nicaragua, Pan American Health Organization, U.S. Department of Agriculture, and the CDC, including J. Amador, J. de los Reyes, A. Gonzalez, C. Jarquin, R. Jimenez, and F. Munoz, Ministry of Health, Nicaragua; M. Jarquin, E. Orosco, F. Zelaya, Hospital EODR, Leon, Nicaragua; C. Castillo, N. Jiron, P. Lamy, and F. Pinheiro, Pan American Health Organization; C. Bolin, U.S. Department of Agriculture; D. Ashford, S. Bragg, L. Coffield, J. Chang, B. Cropp, B. Farrar, C. Goldsmith, P. Greer, N. Karabatsos, T. Ksiazek, D. Martin, E. McClure, S. Nichol, C. J. Peters, J. Rigau, L. Rodriguez, P. Rollin, W.-J. Shieh, R. Spiegel, Y.-C. Sun, T. Tsai, R. Travejo, R. Weyant, and S. Zaki, CDC.

## REFERENCES

1. **Adler, B., A. M. Murphy, S. A. Locarnini, and S. Faine.** 1980. Detection of specific anti-leptospiral immunoglobulins M and G in human serum by solid-phase enzyme-linked immunosorbent assay. *J. Clin. Microbiol.* **11**:452–457.
2. **Bal, A. E., C. Gravekamp, R. A. Hartskeerl, J. De Meza-Brewster, H. Korver, and W. J. Terpstra.** 1994. Detection of leptospires in urine by PCR for early diagnosis of leptospirosis. *J. Clin. Microbiol.* **32**:1894–1898.
3. **Brown, P. D., C. Gravekamp, D. G. Carrington, et al.** 1995. Evaluation of the polymerase chain reaction for early diagnosis of leptospirosis. *J. Med. Microbiol.* **43**:110–114.
4. **Centers for Disease Control and Prevention.** 1995. Outbreak of acute febrile illness and pulmonary hemorrhage—Nicaragua, 1995. *Morbid. Mortal. Weekly Rep.* **44**:841–843.
5. **Centers for Disease Control and Prevention.** 1997. Outbreak of leptospirosis among white-water rafters—Costa Rica, 1996. *Morbid. Mortal. Weekly Rep.* **46**:577–579.
5a. **Centers for Disease Control and Prevention.** Unpublished data.
6. **Faine S.** 1982. *Guidelines for the Control of Leptospirosis.* World Health Organization, Geneva, Switzerland.
7. **Farr, R. W.** Leptospirosis. 1995. CID **21**:1–8.
8. **Feigin, R. D., and D. C. Anderson.** 1975. Human leptospirosis. *Crit. Rev. Clin. Lab. Sci.* **5**:413–167.
9. **Gussenhoven, G. C., M. A. W. G. van der Hoon, M. G. A. Goris, et al.** 1997. LEPTO dipstick: a dipstick assay for the detection of Leptospira-specific immunoglobulin M antibodies in human sera. *J. Clin. Microbiol.* **35**:92–97.
10. **Inada, R., Y. Ido, R. Hoki, R. Kaneko, and H. Ito.** 1916. The etiology, mode of infection and specific therapy of Weil's disease (spirochaetosis icterohaemorrhagica). *J. Exp. Med.* **23**:377–402.

11. **Merien, F., G. Baranton, and P. Perolat.** 1995. Comparison of polymerase chain reaction with microagglutination test and culture for diagnosis of leptospirosis. *J. Infect. Dis.* **172:**281–285.
12. **O'Neil, K. M., L. S. Rickman, and A. A. Lazarus.** 1991. Pulmonary manifestations of leptospirosis. *J. Infect. Dis.* **13:**705–709.
13. **Pappas, M. G., W. R. Ballou, M. R. Gray, E. T. Takafuji, R. N. Miller, and W. T. Hockmeyer.** 1985. Rapid serodiagnosis of leptospirosis using the IgM-specific dot-ELISA: comparison with microscopic agglutination test. *Am. J. Trop. Med. Hyg.* **34:**346–354.
14. **Park, S.-K., S.-H. Lee, and Y.-K. Rhee, et al.** 1989. Leptospirosis in Chonbuk province of Korea in 1987: a study of 93 patients. *Am. J. Trop. Med. Hyg.* **41:**345–351.
15. **Ribeiro, M. A., C. C. Souza, and S. H. Almeida.** 1995. Dot-ELISA for human leptospirosis employing immunodominant antigen. *J. Trop. Med. Hyg.* **98:**452–456.
16. **Rio Goncalves, A. J., J. E. Manhaes de Carvalho, J. B. Guedes de Silva, R. Rozenbaum, and A. R. Machado Vierna.** 1992. Hemoptise/s e sindrome de angustia respiratoria do adulto como causas de morte na leptospirose. Mudancas de padroes clinicos e anatomopatologicos. *Rev. Soc. Brasil. Med. Trop.* **25:**261–270.
17. **Sanders, E. J., H. J. Rigau-Perez, H. Smits, et al.** 1997. Abstract 70. *In Program and Abstracts of the 46th Annual Meeting of the American Society of Tropical Medicine and Hygiene.*
18. **Sanford, J. P.** 1984. Leptospirosis—time for a booster. *N. Engl. J. Med.* **310:**524–525.
19. **Sulzer, C. R., J. W. Glosser, F. Rogers, W. L. Jones, and M. Frix.** 1975. Evaluation of an indirect hemagglutination test for the diagnosis of human leptospirosis. *J. Clin. Microbiol.* **2:**218–221.
20. **Sun-Ho, K., K. Ik-Sang, C. Myung-Sik, and W.-H. Chang.** 1994. Detection of leptospiral DNA by PCR. *J. Clin. Microbiol.* **32:**1035–1039.
21. **Takafuji, E. T., J. W. Kirkpatrick, and R. N. Miller.** 1984. An efficacy trial of doxycycline chemoprophylaxis against leptospirosis. *N. Engl. J. Med.* **310:**497.
22. **Trevejo, R. T., J. G. Rigau-Perez, D. A. Ashford, et al.** Epidemic leptospirosis associated with pulmonary hemorrhage—Nicaragua, 1995. *J. Infect. Dis.*, in press.
23. **Wang, C. N., J. Liu, T. F. Chang, W. J. Cheng, M. Y. Luo, and A. T. Hung.** 1965. Studies on anicteric leptospirosis: I. Clinical manifestations and antibiotic therapy. *Chin. Med. J.* **84:**283–291.
24. **Watt, G., M. L. Tuazon, and E. Santiago.** 1988. Placebo-controlled trial of intravenous penicillin for severe and late leptospirosis. *Lancet* **1:**433–435.
25. **Yasuda, P. H., A. G. Steigerwalt, K. R. Sulzer, A. F. Kaufmann, F. Rogers, and D. J. Brenner.** 1987. Deoxyribonucleic acid relatedness between serogroups and serovars in the family *Leptospiraceae* with proposals for seven new *Leptospira* species. *Int. J. Syst. Bacteriol.* **37:**407–415.
26. **Zaki, S. R., and W. J. Shieh.** 1996. Epidemic Working Group. Leptospirosis associated with outbreak of acute febrile illness and pulmonary haemorrhage, Nicaragua, 1995. *Lancet* **347:**535–536.
27. **Zuerner, R. L., D. Alt, and C. A. Bolin.** 1995. IS*1533*-based PCR assay for identification of *Leptospira interrogans* sensu lato serovars. *J. Clin. Microbiol.* **33:**3284–3289.

*Emerging Infections 2*
Edited by W. M. Scheld, W. A. Craig, and J. M. Hughes
© 1998 ASM Press, Washington, D.C.

*Chapter 9*

# Plague as an Emerging Disease

## *David T. Dennis*

Plague in humans is a severe febrile illness caused by infection with the gram-negative coccobacillus *Yersinia pestis*. It is notorious as a cause of recurring epidemics, at times catastrophic and of pandemic proportion; as such, it is considered a prototypic emerging or reemerging infectious disease. The word plague, derived from the Greek word to beat or to strike, has come in modern use to mean any scourge that threatens the well-being of large numbers of persons, and it carries the connotation of a disaster not easily controllable. It is not surprising, therefore, that plague even today can elicit irrational fear and overreaction (4, 12). Although not widely recognized, plague is maintained continuously in nature as a zoonosis of rodents and their fleas in widely scattered foci over large areas of the world (18). These "silent" natural cycles become manifest when infection spills over into certain highly susceptible rodent populations, resulting in epizootics and consequent rodent die-offs and sometimes in clusters or outbreaks of plague in humans (1). Humans most often become infected by the bite of rodent fleas, less often by handling or ingesting infective animal tissues, and occasionally by airborne (droplet) infection.

Plague is one of three class 1 quarantinable diseases (plague, yellow fever, and cholera) subject to the *International Health Regulations* (37), and the reporting of cases and newly identified foci of infection by national health authorities to the World Health Organization (WHO) is mandatory. From 1981 to 1995, more than 20,000 cases were reported by 25 countries to the WHO (39). Although many countries reported only small numbers of sporadic cases, some reported substantial outbreaks. Outbreaks occurred in several countries that had not reported human plague in recent years or decades. This chapter reviews the changing epidemiology of plague over the past several decades and discusses factors of plague emergence or re-emergence.

---

*David T. Dennis* • Bacterial Zoonoses Branch, Division of Vector-Borne Infectious Diseases, National Center for Infectious Diseases, Centers for Disease Control and Prevention, P.O. Box 2087, Fort Collins, CO 80522.

## EPIDEMIC HISTORY

The Justinian Pandemic (ca. A.D. 542 to 767) began in Egypt and spread to Europe and Asia Minor, causing an estimated 40 million deaths. The second well-documented pandemic began in central Asia in the early 14th century, caused severe epidemics in China and India, moved along caravan routes to Constantinople, and spread through Persia and the Middle East to the Mediterranean region. Entering Sicily at Messina in 1347, it swept across Europe and the British Isles in successive waves over the next three centuries. Known as the "Black Death," medieval plague killed as many as a quarter or more of the affected populations. The latest pandemic, the Third (Modern) Pandemic, arose in southern China in the latter half of the nineteenth century, struck Hong Kong in 1894, and over the next several years spread by rat-infested steamships to major port cities throughout the world. Within 35 years of its appearance in Hong Kong, the Third Pandemic had resulted in an estimated 26 million plague cases and more than 12 million deaths, the vast majority in India (31).

Three biotypes of *Y. pestis*, classified according to their ability to ferment glycerol and reduce nitrate, are correlated with the three major plague pandemics of history (15). The plague strain that spread globally at the time of the Third Pandemic is named the orientalis biotype; the other two are termed the antiqua and mediaevalis biotypes. The orientalis biotype predominates in Asia, and it is the only biotype found in the western hemisphere. The antiqua biotype occurs in parts of Africa, southeastern Russia, and Central Asia; the mediaevalis biotype is found around the Caspian Sea. Gene typing by rRNA profiling (ribotyping) supports these distinctions (20, 30). Wild *Y. pestis* strains have been considered to be uniform and stable in genetic complement and virulence throughout the world; recent studies in Madagascar have, however, documented emergence of genetic deviation from the indigenous orientalis biotype (21).

Effective strategies to prevent and control the spread of plague were made possible by an understanding of its ecology and epidemiology. Alexandre Yersin, working in Hong Kong in 1894, described the plague bacillus in diseased lymph nodes (buboes) of fatal cases. In 1898, Paul-Louis Simond, a French scientist sent to investigate the unfolding epidemics of bubonic plague in Bombay, first provided evidence that the plague bacillus was transmitted from rat to rat, and from rats to humans, by rat fleas. The three principal forms of human plague are bubonic, septicemic, and pneumonic. Epidemiologic investigations revealed that, with rare exception, human-to-human plague transmission occurs only as a result of close (respiratory droplet) contact of persons with a case of pneumonic plague and that contagious spread could be interrupted by isolating plague patients (40).

After 1905, the international spread of plague was largely halted by regulations that controlled rats in ports and required ships to be inspected and rat-proofed, by isolation of cases, and by enhanced plague surveillance with microbiological laboratory support. Nevertheless, by 1910 plague was established in wild rodent populations in all inhabited continents other than Australia, resulting in the many residual enzootic cycles of the plague bacillus that occur throughout the world today (Fig. 1) (31). As an example of pandemic introduction and its subsequent

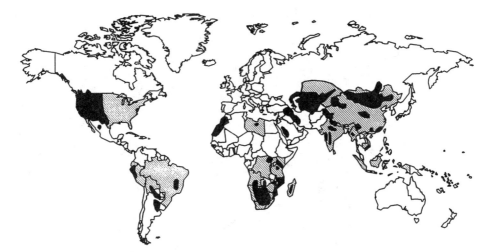

**Figure 1.** Distribution of natural foci of plague. Symbols: ▨, countries reporting plague between 1970 and 1997; ■, probable sylvatic foci. (Compiled from data provided by the WHO, CDC, and other sources.)

establishment and spread, plague was first imported into San Francisco in 1899, followed by major rat-associated outbreaks in the city over the next several years (26). By 1908, however, plague was epizootic in ground squirrels in surrounding counties and in the ensuing decades spread to various wild rodent populations throughout the western third of the United States (16), where it is now entrenched in natural cycles involving various native rodents and their fleas (1, 18).

Insecticidal dusts became widely available to control fleas in the 1940s, and antimicrobials were put into use to treat plague at about the same time. Beginning in about 1950, plague outbreaks worldwide became mostly sporadic events that were contained relatively quickly through surveillance, rat and flea control, and prompt diagnosis, isolation, and treatment of plague patients. The major exception was the recurring rat-borne plague epidemics in war-torn Vietnam between 1962 and 1975.

## EPIDEMIOLOGY AND UPDATED SURVEILLANCE STATISTICS

### *Y. pestis* Life Cycle

*Y. pestis* is nonsaprophytic and dies quickly under conditions of dessication and temperatures exceeding 40°C. As shown in Fig. 2, the plague bacillus is maintained in rodents and their fleas in both wild and domestic rodent cycles. Humans become infected when they intrude into the natural wild cycle or when domestic rat cycles become established. Person-to-person plague occurs as a result of close exposure to patients with respiratory plague and very rarely as a result of direct skin or mucous membrane contact with infectious secretions or exudates. Whether transmission of infection from one person to another by fleas occurs is controversial.

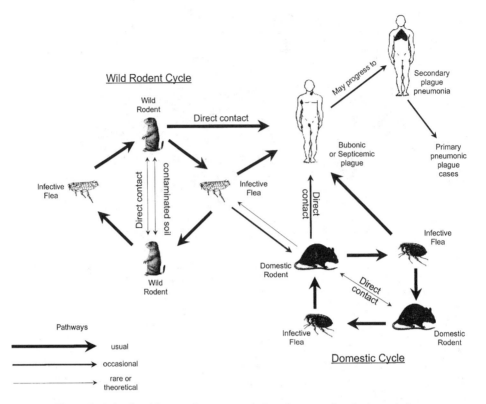

**Figure 2.** Animal and human plague transmission, demonstrating the interrelationship of the wild rodent and domestic rodent cycles and the routes of incidental infection of humans. (Adapted from reference 24.)

## Recent Geographic Distribution and Incidence

Plague foci are widely distributed throughout the world, and human cases are usually identified in some 10 countries each year. The *International Health Regulations* require prompt reporting of plague cases to WHO. From 1981 through 1995, a total of 21,087 human plague cases (mean of 1,406 per year) and 1,931 (11%) deaths were reported by 25 countries to the WHO (Table 1) (39). Sixty percent (12,629) of the total number of cases were reported by countries in eastern and southern Africa, approximately a quarter (5,562) occurred in Asia, and the remaining 2,896 occurred in the Americas. Substantial outbreaks of human plague have occurred recently in Tanzania, the Democratic Republic of Congo (formerly Zaire), Madagascar, Mozambique, India, Vietnam, Myanmar (Burma), and Peru (Fig. 3). Tanzania reported outbreaks involving 1,293 cases in 1991, 444 cases in 1994, and 831 cases in 1995. The Democratic Republic of Congo reported a total of 1,397 cases from 1990 to 1994 and 582 cases in 1995. Zimbabwe experienced outbreak activity involving 392 cases in 1994, after reporting only 1 case in the previous 10 years. Madagascar regularly reports cases, with an average of 167 cases per year from 1990 to 1994 and 1,147 cases in 1995 alone. In 1991, 1995, 1996, and 1997,

**Table 1.** Reported cases of plague in humans, by country, from 1981 to 1995[a]

| Continent(s) | Country | No. of cases | No. of deaths |
|---|---|---|---|
| Africa | Angola | 6 | 0 |
| | Botswana | 173 | 12 |
| | Democratic Republic of Congo (Zaire) | 2,824 | 536 |
| | Kenya | 44 | 8 |
| | Libya | 8 | 0 |
| | Madagascar | 2,526 | 323 |
| | Malawi | 9 | 0 |
| | Mozambique | 216 | 3 |
| | South Africa | 19 | 1 |
| | Tanzania | 5,746 | 482 |
| | Uganda | 660 | 48 |
| | Zambia | 1 | 1 |
| | Zimbabwe | 397 | 31 |
| | Total | 12,629 | 1,445 |
| North and South America | Bolivia | 163 | 25 |
| | Brazil | 611 | 9 |
| | Ecuador | 83 | 3 |
| | Peru | 1,819 | 114 |
| | United States | 220 | 29 |
| | Total | 2,896 | 180 |
| Asia | People's Republic of China | 230 | 56 |
| | India | 876 | 54 |
| | Kazakhstan | 10 | 4 |
| | Mongolia | 58 | 20 |
| | Myanmar (Burma) | 1,087 | 10 |
| | Vietnam | 3,294 | 163 |
| | Total | 5,562 | 307 |
| World total | | 21,087 | 1,932 |

[a]Data are from reference 39.

successive outbreaks of rat-borne bubonic plague occurred in the port city of Mahajanga on the northwestern coast of Madagascar (10). These were the first reports of lowland urban plague in Madagascar in decades. In 1994, India reported its first cases of plague in nearly 30 years, when 876 bubonic and pneumonic plague cases and 54 deaths were reported from the adjacent Maharashtra and Gujarat states in west-central India (38). Vietnam and Myanmar, which experience both urban and rural plague, reported 1,756 and 727 cases, respectively, between period 1990 to 1994.

In the Americas, cases have been reported recently only from Peru, Brazil, and the United States. From 1990 to 1994, Peru reported 1,169 cases; 97 cases were reported in 1995. Brazil reported 57 cases from 1990 to 1994 and 9 cases in 1995. In the 15-year period from 1981 to 1995, the United States reported 220 plague cases (mean of 15 cases per year) and 29 (13%) deaths. Only nine cases and one death were reported in 1995. Although enzootic and epizootic plague occur in 17 of the contiguous western United States, extending from the Pacific coastal states to the Great Plains states and north-central Texas, approximately 80% of U.S. cases

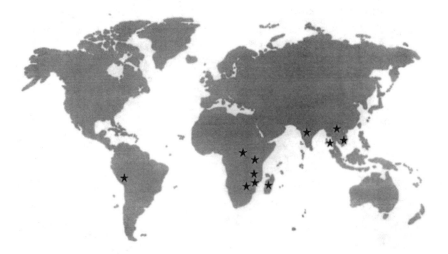

**Figure 3.** Map of the world showing sites of human plague outbreaks in the period from 1991 to 1995.

occur in the southwestern states of New Mexico, Arizona, and Colorado, and another 10% occur in California (11, 18). No plague cases have been reported by Canada or Mexico in recent decades.

## GLOBAL TRENDS IN DISTRIBUTION AND INCIDENCE

As a residual of the Third Pandemic, epidemic plague activity persisted in some regions in lessening intensity into the 1940s. There was, however, a dramatic fall in reported cases of plague worldwide between 1948 and 1956, and an average of only 855 cases were reported annually in the 10-year period from 1956 to 1965 (Fig. 4) (36). In the Third Pandemic, the vast majority of cases globally occurred in the Asian region, and the decrease after 1948 was most marked in Asia, especially India. With the exception of recurring outbreaks of plague in Vietnam in the period from 1965 to 1977, annual numbers of reported cases continued to decrease through 1981, when a low of only 200 cases were reported worldwide (39). Several trends have emerged since 1981: an increase in the annual number of cases to nearly 3,000 cases per year (Fig. 5); an increase in the proportion of all cases reported in the African region; and an increasing influence of just a few countries in each region. The number of cases reported during the 5-year period from 1981 to 1985 was 18% of all cases reported in the 15-year period from 1981 to 1995, compared with 26 and 56%, respectively, for the subsequent two 5-year periods. The proportion of the world's total cases reported in Africa rose from 46% during the period from 1981 to 1985 to 68 and 61%, respectively, for the subsequent two 5-year periods. In the period from 1981 to 1995, only two countries (Madagascar and Tanzania) accounted for 63% of all cases in the African region; Myanmar and

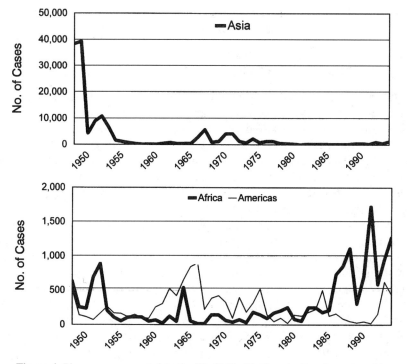

**Figure 4.** Plague cases reported to the World Health Organization, by geographic region, 1948 to 1994, showing marked decrease in cases in Asia and a recent increase in cases in Africa (note difference in scale for cases).

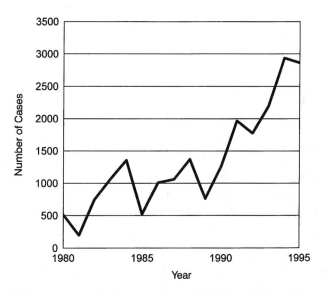

**Figure 5.** Plague cases worldwide reported to the WHO from 1980 to 1995, showing a nearly sixfold increase.

Vietnam accounted for 79% of cases reported in Asia; Peru and Brazil accounted for 84% of cases in the Americas (39).

## CHANGING TRENDS IN THE UNITED STATES

Plague was introduced into a number of Pacific and Gulf Coast states in the early part of this century. Between 1900 and 1908, two notable epidemics of human plague involving several hundred persons occurred in San Francisco, California; later, there were smaller outbreaks in Oakland and Los Angeles, as well as in port cities in Washington, Texas, Louisiana, and Florida (26). Over 500 cases were reported in the United States in the period from 1899 to 1925, and the vast majority of these cases were due to urban, domestic rat-associated exposures. An abrupt change occurred in the period from 1925 to 1964, during which the annual incidence of human plague was static, averaging fewer than two cases per year (range, zero to five), and exposures were almost entirely associated with rural plague among wild rodents and their fleas (24). This long period of quiescence ended in 1965 with an outbreak of seven cases on the Navajo Reservation in New Mexico. A trend of increasing numbers of cases in the Southwest followed, and the overall United States totals of 105 cases from 1970 to 1979 and 179 cases from 1980 to 1989 were the largest numbers of cases reported in any decade since 1900 to 1909 (Fig. 6). Trends beginning in 1965 in the number and geographic location of cases, and in exposure factors, continue to the present and mark important changes in the epidemiology of the disease in the United States (18).

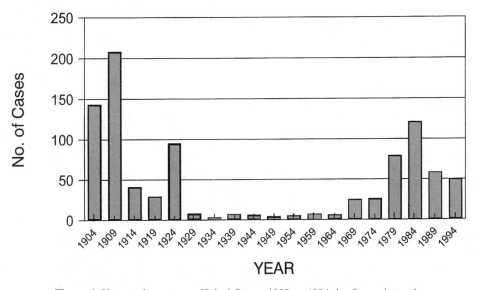

**Figure 6.** Human plague cases, United States, 1900 to 1994, by 5-year intervals, showing peak activity during urban plague outbreaks in the early 20th century, a period of quiescence, and recent resurgence due to increased rural plague in southwestern states.

Prior to 1965, most human cases occurred in California, and although California continues to report sporadic cases (about 10% of the nation's total), the West Coast focus has been superseded by the dramatic shift in plague activity to the southwestern focus. Almost 80% of the 367 cases reported from 1965 to 1995 have occurred in this southwestern focus. Much of the natural plague habitat in this area is comprised of tribal lands, and Native Americans have accounted for nearly 30% of all plague cases since 1965 (3, 6). Trends of plague in the United States have also shown an increasing number of states reporting cases and an eastward movement in human case occurrence toward the 100th meridian (Fig. 7) (7). Plague activity in the southwestern focus and Great Plains states is mostly driven by epizootics involving populations of prairie dogs, rock squirrels, other burrowing rodents, and their fleas (1, 18). A spectacular prairie dog epizootic in the early 1980s resulted in an almost complete die-off of these conspicuous colonial rodents over hundreds of square miles of northern New Mexico, eastern Arizona, and southern Colorado. This epizootic coincided with a burst in human cases in 1983 (40 cases) and in 1984 (31 cases) (2).

An important change in plague epidemiology in the United States is the increasing numbers of cases having infectious exposures in the peridomestic environment, rather than as a result of activities in remote backcountry areas. This is most likely due to the marked increase in home building in natural plague habitats and to the creation of suitable rodent harborage around homes, such as trash piles, old cars, and use of rocks for landscaping and walls. Rock squirrels, with abundant fleas that readily feed on other rodents and on humans, are a principal source of human plague infection in the Southwest and have established themselves around human residences as a direct result of environmental changes (1, 18).

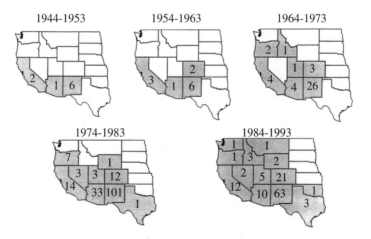

**Figure 7.** Number of human plague cases reported by state and decade in the United States from 1944 to 1993 (total, 362 cases), showing increasing numbers of cases, increasing number of states reporting cases, and an eastward shift in state of occurrence.

Another trend has been an increasing number of human cases associated with plague in domestic cats. Cats that hunt wild rodents in areas where natural plague occurs are at risk of infection. Persons can then be infected by cat bites, scratches, or by direct contact with *Y. pestis*-infected oral lesions, suppurating buboes, saliva, and other tissues or fluids. Further, animals that develop respiratory plague can be a source of primary pneumonic plague in persons who have close contact with them, such as pet owners and veterinary staff. The first documented cat-to-human transmission of infection in the United States occurred in 1977 (25). In the period 1977 to 1997, there were 19 cases of human plague and five deaths in the United States arising from domestic cat exposures; 5 of the 19 cases were of primary pneumonic plague (9a). Although pneumonic plague is highly contagious, it is fortunate that there have been no instances of human-to-human spread from these cat-associated cases or from any of the 36 pneumonic plague cases that have been secondary to bubonic or septicemic plague documented between 1925 and 1995. The last known case of human-to-human transmission of *Y. pestis* in the United states occurred in 1924 during a mixed bubonic and pneumonic plague outbreak in Los Angeles in 1924 and 1925 (26).

Epizootics of plague among urban tree squirrels may lead to a change in the epidemiology of plague in the United States. Epizootic plague in fox squirrels was first identified in 1968 in Denver, Colo., causing a high mortality among squirrels within the city (22). Only one case of human plague was associated with this epizootic, probably because tree squirrel fleas are not likely to feed on humans. However, the large number of dead squirrels found in residential yards and in city parks suggested that the epizootic could spread to urban rat and ground squirrel populations and their fleas and pose a considerable risk to humans. Since then, epizootics in tree squirrels have been recognized in several cities along the front range of Colorado and Wyoming without apparent spread to urban rats or to humans. Studies in Colorado Springs, Colo., suggest that the epizootic in tree squirrels there arose from plague activity in rock squirrels in outlying areas and along parkways (9a).

In 1993, plague was surprisingly found in two tree squirrels and an urban rat in Dallas, Tex. (7). Plague-infected ground squirrels have been found sporadically in recent decades in Los Angeles, Calif., but studies indicate that the likelihood of spread among urban rats (*Rattus rattus*) in the city is low, since infestation of these animals with *Xenopsylla cheopis* fleas has been found to be minimal or absent (35).

## EMERGENCE OF ANTIMICROBIAL RESISTANCE

The development of antimicrobial resistance among pathogenic bacteria is recognized as a pressing emerging infectious disease threat worldwide (23). Untreated, plague is fatal in over 50% of patients with bubonic disease and in nearly all patients with septicemic or pneumonic forms. The overall plague mortality in the United States in the past 25 years has been approximately 15%, and fatalities are almost always due to delayed or incorrect treatment (9, 11). Rapid diagnosis and appropriate antimicrobial therapy are essential in preventing plague deaths. Antibiotics are also used prophylactically to prevent infection in persons at high risk of exposure to infected fleas and to prevent infection and disease in close contacts of pneumonic plague patients (5). Although *Y. pestis* strains have occasionally been found with variable levels of resistance to tetracyclines and to streptomycin (27, 29), treatment failures have not been attributable to antimicrobial resistance. Recently, however, a multidrug-resistant *Y. pestis* strain was isolated from a patient in Madagascar (19). This isolate was resistant at high levels to all first-line antibiotics recommended for treating plague (including tetracycline, streptomycin, and chloramphenicol), as well as to sulfonamides, but it was susceptible to trimethoprim. Genetic characterization of this strain showed that resistance determinants were carried by a plasmid having resistance genes closely related to those commonly found in enterobacteria. This plasmid was highly transferable in vitro to other strains of *Y. pestis* and to *Escherichia coli*, suggesting that this and similar replicons can be transferred among strains of *Y. pestis* in nature, potentially giving rise to further human cases resistant to multiple drugs.

This report of plasmid-mediated multiple-drug-resistant plague raises several questions (14, 19). First, is this an isolated instance of resistance, or is the phenomenon more widespread? The vast majority of human plague occurs under circumstances in which isolation of *Y. pestis* is not feasible, antimicrobial susceptibility testing of plague strains is done in only a few specialized laboratories, and multidrug resistance may easily go unnoticed. Secondly, where did the isolate acquire its resistance plasmid? Did the source patient have multidrug-resistant organisms in the intestinal tract? Do resistant strains of *Y. pestis* occur in rodents and their fleas in Madagascar and elsewhere? How common are plasmid-mediated multidrug-resistant enterobacteria in the gut of rodent hosts of plague? It is not known whether the plasmid for multidrug resistance confers an advantage to *Y. pestis* in its natural cycle; should resistant strains spread among rodents, the public health implications could be substantial. Resistant strains that might arise spontaneously in humans probably would not pose a major public health problem, since infected humans do not contribute to the natural cycle of *Y. pestis* and rarely transmit infection to others through infected respiratory droplets.

Heightened surveillance should be established for detecting antimicrobial-resistant strains of *Y. pestis* from humans and from nature, and alternative antimicrobial agents (such as the fluoroquinolones) should be evaluated for their utility in the prophylaxis and treatment of plague (17).

## CHANGING ENVIRONMENTAL AND SOCIOECONOMIC LANDSCAPES

Many of the natural foci of plague are being increasingly invaded by humans and are undergoing dramatic man-made environmental changes. It is not known how well the rodent and flea reservoirs of plague will adapt to changing habitats, but there are no well-described circumstances where natural foci have been eliminated over large areas. Under some circumstances, a changing rural environment such as suburbanization in the southwestern United States may increase human risk. In another example, investigations of the reported 1994 outbreak of bubonic plague in Maharashtra state, west-central India, identified the Indian gerbil, *Tatera indica*, and its fleas as a likely natural reservoir of plague in that region. This rodent has been described in its natural state as an occupant of arid grassland or open plain habitat. In interface with human activities, it is commonly found on the borders of cultivated areas (32). In plague-affected areas in Maharashtra, large irrigation schemes have allowed cultivation of once-arid land and the creation of a network of villages closely surrounded by crop fields. In this circumstance, *T. indica* burrows were found in dikes between fields and even within the confines of the putative index village itself. *T. indica* collected by trapping within the village had a high index of infestation with *X. cheopis*, which could easily have been acquired from the dense populations of rats in the homes and adjacent fields of the village (13, 34).

Throughout the developing world, massive urbanization has outstripped sanitary and hygienic measures needed to control rats at acceptable levels. Socioeconomic deprivation of recent immigrants, slums, unprotected food stores, uncollected garbage, lack of sewage facilities, and tolerance of rat infestations characterize these rapidly growing urban centers. It is surprising that large epidemics of urban bubonic plague have not happened in the second half of the 20th century, since the environmental conditions appear to be ripe for such occurrences.

## PROSPECTS FOR THE FUTURE

Plague has a long history of unpredicted emerging and reemerging epidemic activity. An important factor today in the epidemiology of plague is its entrenchment in natural rural cycles. In some areas, such as the western United States, plague's geographic range and ecological diversity has slowly expanded; in Indonesia and India, its range has retracted; in many other areas, it has remained stable. Plague's ability to adapt to changing environmental circumstances has created new risks for humans, such as those brought about by suburban development in the southwestern United States and irrigation of once-arid regions for agricultural development. For reasons not well understood, plague has disappeared from Europe and from many cities throughout the world where it once flourished in urban rat cycles, and urban plague outbreaks have been become rare events over the past 50 years. However, the reported outbreak of pneumonic plague in Surat, India, in 1994 and the recurring bubonic plague outbreaks in the port city of Mahajanga in Madagascar from 1991 to 1997 serve as warnings that must not be ignored or met with complacency.

## CONCLUSIONS

The ability to detect, monitor, and respond to plague is based on a solid public health infrastructure. This includes epidemiologic capabilities to detect clusters of new and unusual diseases and syndromes, the ability to identify and characterize infectious agents rapidly in the laboratory, the capacity to analyze and disseminate information promptly, and feedback mechanisms that trigger investigative and control responses. For plague, there must be strong vector and vertebrate host control programs that can quickly respond with operational efficiency. Many parts of the world today are vulnerable to human plague outbreaks because of an eroded and inadequate public health infrastructure; strengthening this infrastructure is a national and international responsibility. The U.S. Centers for Disease and Control Prevention (CDC) has developed a strategy to address emerging infectious disease threats that is both national and international in scope (8). The WHO plays a critical international role in plague surveillance and control, and there is a concerted effort to increase plague preparedness, including rebuilding of the network of WHO Collaborating Centers for Plague. The WHO and the CDC have recently supported regional and global workshops for laboratory diagnosis of plague and programs for improving and standardizing diagnostic methods, especially methods for rapid diagnosis under field conditions. In addition to routine laboratory studies, there is an important role for advanced genetic techniques to define the molecular epidemiology of plague and to detect and characterize newly evolving traits, such as virulence factors and factors associated with antimicrobial resistance. Finally, full advantage must be taken of the advancements in electronic communication, including Internet services linking surveillance, epidemiologic, and laboratory elements for rapid transmission of information nationally and globally on newly identified foci of infection, as well as characteristics of the strain of *Y. pestis* involved, epizootics and human plague outbreaks, and measures taken to prevent and control the disease.

## REFERENCES

1. **Barnes, A. M.** 1982. Surveillance and control of bubonic plague in the United States. *Symp. Zool. Soc. Lond.* **50:**237.
2. **Barnes, A.** 1990. Plague in the U.S.: present and future. *In Proceedings of the 14th Vertebrate Pest Conference.* University of California, Davis.
3. **Barnes, A. M., T. J. Quan, M. L. Beard, and G. O. Maupin.** 1998. Plague in American Indians, 1956–1987. CDC surveillance summaries (July 1988). *Morbid. Mortal. Weekly Rep.* **37**(55-3)**:**11–16.
4. **Campbell, G. L., and J. M. Hughes.** 1995. Plague in India: a new warning from an old nemesis. *Ann. Intern. Med.* **122:**151.
5. **Campbell, G. L., and D. T. Dennis.** 1997. Plague and other *Yersinia* infections, p. 975–983. *In* A. S. Fauci et al. (ed.), *Harrison's Principles of Internal Medicine*, 14th ed. McGraw Hill, New York, N.Y.
6. **Centers for Disease Control and Prevention.** 1992. Plague—United States, 1992. *Morbid. Mortal. Weekly Rep.* **41:**787–790.
7. **Centers for Disease Control and Prevention.** 1994. Human plague—United States, 1993–1994. *Morbid. Mortal. Weekly Rep.* **43:**242–246.
8. **Centers for Disease Control and Prevention.** 1994. *Addressing Emerging Infectious Diseases: A Prevention Strategy for the United States.* Centers for Disease Control and Prevention, Atlanta, Ga.
9. **Centers for Disease Control and Prevention.** 1997. Fatal human plague—Arizona and Colorado, 1996. *Morbid. Mortal. Weekly Rep.* **46:**617–620.
9a. **Centers for Disease Control and Prevention.** Unpublished data.
10. **Chanteau, S., L. Ratsifasoamanana, B. Rasoamanana, L. Rahalison, J. Randriambelosoa, J. Roux, and D. Rabeson.** 1998. Plague, a reemerging disease in Madagascar. *Emerg. Infect. Dis.* **4:**101–104.
11. **Craven, R. B., G. O. Maupin, M. L. Beard, T. J. Quan, and A. M. Barnes.** 1993. Reported cases of human plague infections in the United States, 1970–1991. *J. Med. Entomol.* **30:**758.
12. **Dennis, D. T.** 1994. Plague in India. *Br. Med. J.* **309:**893.

13. **Dennis, D. T., and K. Orloski.** 1996. Plague!, p. 160. *In 1996 Medical and Health Annual.* Encyclopaedia Britannica, Chicago, Ill.

14. **Dennis, D. T., and J. M. Hughes.** 1997. Multidrug resistance in plague. (Editorial.). *N. Engl. J. Med.* **337:**702–703.

15. **Devignat, R.** 1951. Variétés de l'espèce *Pastuerella pestis.* Nouvelle hypothese. *Bull. W. H. O.* **4:** 247.

16. **Eskey, C. R., and V. H. Haas.** 1940. Plague in the western part of the United States. *Public Health Bull.* **254:**1.

17. **Frean, J. A., L. Arntzen, T. Capper, A. Bryskier, and K. P. Klugman.** 1996. In vitro activities of 14 antibiotics against 100 human isolates of *Yersinia pestis* from a southern African plague focus. *Antimicrob. Agents. Chemother.* **40:**2646–2647.

18. **Gage, K. L.** 1998. Plague, p. 885–904. *In* L. Collier, A. Balows, M. Sussman, and W. L. Hausler (ed.), *Topley and Wilson's Microbiology and Microbial Infections,* 9th ed., vol. 3. *Bacterial Infections.* Edward Arnold, London, England.

19. **Galimand, M., A. Guiyole, G. Gerbaud, B. Rasoamanana, S. Chanteau, E. Carniel, and P. Courvalin.** 1997. Multidrug resistance in *Yersinia pestis* mediated by a transferable plasmid. *N. Engl. J. Med.* **337:**677–680.

20. **Guiyoule, A., F. Grimont, I. Iteman, P. A. D. Brimont, M. Lefevre, and E. Carniel.** 1994. Plague pandemics investigated by ribotyping of *Yersinia pestis* strains. *J. Clin. Microbiol.* **32:**634–641.

21. **Guiyoule, A., B. Rasoamanana, C. Buchrieser, P. Michel, S. Chanteau, and E. Carniel.** 1997. Recent emergence of new variants of *Yersinia pestis* in Madagascar. *J. Clin. Microbiol.* **35:**2826–2833.

22. **Hudson, B. W., M. I. Goldenberg, J. D. McCluskie, H. E. Larson, C. D. McGuire, A. M. Barnes, and J. D. Poland.** 1971. Serological and bacteriological investigations of an outbreak of plague in an urban tree squirrel population. *Am. J. Trop. Med. Hyg.* **20:**255–263.

23. **Institute of Medicine.** 1992. *Emerging Infections: Microbial Threats to Health in the United States.* National Academy Press, Washington, D.C.

24. **Kartman, L., M. I. Goldenberg, and W. T. Hubbert.** 1966. Recent observations on the epidemiology of plague in the United States. *Am. J. Public Health* **56:**1554.

25. **Kaufman, A. F., J. M. Mann, T. M. Gardiner, F. Heaton, J. D. Poland, A. M. Barnes, and G. O. Maupin.** 1981. Public health implications of plague in domestic cats. *J. Am. Vet. Med. Assoc.* **179:**875–878.

26. **Link, V. B.** 1955. *A History of Plague in the United States of America.* Public Health Monograph 26. U.S. Government Printing Office, Washington, D.C.

27. **Louis, J.** 1967. Sensibilité "in vitro" de *Yersinia pestis* a quelques antibiotiques et sulfanamides. *Med. Trop.* **27:**313–317.

28. **Mann, J. M., W. J. Martone, J. M. Boyce, A. F. Kaufman, A. M. Barnes, and N. S. Weber.** 1979. Endemic human plague in New Mexico: risk factors associated with infection. *J. Infect. Dis.* **140:**397.

29. **Marshall, J. D., D. V. Ouy, F. L. Gibson, T. C. Dung, and D. C. Cavanaugh.** 1977. Ecology of plague in Vietnam: commensal rodents and their fleas. *Mil. Med.* **132:**896–903.

30. **Perry, R. D., and J. D. Fetherston.** 1997. *Yersinia pestis*—etiologic agent of plague. *Clin. Microbiol. Rev.* **10:**35.

31. **Pollitzer, R.** 1954. *WHO Monograph Series 22:1. Plague.* World Health Organization, Geneva, Switzerland.

32. **Prater, S. H.** 1971. *The Book of Indian Mammals,* p. 203–205. Bombay Natural History Society, Bombay, India.

33. **Rasoamanana, B., P. Coulanges, P. Michel, and N. Rasolofonirina.** 1989. Sensibilité de *Yersinia pestis* aux antibiotiques: 277 souches isolées a Madagascar entre 1926 et 1989. *Arch. Inst. Pasteur Madagascar* **56:**37–53.

34. **Saxena, V. K., and T. Verghese.** 1990. Ecology of flea-transmitted zoonotic infection in village Mamla, District Beed. *Curr. Sci.* **71:**800–802.

35. **Schwann, T. G., D. Thompson, and B. C. Nelson.** 1985. Fleas on roof rats in six areas of Los Angeles County, California: their potential role in the transmission of plague and murine typhus in humans. *Am. J. Trop. Med. Hyg.* **34:**372–379.

36. **Vessereau, A.** 1988. Le règlement sanitaire international bilan et perspectives. *World Health Stat. Q.* **41:**37–45.
37. **World Health Organization.** 1983. *International Health Regulations (1969).* World Health Organization, Geneva, Switzerland.
38. **World Health Organization.** 1996. Human plague in 1994. *Weekly Epidemiol. Rec.* **22:**165.
39. **World Health Organization.** 1997. Human plague in 1995. *Weekly Epidemiol. Rec.* **46:**344–347.
40. **Wu Lien-Teh.** 1926. *A Treatise on Pneumonic Plague.* League of Nations Health Organization, Geneva, Switzerland.

*Emerging Infections 2*
Edited by W. M. Scheld, W. A. Craig, and J. M. Hughes
© 1998 ASM Press, Washington, D.C.

Chapter 10

# *Cyclospora:* Whence and Where to?

## David A. Relman

To the casual reader of the lay press and to the nonparasitologist, *Cyclospora* appears to have come "out of nowhere" (5). The organism, referred to by name, was first associated with human disease in 1993 (31). In the developed world, significant numbers of cases and major issues of public health first came to light in dramatic fashion during the summer of 1996. But when the story is examined in more detail, one finds that this organism is probably the same that masqueraded for nearly 15 years under a variety of false names and that the organism has probably infected a large number of humans in widespread regions of the world for a much longer period of time. These issues of microbial detection and identification, taxonomic assignment, and recognition of infection and clinical disease are critical to many "emerging" microbial pathogens. A discussion of this apparently changing *Cyclospora* dynamic teaches us about how we recognize and come to understand new microbial threats to our health.

### HISTORY: WHAT'S IN A NAME?

The organism that we now identify as *Cyclospora* in humans was probably first described by Ashford in 1979 (1). It was detected in fecal specimens from three unrelated individuals in Papua New Guinea (two of whom had diarrhea at the time) in the absence of any other known diarrheal disease agents. Ashford recognized the structures as coccidian oocysts but could not make a specific identification. Their size, general morphology, and internal structure suggested that they might be related to members of the *Isospora* genus. Morphology in situ, accompanied by only clinical findings, was insufficient for specific microbial identification.

Over the following 10 to 15 years, a number of independent observations and studies in diverse human populations and geographic settings suggested that these organisms were widely distributed around the globe and associated with both symptomatic and asymptomatic infection in humans (37, 41). With greater numbers of

---

***David A. Relman*** • Veterans Affairs Palo Alto Health Care System 154T, 3801 Miranda Ave. Palo Alto, CA 94304.

available organisms, a variety of staining and imaging procedures became more practical. Based upon size (8 to 10 $\mu$m in diameter) and shape and other features (spherical, refractile wall, internal granular material), the possibility of a fungal spore could not be ruled out (41). The variable reactivity of these coccidian-like organisms with modified acid-fast stains prompted comparisons with the *Cryptosporidium* genus (37), although the latter (4 to 6 $\mu$m in diameter) are one-half the size of the former. Electron microscopy revealed internal organelles that resembled the thylakoid photosynthesizing organelles of blue-green algae (20, 21). Pronounced bluish autofluorescence under UV illumination supported this comparison, as well as comparison to the cyanobacteria (6, 20, 21). Morphology and staining properties suggested a number of mutually inconsistent taxonomic assignments (Table 1).

Early observers of sporulation by this organism noted the similarity of the two internal sausage-shaped sporocysts to those of the isosporid coccidians (21). But it was not until 1993 that Ortega and colleagues reported the results of definitive sporulation and excystation experiments (two sporocysts per oocyst and two sporozoites per sporocyst) that permitted assignment of this organism to the *Cyclospora* genus; they proposed a new species designation, *Cyclospora cayetanensis* (28, 31). Despite its genus assignment, the evolutionary relationships of the human-associated *Cyclospora* were unclear at that time.

## PHYLOGENY AND BIOLOGY

Molecular, or sequence-based analysis, has proven particularly helpful in resolving relationships among the intestinal coccidians. Eimer first described cyclosporan organisms over a century ago, and their association with the "eimeriids" was tacitly assumed. In fact, phylogenetic analysis based upon 18S rDNA sequence comparisons indicates that the human-associated *Cyclospora* (*C. cayetanensis*) is more closely related to members of the *Eimeria* genus than to any other characterized organisms, and it is not closely related to *Cryptosporidium* (36). A more recent analysis with sequence data from additional *Eimeria* species suggests that this human-associated coccidian is as closely related to some *Eimeria* species as many *Eimeria* species are to each other (Fig. 1). The limited number of eimeriids from which 18S rDNA sequence is available restricts the types of statements one might make about relationships within this group of organisms, but it is safe to

**Table 1.** Designations previously given to the human-associated *Cyclospora*

| Designation | Yr | Reference(s) |
| --- | --- | --- |
| Coccidian related to *Isospora* | 1979 | 1 |
| Fungal spore | 1986 | 41 |
| Cyanobacterium-like body | 1990–1991 | 6, 21, 34, 37 |
| Blue-green alga | 1990–1991 | 6, 20, 37 |
| Large *Cryptosporidium* | 1991 | 37, 40, 44 |
| Coccidian-like body/organism | 1993 | 3, 14 |
| *Cyclospora cayetanensis* | 1993 | 28, 31 |

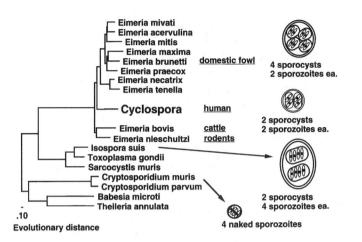

**Figure 1.** Evolutionary relationships of *Cyclospora*. The dendrogram was generated from 18S rDNA sequence analysis using parsimony methods. The hosts for the eimeriids are indicated to the right in underlined text. Morphologic features for some of the coccidians are shown in schematic form at the far right.

conclude that the human-associated *Cyclospora* shares a common ancestor with the *Eimeria* species. At the same time, the distinct oocyst morphologies and sporulation characteristics of these two genera together with the topology of currently established evolutionary trees argues for fragmentation of the *Eimeria* genus into at least three subgroups, with one of these defined by the human-associated *Cyclospora*. Interestingly, 18S rDNA sequence analysis predicts that the *Isospora* genus should not be grouped with *Eimeria* and *Cyclospora* and is more closely related to the family *Sarcocystidae*.

The *Eimeria* species are each restricted to either one or a few host species. In fact, speciation of these organisms often predicts a localized anatomic region of colonization within the host intestinal tract (2). The phylogenetic relationships between the human-associated *Cyclospora* and the *Eimeria* suggest that the former may also exhibit restricted host species range. So far, humans are the only known host for this organism. The eimerias and the human-associated cyclosporas, as well as *Cryptosporidium*, complete their life cycles within their respective hosts. All of the expected asexual and sexual stages for *Cyclospora* have been observed within intracytoplasmic parasitophorous vacuoles of small intestinal epithelial cells in infected patients (27, 29, 42). These forms resemble more closely the corresponding forms of *Isospora* development than those of *Cryptosporidium* (25). Unlike the oocysts of *Cryptosporidium*, *Cyclospora* oocysts are not immediately infective upon excretion by the human host; they require 7 to 10 days in the external environment before they become capable of causing infection.

## EPIDEMIOLOGY

Human cyclosporiasis is endemic in Southeast Asia, Central and South America, the Caribbean region, and parts of Africa. Infection is relatively more common among children than adults, and children are more likely to have symptoms when infected. Much of our understanding of *Cyclospora* epidemiology has been established by studies conducted in Peru and Nepal. In the region surrounding Lima, Peru, 1.1% of children less than 18 years of age are infected (24); there does not appear to be any gender predilection. The highest prevalence is found among children between the ages of 2 and 4 years. *Cyclospora* could not be detected in approximately 500 adults from the same region. Thirty-two percent of those infected were symptomatic; diarrhea lasted an average of 5 to 6 days in untreated children. In a study of Nepalese children with diarrhea, *Cyclospora* was detected in 12% of those between the ages of 18 and 60 months, as compared to 2% of the age-matched asymptomatic children and none of the symptomatic children less than 18 months old (12). In Guatemala, unpublished data indicate that approximately 3 to 4% of the general population is infected in some regions (4). Children between 18 and 48 months of age have the highest prevalence of infection.

The impression of investigators in these regions where *Cyclospora* is endemic is that age-dependent immunity may protect older children and adults from more severe disease (24). Thus, it is not surprising that immunologically naive adults, (travelers or foreign residents from zones where *Cyclospora* is not endemic) who visit or live in regions of endemicity are at much higher risk of developing symptomatic infections. Many of the first descriptions of *Cyclospora* were prompted by outbreaks or high rates of disease among these special subsets of the population (20, 34, 37). One study found *Cyclospora* in 1.1% of all travelers returning with diarrhea from developing countries (16). The disproportionate susceptibility of immunologically naive animals to *Eimeria*-associated disease (coccidiosis) is well-known (18, 19). Immunologically compromised hosts also appear to be at greater risk of disease from both *Cyclospora* and *Eimeria*, persons infected with human immunodeficiency virus (HIV) are well-represented among the reported cases of cyclosporiasis (10, 32).

Cyclosporiasis is seasonal. In Peru, infection is most common from December to May; in Guatemala and in Nepal, it is most frequent from May to August.

*Cyclospora* is transmitted from person to person via ingestion of contaminated water and food. Water has been a consistently identified risk factor for cyclosporiasis in most regions of the world where *Cyclospora* is endemic, although it has rarely been detected in the incriminated water supply (4, 14, 35). As noted below, raspberries have been an important vehicle for disease transmission to the United States. In a recently published investigation, a wide variety of vegetables and fruits from 13 markets in a periurban setting outside of Lima, Peru, were tested for *Cyclospora* (30). Of the 21 types tested, only lettuce and herbs were positive. *Cyclospora* may adhere tenaciously to vegetables and fruits, thereby thwarting attempts to wash the oocysts off these foods (30).

Widespread outbreaks of cyclosporiasis occurred throughout the United States and Canada in 1996 and 1997. Although they were unanticipated, perhaps their occurrence should not have been so surprising. During May and June 1996, 1,465 cases were reported; most of these cases were associated with ingestion of raspberries imported from Guatemala. The mechanism(s) by which these berries became contaminated remains unclear. One hypothesis holds that contaminated water was used to prepare insecticide or fungicide solutions that were then sprayed on the produce prior to harvesting. As noted above, this is the time of the year during which *Cyclospora* is most prevalent in Guatemala. At least as many cases of cyclosporiasis were reported in the United States and Canada in 1997 beginning in March. However, in 1997 the vehicles incriminated in transmission included mesclun lettuce (Florida, March and April), Guatemalan raspberries (United States, and Canada, April and May), and basil (Washington, D.C., July). The 1996 and 1997 outbreaks can be largely explained in the context of significant increases in importation of produce from regions of the world where *Cyclospora* is endemic. Nevertheless, some observations are less well understood. In 1990, an outbreak of cyclosporiasis occurred among immunocompetent individuals in a hospital dormitory in Chicago and was associated with ingestion of tap water (15). A separate but unrelated case occurred during the same period of time in the same region of Chicago (15). It is also curious that the patient reported by Hart in 1990 was from Chicago and became ill during the previous year (10). However, *Cyclospora* has not been definitely linked to a reservoir of the disease in the United States.

## CLINICAL MANIFESTATIONS, DETECTION, AND TREATMENT

The infectious dose of *Cyclospora* for humans is unknown. Estimates based upon well-characterized inocula in an epidemic setting indicate that as few as 10 to 100 oocysts may be sufficient. After an incubation period of 7 days on average, cyclosporiasis begins with a flu-like syndrome, followed by watery diarrhea, bloating, nausea, anorexia, and abdominal pain (Table 2) (11, 15, 29, 37). In contrast to cryptosporidiosis and other intestinal infections with similar features, cyclosporiasis in the immunologically naive host is frequently accompanied by profound fatigue and weight loss. The disease lasts for at least 1 to 2 weeks and often assumes a relapsing remitting course (15); in some studies, the median duration of illness is 6 to 7 weeks (14, 37). Cyclosporiasis is more severe in children and in immunocompromised hosts. In the individual infected with human immunodeficiency virus (HIV), cyclosporiasis is more prolonged. It relapses more often, results in greater weight loss, and sometimes involves the biliary tract (32, 38, 44). Disease is accompanied by villus blunting and intramucosal lymphocytic infiltrates. The clinical

**Table 2.** Clinical features of human cyclosporiasis[a]

| Sign or symptom | Frequency among patients (%) |
| --- | --- |
| Diarrhea | 99–100 |
| Weight loss | 81–96 |
| Anorexia | 48–93 |
| Fatigue | 90–92 |
| Abdominal pain | 71–76 |
| Vomiting | 22–29 |

[a]These features refer primarily to immunocompetent but naive individuals living in regions where the disease is not endemic and who develop symptomatic infection with *Cyclospora*. Infection among persons living in regions where the disease is endemic is most often asymptomatic or milder. Data are from references 11, 15, 29, and 37.

and histological findings are similar in general to those of coccidiosis in animals and birds.

The detection and diagnosis of *Cyclospora* infection have relied heavily upon light microscopic examination of stool specimens. Discontinuous Percoll gradient centrifugation, which facilitates purification and concentration of the oocysts, can be used in simple laboratory settings (26). Phase contrast or differential interference techniques may enhance the ability to discriminate true oocysts from other similar-appearing structures. Many investigators have emphasized the utility of epifluorescence microscopy for improving the detection of the autofluorescent *Cyclospora* oocysts in rapid screening of fecal samples (8). The modified Kinyoun's acid-fast stain, on the other hand, produces variable results with oocysts in fecal smears. More uniform staining of oocysts in fecal smears has been reported by subjecting the slide to microwave heating while immersed in 1% safranin solution, pH 6.5, followed by malachite green counterstain (43). Proper interpretation of an inspected smear requires experience; a pseudoepidemic of cyclosporiasis was attributed to misinterpretation of the microscopy findings (7). Molecular detection methods for *Cyclospora* based upon PCR offer significant theoretical advantages in terms of sensitivity and specificity (36); however, these methods have been hampered in practice by inhibitory factors in stool and inefficient DNA extraction (33).

Effective treatment for cyclosporiasis exists in the form of trimethoprim-sulfamethoxazole (13, 23, 24). A 7-day course of this antibiotic combination was shown in a placebo-controlled trial to reduce oocyst carriage in adults and lead to clinical improvement (13). This same combination is also effective in decreasing the duration of oocyst excretion in children (24). There are no known effective treatment alternatives for individuals who are intolerant of these drugs. Prevention of disease hinges on early detection of the organism, early recognition of disease clusters, improved safety measures within the food industry, and the potential use of food irradiation (17).

## FACTORS INVOLVED IN EMERGENCE

Increasing recognition or emergence of a microbial pathogen usually reflects an interplay between the genetic capabilities of a microorganism and the susceptibilities of a host, viewed within the context of societal and environmental factors. The sudden increase in recognized cases of cyclosporiasis in North America has its origins in some easily defined host and societal factors (Fig. 2). A dramatic increase in raspberry imports from Guatemala into North America during the 1990s played a considerable role in the 1996 and 1997 outbreaks. The coincident seasonality of berry export and endemic cyclosporiasis in Guatemala directly determined the timing of many of these cases. In addition, the susceptibility of previously unexposed but immunocompetent North Americans and the particular socioeconomic groups affected made these disease events more visible. The immunologically naive, i.e., travelers, foreign residents within regions of endemicity (14, 34, 37, 41), and the immunocompromised (10, 20), have dominated reports of clinical-evident disease. Many of the same issues explain the occurrence of coccidiosis: immunological naivete, crowding, and other forms of stress. In the case of *Cyclospora*, with rec-

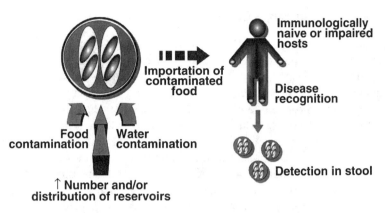

**Figure 2.** Factors involved in the emergence of *Cyclospora*.

ognition of the agent early in the course of events and the somewhat "exotic" nature of the organism, came enhanced disease awareness and improved surveillance. Methods for *Cyclospora* detection and identification were improved and disseminated after the first 1996 outbreaks. Detection certainly plays some part in the perception that cyclosporiasis is new to North America; some cases in past years are likely to have been missed or confused with other coccidians such as *Cryptosporidium*. However, there are potential additional factors concerning the microorganism that are more difficult to address.

We know very little about the natural reservoirs for the human-associated *Cyclospora* and the possibility that this organism may have recently expanded its niche in nature by adapting to new hosts. The host species specificity of the *Eimeria* suggests that humans may be the only (or major) reservoir for *C. cayetanensis*; however, there are reports in the literature that this same organism can be detected in poultry in Mexico and Peru (9, 45). The difficulty in species-specific identification of the eimeriids, in the absence of sequence information, renders interpretation of reports based on visual detection problematic. And the recent study by Ortega and colleagues raises questions about these reports since a thorough evaluation by this group of numerous species of animals, birds, and insects in the Lima environs found no evidence of *Cyclospora* (30). A publication in 1996 by Smith and colleagues again illustrates the problem of reliance on coccidian morphology for identification. They described finding oocysts in baboons and chimpanzees in Tanzania that were identical in appearance to *Cyclospora* oocysts found in humans (39). However, data based on 18S rDNA sequence analysis indicate that these baboon-associated organisms are not identical to the human-associated *Cyclospora* (22). The possibility of *Cyclospora* reservoirs in North America has not been ruled out. As discussed above, the group of cyclosporiasis cases in Chicago in 1989 and 1990 raise questions about the local water supply, birds, other animals, and the local ecosystem as a whole. Nevertheless, without a better understanding of where the human-associated *Cyclospora* is normally found in nature, it is difficult to determine whether there has been a change in the numbers and/or distribution of hosts and an increase in oocyst numbers within water and food sources.

## CONCLUSIONS AND DIRECTIONS FOR THE FUTURE

Questions have been raised about the natural ecology of *Cyclospora* and the pathogenicity of this organism. Two formal possibilities must be entertained: (i) that the human-associated *Cyclospora* isolates in current human circulation are more capable of causing disease than those that may have been present in the past and (ii) that *Cyclospora* has only recently "jumped species" (i.e., become introduced into humans, and without adequate adaptation). In order to address these issues we will need precise methods for "strain" identification. Although very reliable for taxonomic assignment at the genus and sometimes species levels, 18S rDNA sequence is not sufficiently variable to discriminate among strains. More variable genetic loci, such as the ribosomal RNA operon intergenic transcribed spacers, provide this degree of variability. With the ability to "fingerprint" *Cyclospora* strains will come the means to determine whether the population of extant *Cyclospora* strains is clonal, whether certain strains cause a disproportionate amount of human disease, and whether humans are sometimes infected with multiple strains. Outbreaks can then be associated with specific strains, and transmission patterns can be established. Ultimately, we will require a means of propagating the human-associated *Cyclospora*, a reliable and relevant disease model, and a system for genetic manipulation. The emergence of this particular organism has emphasized our state of relative ignorance, but at the same time, it has also revealed a number of important principles and a potentially exciting new biological system for further study.

### REFERENCES

1. **Ashford, R. W.** 1979. Occurrence of an undescribed coccidian in man in Papua New Guinea. *Ann. Trop. Med. Parasitol.* **73:**497–500.
2. **Barta, J. R., D. S. Martin, P. A. Liberator, M. Dashkevicz, J. W. Anderson, S. D. Feighner, A. Elbrecht, A. Perkins-Barrow, M. C. Jenkins, H. D. Danforth, M. D. Ruff, and H. Profous-Juchelka.** 1997. Phylogenetic relationships among eight *Eimeria* species infecting domestic fowl inferred using complete small subunit ribosomal DNA sequences. *J. Parasitol.* **83:**262–271.
3. **Bendall, R. P., S. Lucas, A. Moody, G. Tovey, and P. L. Chiodini.** 1993. Diarrhoea associated with cyanobacterium-like bodies: a new coccidian enteritis of man. *Lancet* 341:590–592.
4. **Bern, C., D. B. Hernandez, M. J. Arrowood, M. B. Lopez, A. M. De Merida, B. L. Herwaldt, and R. Klein.** 1998. Epidemiology of *Cyclospora cayetanensis* infection among outpatients in Guatemala, p. 47. *In International Conference on Emerging Infectious Diseases, Program & Abstracts Book.*
5. **Brown, J. W.** 1997. New and emerging pathogens—Part 8. From out of nowhere: *Cyclospora cayetanensis. Mlo. Med. Lab. Obs.* **29:**32–34.
6. **Centers for Disease Control and Prevention.** 1991. Outbreaks of diarrheal illness associated with cyanobacteria (blue-green algae)-like bodies—Chicago and Nepal, 1989 and 1990. *Morbid. Mortal. Weekly Rep.* **40:**325–327.
7. **Centers for Disease Control and Prevention.** 1997. Outbreaks of pseudo-infection with *Cyclospora* and *Cryptosporidium*—Florida and New York City, 1995. *Morbid. Mortal. Weekly Rep.* **46:**354–358.
8. **Eberhard, M. L., N. J. Pieniazek, and M. J. Arrowood.** 1997. Laboratory diagnosis of *Cyclospora* infections. *Arch. Pathol. Lab. Med.* **121:**792–797.
9. **Garcia-Lopez, H. L., L. E. Rodriguez-Tovar, and C. E. Medina-DelaGarza.** 1996. Identification of *Cyclospora* in poultry. *Emerg. Infect. Dis.* **2:**356–357. (Letter.)

10. **Hart, A. S., M. T. Ridinger, R. Soundarajan, C. S. Peters, A. L. Swiatlo, and F. E. Kocka.** 1990. Novel organism associated with chronic diarrhoea in AIDS. *Lancet* **335:**169–170. (Letter.)

11. **Herwaldt, B. L., and M. L. Ackers.** 1997. An outbreak in 1996 of cyclosporiasis associated with imported raspberries. The Cyclospora Working Group. *N. Engl. J. Med.* **336:**1548–1556.

12. **Hoge, C. W., P. Echeverria, R. Rajah, J. Jacobs, S. Malthouse, E. Chapman, L. M. Jimenez, and D. R. Shlim.** 1995. Prevalence of *Cyclospora* species and other enteric pathogens among children less than 5 years of age in Nepal. *J. Clin. Microbiol.* **33:**3058-3060.

13. **Hoge, C. W., D. R. Shlim, M. Ghimire, J. G. Rabold, P. Pandey, A. Walch, R. Rajah, P. Gaudio, and P. Echeverria.** 1995. Placebo-controlled trial of co-trimoxazole for cyclospora infections among travellers and foreign residents in Nepal. *Lancet* **345:**691–693.

14. **Hoge, C. W., D. R. Shlim, R. Rajah, J. Triplett, M. Shear, J. G. Rabold, and P. Echeverria.** 1993. Epidemiology of diarrhoeal illness associated with coccidian-like organism among travellers and foreign residents in Nepal. *Lancet* **341:**1175–1179.

15. **Huang, P., J. T. Weber, D. M. Sosin, P. M. Griffin, E. G. Long, J. J. Murphy, F. Kocka, C. Peters, and C. Kallick.** 1995. The first reported outbreak of diarrheal illness associated with *Cyclospora* in the United States. *Ann. Intern. Med.* **123:**409–414.

16. **Jelinek, T., M. Lotze, S. Eichenlaub, T. Loscher, and H. D. Nothdurft.** 1997. Prevalence of infection with *Cryptosporidium parvum* and *Cyclospora cayetanensis* among international travellers. *Gut* **41:**801–804.

17. **Jenkins, M. C., M. B. Chute, and H. D. Danforth.** 1997. Protection against coccidiosis in outbred chickens elicited by gamma-irradiated *Eimeria maxima*. *Avian. Dis.* **41:**702–708.

18. **Levine, N. D.** 1973. *Protozoan Parasites of Domestic Animals and of Man.* Burgess Publishing Co., Minneapolis, Minn.

19. **Lindsay, D. S., and K. S. J. Todd.** 1993. Coccidia of mammals, p. 89–131. *In* J. P. Kreier (ed.), *Parasitic Protozoa*. Academic Press, Inc., San Diego, Calif.

20. **Long, E. G., A. Ebrahimzadeh, E. H. White, B. Swisher, and C. S. Callaway.** 1990. Alga associated with diarrhea in patients with acquired immunodeficiency syndrome and in travelers. *J. Clin. Microbiol.* **28:**1101–1104.

21. **Long, E. G., E. H. White, W. W. Carmichael, P. M. Quinlisk, R. Raja, B. L. Swisher, H. Daugharty, and M. T. Cohen.** 1991. Morphologic and staining characteristics of a cyanobacterium-like organism associated with diarrhea. *J. Infect. Dis.* **164:**199–202.

22. **Lopez, F., J. Manglicmot, H. Smith, and D. A. Relman.** Unpublished data.

23. **Madico, G., R. H. Gilman, E. Miranda, L. Cabrera, and C. R. Sterling.** 1993. Treatment of cyclospora infections with co-trimoxazole. *Lancet* **342:**122–123. (Letter.)

24. **Madico, G., J. McDonald, R. H. Gilman, L. Cabrera, and C. R. Sterling.** 1997. Epidemiology and treatment of Cyclospora cayetanensis infection in Peruvian children. *Clin. Infect. Dis.* **24:**977–981.

25. **Marshall, M. M., D. Naumovitz, Y. Ortega, and C. R. Sterling.** 1997. Waterborne protozoan pathogens. *Clin. Microbiol. Rev.* **10:**67–85.

26. **Medina-De La Garza, C. E., H. L. Garcia-Lopez, M. C. Salinas-Carmona, and D. J. Gonzalez-Spencer.** 1997. Use of discontinuous Percoll gradients to isolate *Cyclospora* oocysts. *Ann. Trop. Med. Parasitol.* **91:**319–321.

27. **Nhieu, J. T., F. Nin, J. Fleury-Feith, M. T. Chaumette, A. Schaeffer, and S. Bretagne.** 1996. Identification of intracellular stages of *Cyclospora* species by light microscopy of thick sections using hematoxylin. *Hum. Pathol.* **27:**1107–1109.

28. **Ortega, Y. R., R. H. Gilman, and C. R. Sterling.** 1994. A new coccidian parasite (Apicomplexa: Eimeriidae) from humans. *J. Parasitol.* **80:**625–629.

29. **Ortega, Y. R., R. Nagle, R. H. Gilman, J. Watanabe, J. Miyagui, H. Quispe, P. Kanagusuku, C. Roxas, and C. R. Sterling.** 1997. Pathologic and clinical findings in patients with cyclosporiasis and a description of intracellular parasite life-cycle stages. *J. Infect. Dis.* **176:**1584–1589.

30. **Ortega, Y. R., C. R. Roxas, R. H. Gilman, N. J. Miller, L. Cabrera, C. Taquiri, and C. R. Sterling.** 1997. Isolation of *Cryptosporidium parvum* and *Cyclospora cayetanensis* from vegetables collected in markets of an endemic region in Peru. *Am. J. Trop. Med. Hyg.* **57:**683–686.

31. **Ortega, Y. R., C. R. Sterling, R. H. Gilman, V. A. Cama, and F. Diaz.** 1993. *Cyclospora* species—a new protozoan pathogen of humans. *N. Engl. J. Med.* **328:**1308–1312.

32. **Pape, J. W., R. I. Verdier, M. Boncy, J. Boncy, and W. D. J. Johnson.** 1994. *Cyclospora* infection in adults infected with HIV: Clinical manifestations, treatment, and prophylaxis. *Ann. Intern. Med.* **121:**654–657.

33. **Pieniazek, N. J., S. B. Slemenda, A. J. da Silva, E. M. Alfano, and M. J. Arrowood.** 1996. PCR confirmation of infection with *Cyclospora cayetanensis. Emerg. Infect. Dis.* **2:**357–359. (Letter.)

34. **Pollok, R. C., R. P. Bendall, A. Moody, P. L. Chiodini, and D. R. Churchill.** 1992. Traveller's diarrhoea associated with cyanobacterium-like bodies. *Lancet* **340:**556–557. (Letter.)

35. **Rabold, J. G., C. W. Hoge, D. R. Shlim, C. Kefford, R. Rajah, and P. Echeverria.** 1994. *Cyclospora* outbreak associated with chlorinated drinking water. *Lancet* **344:**1360–1361. (Letter.)

36. **Relman, D. A., T. M. Schmidt, A. Gajadhar, M. Sogin, J. Cross, K. Yoder, O. Sethabutr, and P. Echeverria.** 1996. Molecular phylogenetic analysis of *Cyclospora*, the human intestinal pathogen, suggests that it is closely related to *Eimeria* species. *J. Infect. Dis.* **173:**440–445.

37. **Shlim, D. R., M. T. Cohen, M. Eaton, R. Rajah, E. G. Long, and B. L. Ungar.** 1991. An alga-like organism associated with an outbreak of prolonged diarrhea among foreigners in Nepal. *Am. J. Trop. Med. Hyg.* **45:**383–389.

38. **Sifuentes-Osornio, J., G. Porras-Cortes, R. P. Bendall, F. Morales-Villarreal, G. Reyes-Teran, and G. M. Ruiz-Palacios.** 1995. *Cyclospora cayetanensis* infection in patients with and without AIDS: biliary disease as another clinical manifestation. *Clin. Infect. Dis.* **21:**1092–1097.

39. **Smith, H. V., C. A. Paton, R. W. Girdwood, and M. M. Mtambo.** 1996. *Cyclospora* in non-human primates in Gombe, Tanzania. *Vet. Rec.* **138:**528. (Letter.)

40. **Soave, R.** 1996. *Cyclospora:* an overview. *Clin. Infect. Dis.* **23:**429–435.

41. **Soave, R., J. P. Dubey, L. J. Ramos, and M. Tummings.** 1986. A new intestinal pathogen? *Clin. Res.* **34:**533A. (Abstract.)

42. **Sun, T., C. F. Ilardi, D. Asnis, A. R. Bresciani, S. Goldenberg, B. Roberts, and S. Teichberg.** 1996. Light and electron microscopic identification of *Cyclospora* species in the small intestine. Evidence of the presence of asexual life cycle in human host. *Am. J. Clin. Pathol.* **105:**216–220.

43. **Visvesvara, G. S., H. Moura, E. Kovacs-Nace, S. Wallace, and M. L. Eberhard.** 1997. Uniform staining of *Cyclospora* oocysts in fecal smears by a modified safranin technique with microwave heating. *J. Clin. Microbiol.* **35:**730–733.

44. **Wurtz, R. M., F. E. Kocka, C. S. Peters, C. M. Weldon-Linne, A. Kuritza, and P. Yungbluth.** 1993. Clinical characteristics of seven cases of diarrhea associated with a novel acid-fast organism in the stool. *Clin. Infect. Dis.* **16:**136–138.

45. **Zerpa, R., N. Uchima, and L. Huicho.** 1995. *Cyclospora cayetanensis* associated with watery diarrhoea in Peruvian patients. *J. Trop. Med. Hyg.* **98:**325–329.

*Chapter 11*

# The Resurgence of Malaria

## Yao-Lung Tsai and Donald J. Krogstad

### OVERVIEW

In contrast to most resurgent diseases, malaria has been known for millennia (42). Today the life cycle of the parasite is understood, the parasite can be grown in vitro, and the molecular basis of its antigenic variation has been clarified (79, 107). Despite these advances and a worldwide malaria eradication campaign that began in the 1950s and continued for more than 20 years (13), the malaria situation is worsening (54, 97). There are now more than 300 to 500 million cases of malaria worldwide, 1 to 2 million children die from malaria each year (124), and drug resistance is increasing (21, 62).

Although the recent experience with bednets has been encouraging (24), there are at least six factors that interfere with effective malaria control: (i) the lack of effective (sterile) immunity among repetitively exposed humans (43, 50), (ii) the lack of recombinant parasite antigens which protect and provide boosting with natural reexposure as well as an inadequate number of adjuvants available for human use (23), (iii) inadequate information about the pathogenesis of severe malaria (66, 73), (iv) inadequate information about the basis of antimalarial resistance (56, 100), (v) the paucity of effective new antimalarials (55), and (vi) the limited number of interventions that reduce transmission under field conditions, such as insecticide-impregnated bednets (24). The major successes of the malaria eradication campaign were in isolated (island) locations such as Madagascar (77), and in areas of North America, Europe, Asia, and Latin America where development had a major impact because of better housing and greater access to medical care (83). Although the malaria eradication campaign did not eradicate malaria, it did substantially reduce the number of countries where malaria is endemic (104). These changes and the changes produced by increasing drug resistance have fundamentally altered the epidemiology of malaria. As a result, the epidemiology of resurgent malaria is qualitatively different from the previous epidemiology of malaria (10, 52, 64). This is because resurgent malaria affects not only the semi-immune resident

*Yao-Lung Tsai and Donald J. Krogstad* • Department of Tropical Medicine, Tulane School of Public Health and Tropical Medicine, New Orleans, LA 70112.

populations of Asia, Latin America, and sub-Saharan Africa, but also nonimmune adults and children driven by civil strife, famine, and other emergencies from areas without transmission to areas with transmission in Somalia, Eritrea, Rwanda, Burundi, Cambodia, Thailand, Vietnam and elsewhere (4, 6, 16, 61, 65, 86, 89, 92, 114, 117, 120). Despite these changes, persistent transmission in sub-Saharan Africa, Asia, and Latin America continues to account for the majority of the world's cases. Thus, changes in the global epidemiology of malaria are linked not only to traditional (established) factors such as distribution of suitable anopheline vectors but also to civil strife and the movement of refugees, which have rarely been recognized as important factors in the epidemiology of malaria in the past.

## INTRODUCTION

Malaria has been a threat to human health since prehistoric times (14). Its clinical features have been described in both the ancient and the recent literature. Malaria has played a decisive role in the outcome of military conflicts from the time of Hannibal's invasion of Europe 2000 years ago to more recent conflicts in Vietnam and Somalia (34). However, until the early 20th century, malaria was known only by its symptoms and signs. In this century, there have been three major stages in our understanding of malaria: (i) a period of discovery, beginning in the late 19th century, which defined the parasite life cycle and identified the parasites that infect humans; (ii) a worldwide malaria eradication program, based on massive use of chloroquine (CQ) and DDT, which began in the 1950s and continued for 20 years until it was acknowledged as a failure in the 1970s (14); and (iii) an era of active scientific investigation that began with development of the in vitro culture system for *Plasmodium falciparum* (112) and permitted the application of advances in molecular biology, cell biology, and immunology to malaria in the 1980s and 1990s (96).

This chapter begins by reviewing these three stages in our understanding of malaria. It then examines the biologic and public health reasons that malaria remains a major problem in Southeast Asia, South America, and sub-Saharan Africa at a time when it has been possible to eradicate or control smallpox (32, 33, 41), polio (27, 30, 36, 47, 78, 81, 85), yellow fever (18, 35, 74, 94), and guinea worm (dracunculiasis) (45). The chapter then concludes by examining the global impact of increasing resistance to antimalarials and by highlighting recent work which may permit the development of long-term strategies for successful malaria control.

### The Late 19th and Early 20th Centuries: Initial Discovery of the Parasite Life Cycle

Although malaria was known as a syndrome with fever and chills (see above), its cause was a matter of debate until the pioneering studies of Ross and Laveran, who identified parasites in the blood of symptomatic patients (Laveran) and in the salivary glands of mosquitoes (Ross). For these discoveries, they received the Nobel Prize in 1902 and 1907, respectively. Subsequently, a number of investigators have identified parasites in anopheline mosquitoes. Of the approximately 500 known anophelines, only 45 to 50 have been shown to function as malaria vectors (8). In the late 1940s, Shortt and his colleagues completed our understanding of the parasite life cycle by identifying the initial exo-erythrocytic stage of the parasite in the liver (98) (Fig. 1).

## Present-Day Understanding of the Parasite Life Cycle

More recently, Krotoski et al. identified a dormant parasite form (the hypnozoite) in the liver of subjects with relapsing malarias such as *Plasmodium vivax* (59). Thus, our present understanding of the parasite life cycle is that natural transmission is based on the sporozoite, which is injected under the epidermis by female anophelines as they probe prior to feeding. Once in the circulation, sporozoites adhere to the surface of hepatocytes in the liver, enter the hepatocyte, and then either mature to tissue schizonts or remain dormant as hypnozoites. Tissue schizonts in the liver release 10,000 to 30,000 merozoites between 8 and 25 days after the initial sporozoite infection depending on the species. Each merozoite is capable of infecting a red blood cell (RBC) and initiating a new cycle of asexual replication. Within the RBC, asexual replication typically produces from 16 to 32 merozoites 48 to 72 hours later. These merozoites then rupture (lyse) the host RBC and enter the bloodstream to infect other RBCs. In addition, some intraerythrocytic parasites differentiate to sexual stage parasites (gametocytes) rather than asexual forms (merozoites). Important unresolved issues include the factors that stimulate the sexual differentiation necessary for transmission from humans to mosquitoes. From the genetic perspective, the parasite is haploid for the majority of its life cycle. It is transiently diploid in the mosquito after the male and female gametes unite to form a zygote. However, shortly after that fertilization, the diploid zygote undergoes a meiotic reduction division and transforms to an ookinete, which ultimately yields the haploid sporozoites that migrate to the mosquito salivary gland and complete the life cycle by reinfecting humans.

## The Rationale for Malaria Eradication

When the malaria eradication campaign was begun in the 1950s (11, 14), smallpox eradication had not even been considered. Thus the rationales that were used for smallpox eradication and have since been used to plan the eradication of other diseases (Table 1) were not available. The approach to malaria eradication was based almost entirely on the use of two drugs: (i) chloroquine to eliminate human bloodstream infection (parasitemia), thus preventing human disease due to malaria and reinfection of the anopheline mosquito pool (transmission); and (ii) a residual insecticide (DDT [dichlorodiphenyltrichloroethane]) to kill anopheline mosquitoes as they rested under the eaves of houses after obtaining their blood meal from persons sleeping in those houses.

## The Failure of Malaria Eradication

In fact, chloroquine was added to table salt in both South America and Southeast Asia at a concentration thought sufficient to provide effective chemoprophylaxis

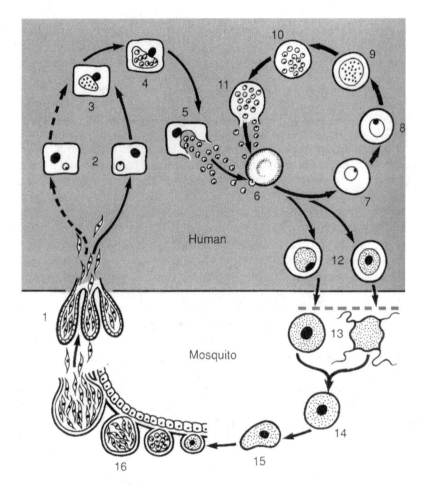

**Figure 1.** Malaria parasite life cycle. Sporozoites released from the salivary gland of the female anopheles mosquito are injected under the skin when the mosquito bites a human (step 1). They then travel through the bloodstream to the liver and enter hepatocytes (2). Within hepatocytes, parasites mature to tissue schizonts (4). They are then released into the bloodstream as merozoites (5) and produce symptomatic infection as they invade and destroy RBCs (6 to 11). However, some parasites remain dormant in the liver as hypnozoites (2, dashed line from 1 to 3). These parasites (in *P. vivax* and *P. ovale* infections) cause relapsing malaria when they mature and produce merozoites 6 to 11 months or more later. Once within the bloodstream, merozoites (5) invade RBCs (6), and mature to ring (7, 8), trophozoite (9) and schizont (10) asexual-stage parasites. Schizonts lyse their host RBCs as they complete their maturation and release the next generation of merozoites (11), which then invade previously uninfected RBCs. Within RBCs, some parasites differentiate to sexual forms (male and female gametocytes) (12). When gametocytes are taken up by a female anopheles mosquito, the male gametocyte loses its flagellum to produce male gametes which fertilize the female gamete (13) to produce a zygote (14). The zygote invades the gut of the mosquito (15) and develops into an oocyst (16). Mature oocysts produce sporozoites, which migrate to the salivary gland of the mosquito (1) and repeat the cycle. The dashed line between 12 and 13 indicates that absence of the mosquito vector precludes natural (mosquito-borne) transmission via this cycle. Note, however, that the injection of infected blood bypasses this constraint and permits transmission among intravenous drug addicts and to persons who receive blood transfusions from infected donors. (Reproduced from reference 53a with permission from Williams and Wilkins.)

**Table 1.** Criteria that favor disease eradication relative to malaria

| Criteria that favor eradicability | Malaria |
| --- | --- |
| Sterile immunity after natural infection......... | No; repetitive reinfection is common |
| Effective vaccine available.................... | No effective vaccine is available at present |
| Characteristic (typical) clinical presentation ..... | Anomalous presentations are common, especially among semi-immune residents of areas of endemicity and persons on chemoprophylaxis |
| No evidence for subclinical illness............. | Subclinical illness is common among semi-immune residents of areas of endemicity and among persons on chemoprophylaxis |
| No nonhuman (vertebrate) reservoir of infection | No nonhuman vertebrate reservoirs are known for *P. falciparum, P. vivax, P. ovale* or *P. malariae* |
| Transmission only from human to human....... | No; transmission is typically vector borne by infection of anopheline mosquitoes from one infected person and transmission to another at least 8 to 10 days later |
| Homogeneity among strains.................. | Marked heterogeneity, especially in *P. falciparum* |
| Drug susceptibility ......................... | No; drug resistance is a major problem |

based on the average consumption of table salt. Perhaps because of the selective pressure exerted by the addition of chloroquine to table salt (87, 88), chloroquine resistance emerged in the late 1950s and early 1960s in both South America and Southeast Asia (40, 76). Likewise, DDT was sprayed extensively under the eaves of houses in South America and Southeast Asia. Subsequently, DDT resistance appeared in the 1960s and became established in South America, Southeast Asia, and parts of Africa by the 1970s (21, 87, 108). The extensive use of chloroquine and DDT selected for the chloroquine-resistant parasites and DDT-resistant mosquitoes, which were ultimately the reason for the failure of malaria eradication in South America and Southeast Asia. In addition, the malaria eradication campaign formulated by the World Bank and the World Health Organization did not include sub-Saharan Africa (14). Thus, the malaria eradication campaign did not even consider the continent with the most intense malaria transmission and the greatest morbidity and mortality.

Despite its shortcomings, the malaria eradication campaign had important positive effects. It accelerated the eradication of malaria in the United States and Europe and in parts of the Near East and the Far East (19, 84, 104). It also temporarily eradicated malaria from islands such as Madagascar and Sardinia (28, 70, 77, 99) and almost eradicated malaria from Sri Lanka (12, 99). Unfortunately, the resurgence of malaria was observed first in these tropical island environments, where it rapidly became apparent that the reintroduction of malaria could produce enormous morbidity and mortality (77). As a result of this experience, most malaria control programs are now extremely concerned about the risk of subsequent resurgence, after reducing transmission with control programs.

## Recent Scientific Advances

### In Vitro Culture

In malaria, the most important scientific advance in the past 30 years has been development of the in vitro culture system for *P. falciparum* (112). This system has been used by hundreds (perhaps thousands) of investigators to study *P. falciparum* parasites from all areas of endemicity and has been adapted to permit the growth and study of *P. vivax* (75), *P. knowlesi* (15, 121), *P. coatneyi* (111), *P. fragile*, and other human and nonhuman primate malaria parasites. Without this system, the molecular biology of the parasite would never have been dissected as it has been during the past 10 to 15 years.

### Receptor-Ligand Relationships Involved in Parasite Invasion of the Hepatocyte and the RBC

For example, sporozoite entry into the hepatocyte results from a receptor-ligand interaction in which region II of circumsporozoite protein (CSP) on the parasite surface is the ligand and binds to heparan sulfate glycoproteins and low-density lipoprotein receptor on the hepatocyte surface (17, 95). Likewise, after merozoites are released from the liver, they bind to molecules on the RBC surface which function as receptors for RBC invasion (Table 2).

### Receptor-Ligand Relationships Involved in Cytoadherence to the Microvascular Endothelium

Unlike the receptor-ligand relationships involved in parasite entry into mammalian cells (which are generalizable to all malaria parasites), cytoadherence to the peripheral microvascular endothelium occurs only with *P. falciparum* (20, 73) and is mediated by a family of variable (*var*) genes which contain conserved sequences responsible for binding to receptors on the endothelial surface and variable sequences responsible for evasion of the host immune response (107).

### Immune Responses to Plasmodial Infection

As with other pathogens, infected humans produce both humoral and cellular responses to plasmodial infection. These responses include antibodies directed

**Table 2.** Ligands and receptors involved in parasite entry and cytoadherence in humans

| Parasite stage | Species | Parasite ligand | Human cell type | Receptor(s) |
|---|---|---|---|---|
| Sporozoite | *P. falciparum* | CSP | Hepatocyte | Heparan sulfate proteoglycan, low-density lipoprotein receptor |
| Merozoite | *P. falciparum* | EBA-175 | RBC | Glycophorin A |
| Merozoite | *P. vivax* | Duffy-binding protein | RBC | Duffy factor |
| Merozoite | *P. vivax* | Reticulocyte-binding protein | RBC (reticulocytes) | Protein on reticulocyte surface |
| Parasitized RBC | *P. falciparum* | PfEMP1 | Endothelial cells | Intercellular adhesion molecule 1, CD36, endothelial leukocyte adhesion molecule, thrombospondin, vascular cell adhesion molecule 1 |

against surface determinants such as CSP on the sporozoite (44); merozoite surface protein 1 (MSP-1) (2), merozoite surface protein 2 (MSP-2) (1), apical merozoite antigen 1 (AMA-1) (68), and rhoptry-associated protein 1 (RAP-1) (48, 106) on the merozoite; and 25- and 230-kDa antigens on the surface of the gametocyte (51, 122). They also include cell-mediated responses directed against such antigens as measured by [$^3$H]thymidine incorporation, cytokine production, the production of cytokine mRNA, and the production of intermediates such as nitric oxide (3, 31, 46, 60, 93).

## FACTORS THAT PREVENT EFFECTIVE MALARIA CONTROL

### Lack of Sterile Immunity among Repetitively Exposed Humans

Unlike other tropical infectious diseases, recovery from natural malaria infection does not protect against subsequent reinfection. As noted above, this is not because there is no immune response. A number of investigators have demonstrated vigorous humoral and cellular responses to plasmodial infection in humans (115). However, those responses do not provide sterile immunity. For example, antibodies directed against the dominant antigen on the sporozoite surface (CSP) do not prevent reinfection with sporozoites bearing the same dominant repetitive antigen (44). This is a problem from both the public health perspective and the investigational perspective. From the public health perspective, it means that the burden of infection and reinfection is enormous and is an issue for all age groups in the population. From the investigational perspective, it means that there is no model of sterile immunity in humans (i.e., there is no model to study for the development of a vaccine).

### Lack of Recombinant Antigens That Elicit Boosting with Natural Reinfection and Inadequate Number of Adjuvants Available for Human Use

Because the persons at greatest risk of complications and death are young children, most investigators expect that the initial immune responses elicited will be suboptimal. In addition, because the costs of vaccine delivery are substantial (even for vaccines that do not require a cold chain), the ideal malaria vaccine should require only one administration and should then be boosted subsequently by natural reinfection (50). Thus the intense transmission in areas such as sub-Saharan Africa would in fact increase the efficacy of the vaccine. A second important and unsolved problem is the limited number of adjuvants available for human use. Although the adjuvant often has an important role in driving the host immune response (25), alum (aluminum hydroxide) remains the only adjuvant approved for human use (23). Alternative adjuvants such as modified endotoxin (29) are safe in humans and have recently been shown to be effective with a wide variety of antigens (82). They represent a potentially exciting and novel approach to this problem. This view is also consistent with recent experience using another adjuvant, which may elicit protective immune responses to CSP fused with hepatitis B surface antigen (105).

## Inadequate Understanding of the Pathogenesis of Severe Malaria

The goal of most investigators is to prevent severe and cerebral malaria by immunization or to treat those at risk sufficiently early to prevent complications and death. However, there is a fundamental problem with the approaches that have been used in the laboratory. Although their goal is to prevent severe disease, the in vitro and in vivo studies performed typically assess the prevention of infection, not disease. This conundrum is compounded by the fact that we simply do not understand why one child develops life-threatening complications while another child with a similar parasitemia remains well and continues to play with friends despite a similar parasitemia (66, 67, 73). This basic ignorance is at the heart of the problem. Until we understand why one child is at risk of severe disease and another is not, we are unlikely to develop an effective malaria vaccine to prevent life-threatening complications such as cerebral malaria. Indeed, if cerebral malaria in part represents an excessive immune response to the parasite (consistent with the elevated TNF-$\alpha$ levels that are observed in severe malaria) (38, 39), it is possible that some vaccine constructs could actually increase the incidence of complications such as cerebral malaria.

## Insufficient Information about the Basis of Antimalarial Resistance

At least four important groups of antimalarials are in use today: (i) aminoquinolines such as CQ (to which there is now widespread resistance), with analogs such as mefloquine and halofantrine that are active against many CQ-resistant *P. falciparum* (110, 113); (ii) cinchona alkaloids such as quinine and quinidine, which are active against most CQ-resistant *P. falciparum*; (iii) antifolates such as pyrimethamine and sulfadoxine, which are now inactive against many CQ-resistant strains of *P. falciparum* (80, 123); and (iv) artemisinin compounds, which are active against most CQ-resistant *P. falciparum* (49). It should be possible to design alternative antimalarials which retain the biologic (antiplasmodial) activity of the original compounds and are also active against otherwise resistant parasites if enough is known about the basis of their antimalarial resistance (26).

## Mechanism of Resistance to AQs

### CQ

Although CQ resistance has been established in *P. falciparum* for more than 30 years, the mechanism(s) responsible for CQ resistance remains controversial. There is, however, general agreement that there are multiple potential sites of CQ action within the parasite food vacuole (heme polymerase activity, aspartic and cysteine proteases [plasmepsins, falcipain], intravesicular pH) (100, 109), that CQ resistance involves decreased CQ accumulation within the food vacuole (and may involve active CQ efflux) (7, 9, 119), and that there is no evidence of CQ inactivation by resistant parasites (37). Despite the lack of consensus about the mechanism of CQ resistance, it has recently been possible to develop a series of 4-aminoquinolines (4-AQs) which are active against CQ-resistant *P. falciparum* (26).

## Mefloquine and Halofantrine

Mefloquine and halofantrine are quinoline methanols active against most CQ-resistant *P. falciparum* (110, 113). Although they both produce morphologic changes in the parasite food vacuole (as does CQ), the mechanism(s) by which they inhibit parasite growth is unclear. Likewise, the mechanism(s) responsible for resistance to mefloquine and halofantrine are undefined. However, the fact that mefloquine-resistant parasites are also resistant to halofantrine (22) suggests that they may share a similar mechanism of resistance.

## Quinine and Quinidine

Quinine and quinidine are cinchona alkaloids which are also active against most CQ-resistant *P. falciparum* (63). Because they inhibit heme polymerase activity in vitro (101), it is thought that they also act on the parasite food vacuole. However, the mechanism(s) responsible for quinine and quinidine resistance is undefined.

## Antifolates

Antifolates have been important drugs for the prevention and treatment of malaria. These include both sulfonamides (which inhibit dihydropteroate synthase) and pyrimethamine and cycloguanil (which inhibit dihydrofolate reductase) (53). Studies by several investigators have shown that resistant parasites contain point mutations in these enzymes (90) and suggest that altered transport may also play a role in sulfonamide resistance (118). Unfortunately, although the mechanism of resistance has been defined at the molecular level, new compounds which take advantage of this information have not yet been developed.

## Artemisinin

Artemisinin compounds act against the parasite by binding to heme and releasing free radicals that alkylate parasite proteins (5). The work of Meshnick and his colleagues suggests that the unstable endoperoxide bridge of artemisinin is essential for drug action (72). Analogs in which the endoperoxide linkage has been replaced by an ether linkage are biologically inactive. Although resistance may become a problem, the initial problem has been recrudescences, which can be prevented by adding a longer-acting compound such as mefloquine (49, 116).

## Paucity of Effective New Antimalarials

Although a malaria vaccine is the ultimate goal, most investigators expect that 10 to 20 years are likely to pass before that goal is realized. Therefore, the development of new antimalarials effective against multiply resistant parasites is an important interim goal to reduce the annual toll of deaths and complications from malaria. Barriers to the development of new antimalarials include insufficient information about mechanisms of resistance (above), but they also include the lack of financial incentives for pharmaceutical companies which view such drugs as loss leaders. Although there are important economically viable markets in a number of countries where malaria is endemic, such as China, India, Kenya, Nigeria, Colombia, and Brazil (55), the industry perspective is not likely to change in the short term. Therefore, in the short term, it may be necessary to rely primarily on strategies such as the Product Development Programme of the World Health Organization and the Drug Development Program of the National Institute of Allergy and Infectious Diseases, which was developed to provide AIDS drugs but has been made available for the synthesis and preclinical testing of promising antimalarials developed by investigators funded by the National Institutes of Health (NIH).

## Limited Number of Strategies To Reduce Transmission under Field Conditions

Vector eradication has been particularly effective when the vector was not indigenous (e.g., eradication of *Anopheles gambiae* in Brazil and Egypt) (84, 102). However, it is not a practical alternative in sub-Saharan Africa or in most malarious areas of Latin America and Southeast Asia because those vectors typically breed in microhabitats (Africa) or in forested or grassland areas (Latin America and southeast Asia). The most promising approach at the present time is the use of bednets impregnated with permethrin insecticides. When used properly, insecticide-impregnated bednets may reduce the entomologic inoculation rate by ≥90% and the prevalence of infection by more than 50%. However, their impact on disease has been less clear. It has been less in areas with the most intense transmission (24) and had no impact on the incidence of severe disease in one study (71). In addition, the effectiveness of permethrin insecticides may be compromised by their extensive agricultural use in the same or nearby communities. Although they have been shown to reduce the entomologic inoculation rate, insecticide-impregnated bednets remain an experimental strategy for the reduction of severe disease.

## GLOBAL IMPACT OF ANTIMALARIAL RESISTANCE

Antimalarial resistance has had a devastating impact on malaria control (55). Because of CQ resistance, residents of areas of endemicity no longer have effective treatment available to them at a price that they can afford. Although pyrimethamine-sulfadoxine (Fansidar) is relatively economical, experience in Malawi suggests that resistance develops within 2 to 3 years of widespread use as a first-line drug (91). Thus, most of the drugs that remain are beyond the resources of the people who live in malarious areas. Economically feasible alternatives include AQs effective against CQ-resistant *P. falciparum* in vitro and in vivo (26), the addition of antihistamines to CQ to inhibit the efflux process and thus enhance CQ accumulation and CQ activity (103), and the use of production facilities in developing nations for more economical synthesis of CQ, other AQs, artemisinin, and other antimalarials.

## DEVELOPMENTS THAT MAY PERMIT SUCCESSFUL MALARIA CONTROL

As in North America, Europe, and the malaria-free regions of Asia, economic development is likely to play an important role in the control and ultimate eradication of malaria from Southeast Asia, Latin America, and sub-Saharan Africa

**Table 3.** Global heterogeneity of malaria

| Region | Drug resistance | Intensity of transmission |
|---|---|---|
| South America | CQ, pyrimethamine-sulfadoxine (Fansidar) | Varying |
| Africa | CQ | High |
| Southeast Asia | High-level multidrug | Low |

(Table 3). Even in the absence of scientific progress, it is likely that the prevalence of malaria in Southeast Asia will be greatly reduced in 10 to 15 years by reduction or elimination of the forest habitat of the principal vector, *Anopheles dirus*. In contrast, major scientific progress will be necessary to reduce the prevalence of malaria in rural Africa within the next 10 to 15 years. Feasible scientific advances include the development of new antimalarials, especially practical trials with existing drugs or analogs (AQ analogs, CQ plus antihistamines) (26, 103), testing of candidate vaccines using proxy immunologic or molecular markers (69) to reduce the need for expensive studies with large numbers of subjects, and novel strategies such as new adjuvants (23, 29) and transmission-blocking vaccines (51, 122).

## CONCLUSIONS

The reduction of malaria complications and deaths in the near future is likely to depend most heavily on the development of economical antimalarials which are effective against CQ-resistant and multiply resistant *P. falciparum*. Although insecticide-impregnated bednets reduce the incidence of infection, their effect on mortality is less clear (24). Therefore, the resurgence of malaria (Table 4) is likely to continue for at least the next 3 to 5 years. Conversely, the development of effective immunization strategies, which may require another 10 to 15 years, holds long-term promise for malaria control, especially if antigen-adjuvant combinations can be identified which provide boosting with the reexposures that occur repeti-

**Table 4.** Reasons for the resurgence of malaria

| Factor(s) responsible for resurgence | Affected region(s) | Most important species |
|---|---|---|
| Insecticide resistance in the vector | South and Latin America, southeast Asia, less in sub-Saharan Africa | Affects transmission of all species |
| Drug resistance in the parasite | South America, southeast Asia, less in sub-Saharan Africa | Most important in *P. falciparum*, now also present in *P. vivax* |
| Inadequate funding for malaria control | All areas of endemicity | Affects control of all species |
| Civil strife and movement of refugee populations | Sub-Saharan Africa | Predominantly *P. falciparum* |
| Increased travel by nonimmune expatriates | Especially sub-Saharan Africa | *P. falciparum* |

tively with natural reinfection under field conditions. In basic scientific terms, there are fundamental problems (the lack of sterile immunity after natural infection) and a limited understanding (we do not know why some children develop severe disease such as cerebral malaria) which limit our approach to this problem.

**Acknowledgments.** Our studies have been supported by the National Institute of Allergy and Infectious Diseases (grants AI 25136, AI 39479, and AI 39496), the Burroughs Wellcome Fund (New Initiatives in Malaria Research), the UNDP/World Bank/World Health Organization Special Programme for Research and Training in Tropical Diseases (TDR 900131, TDR 940622), the U.S. Agency for International Development, and the Paul C. Beaver Fellowship Fund (Y.-L.T.).

## REFERENCES

1. **al Yaman, F., B. Genton, R. Anders, J. Taraika, M. Ginny, S. Mellor, and M. P. Alpers.** 1995. Assessment of the role of the humoral response to *Plasmodium falciparum* MSP2 compared to RESA and SPf66 in protecting Papua New Guinean children from clinical malaria. *Parasite Immunol.* **17:**493–501.

2. **al Yaman, F., B. Genton, K. J. Kramer, S. P. Chang, G. S. Hui, M. Baisor, and M. P. Alpers.** 1996. Assessment of the role of naturally acquired antibody levels to *Plasmodium falciparum* merozoite surface protein-1 in protecting Papua New Guinean children from malaria morbidity. *Am. J. Trop. Med. Hyg.* **54:**443–448.

3. **al Yaman, F., B. Genton, J. Taraika, R. Anders, and M. P. Alpers.** 1997. Cellular immunity to merozoite surface protein 2 (FC27 and 3D7) in Papua New Guinean children: temporal variation and relation to clinical and parasitological status. *Parasite Immunol.* **19:**207–214.

4. **Andersen, E., T. R. Jones, Purnomo, S. Masbar, I. Wiady, S. Tirtolusumo, M. J. Bangs, Y. Charoenvit, S. Gunawan, and S. L. Hoffman.** 1997. Assessment of age-dependent immunity to malaria in transmigrants. *Am. J. Trop. Med. Hyg.* **56:**647–649.

5. **Asawamahasakda, W., I. Ittarat, Y. M. Pu, H. Ziffer, and S. R. Meshnick.** 1994. Reaction of antimalarial endoperoxides with specific parasite proteins. *Antimicrob. Agents Chemother.* **38:**1854–1858.

6. **Bawden, M. P., D. Slaten, and J. D. Malone.** 1995. Falciparum malaria in a displaced Haitian population. *Trans. R. Soc. Trop. Med. Hyg.* **89:**600–603.

7. **Bayoumi, R. A., H. A. Babiker, and D. E. Arnot.** 1995. Uptake and efflux of chloroquine by chloroquine-resistant *Plasmodium falciparum* clones recently isolated in Africa. *Acta Trop.* **58:**141–149.

8. **Boyd, M. F.** 1949. Historical review, p. 3–25. *In* M. F. Boyd (ed.), *Malariology.* The W. B. Saunders Co., Philadelphia, Pa.

9. **Bray, P. G., R. E. Howells, G. Y. Ritchie, and S. A. Ward.** 1992. Rapid chloroquine efflux phenotype in both chloroquine-sensitive and chloroquine-resistant *Plasmodium falciparum*: a correlation of chloroquine sensitivity with energy-dependent drug accumulation. *Biochem. Pharmacol.* **44:**1317–1324.

10. **Brinkmann, U., and A. Brinkmann.** 1991. Malaria and health in Africa: the present situation and epidemiological trends. *Trop. Med. Parasitol.* **42:**204–213.

11. **Brown, A. W.** 1976. Malaria eradication and control from a global standpoint. 1976. *J. Med. Entomol.* **13:**1–25.

12. **Brown, P. J.** 1986. Socioeconomic and demographic effects of malaria eradication: a comparison of Sri Lanka and Sardinia. *Soc. Sci. Med.* **2:**847–859.

13. **Bruce-Chwatt, L. J.** 1984. Lessons learned from applied field research activities in Africa during the malaria eradication era. *Bull. W. H. O.* **62**(Suppl.)**:**S19–S29.

14. **Bruce-Chwatt, L. J.** 1988. History of malaria from prehistory to eradication, p. 1–60. *In* W. H. Wernsdorfer and I. A. McGregor (ed.). *Malaria: Principles and Practice of Malariology*, Churchill Livingstone, New York, N.Y.

15. **Butcher, G. A.** 1979. Factors affecting the *in vitro* culture of *Plasmodium falciparum* and *Plasmodium knowlesi*. *Bull. W. H. O.* **57**(Suppl. 1)**:**17–26.

16. **Cali, G.** 1996. The Italian Army Medical Corps in the United Nations "peace-keeping" operations: Somalia and Mozambique, December 1992–December 1994. *Med. Trop.* **56:**400–403.

17. **Cerami, C., U. Frevert, P. Sinnis, B. Takacs, P. Clavijo, M. J. Santos, and V. Nussenzweig.** 1992. The basolateral domain of the hepatocyte plasma membrane bears receptors for the circumsporozoite protein of *Plasmodium falciparum* sporozoites. *Cell* **70:**1021–1033.

18. **Chastel, C.** 1997. Reflections on two current viral diseases: yellow fever and dengue. *Ann. Biol. Clin.* **55:**415–424.

19. **Chuang, C. H.** 1991. Current status of malaria in Taiwan from 1966 to 1990. *Kao Hsiung I Hsueh Ko Hsueh Tsa Chih* **7:**233–242.

20. **Chulay, J. D., and C. F. Ockenhouse.** 1990. Host receptors for malaria-infected erythrocytes. *Am. J. Trop. Med. Hyg.* **43:**6–14.

21. **Clyde, D. F.** 1987. Recent trends in the epidemiology and control of malaria. *Epidemiol. Rev.* **9:** 219–243.

22. **Cowman, A. F., D. Galatis, and J. K. Thompson.** 1994. Selection for mefloquine resistance in *Plasmodium falciparum* is linked to amplification of the *pfmdr1* gene and cross-resistance to halofantrine and quinine. *Proc. Natl. Acad. Sci. USA* **91:**1143–1147.

23. **Cox, J. C., and A. R. Coulter.** 1997. Adjuvants—a classification and review of their modes of action. *Vaccine* **15:**248–256.

24. **Curtis, C. F.** 1996. Impregnated bednets, malaria control and child mortality. *Trop. Med. Int. Health* **1:**137–138.

25. **Daly, T. M., and C. A. Long.** 1996. Influence of adjuvants on protection induced by a recombinant fusion protein against malarial infection. *Infect. Immun.* **64:**2602–2608.

26. **De, D., F. M. Krogstad, F. B. Cogswell, and D. J. Krogstad.** 1996. Aminoquinolines that circumvent resistance in *P. falciparum in vitro. Am. J. Trop. Med. Hyg.* **55:**579–583.

27. **de Quadros, C. A., B. S. Hersh, J. M. Olive, J. K. Andrus, C. M. da Silveira, and P. A. Carrasco.** 1997. Eradication of wild poliovirus from the Americas: acute flaccid paralysis surveillance. *J. Infect. Dis.* **175**(Suppl.)**:**S37–S42.

28. **de Zulueta, J.** 1990. Forty years of malaria eradication in Sardinia: a new appraisal of a great enterprise. *Parassitologia* **32:**231–236.

29. **Dickinson, B. L., and J. D. Clements.** 1995. Dissociation of *Escherichia coli* heat-labile enterotoxin adjuvanticity from ADP-ribosyltransferase activity. *Infect. Immun.* **63:**1617–1623.

30. **Dowdle, W. R., and M. E. Birmingham.** 1997. The biologic principles of poliovirus eradication. *J. Infect. Dis.* **175**(Suppl.)**:**S286–S292.

31. **Egan. A., M. Waterfall, M. Pinder, A. Holder, and E. Riley.** 1997. Characterization of human T- and B-cell epitopes in the C terminus of *Plasmodium falciparum* merozoite surface protein 1: evidence for poor T cell recognition of polypeptides with numerous disulfide bonds. *Infect. Immun.* **65:**3024–3031.

32. **Fenner, F.** 1982. A successful eradication campaign: global eradication of smallpox. *Rev. Infect. Dis.* **4:**916–930.

33. **Fenner, F., D. A. Henderson, D. I. Arita, et al.** 1988. *Smallpox and Its Eradication.* World health Organization, Geneva, Switzerland.

34. **Gabriel, R. A., and K. S. Metz.** 1992. *A History of Military Medicine: from the Renaissance Through Modern Times.* Greenwood Press, New York, N.Y.

35. **Galata, G., and A. Galata-Luong.** 1997. Circulation des virus en milieu tropical, socio-ecologie des primates et equilibre des ecosystemes. *Sante* **7:**81–87.

36. **Ghendon, Y., and S. E. Robertson.** 1994. Interrupting the transmission of wild polioviruses with vaccines: immunologic considerations. *Bull. W. H. O.* **72:**973–984.

37. **Gluzman, I. Y., P. H. Schlesinger, and D. J. Krogstad.** 1987. The inoculum effect with chloroquine and *Plasmodium falciparum. Antimicrob. Agents Chemother.* **31:**32–36.

38. **Grau, G. E., P. F. Piguet, P. Vassalli, and P. H. Lambert.** 1989a. Tumor necrosis factor and other cytokines in cerebral malaria: experimental and clinical data. *Immunol. Rev.* **112:**49–70.

39. **Grau, G. E., T. E. Taylor, M. E. Molyneux, J. J. Wirima, P. Vassalli, M. Hommel, and P. H. Lambert.** 1989b. Tumor necrosis factor and disease severity in children with falciparum malaria. *N. Engl. J. Med.* **320:**1586–1591.

40. **Harinasuta, T., S. Migasen, and D. Bunnag.** 1962. Pages 143–153. *In UNESCO 1st Regional Symposium on Scientific Knowledge of Tropical Parasites.* University of Singapore, Singapore.

41. **Henderson, D. A.,** 1987. Principles and lessons from the smallpox eradication programme: *Bull. W. H. O.* **65:**535–546.

42. **Hoeppli, R.** 1959. *Parasites and Parasitic Infections in Early Medicine and Science.* University of Malaysia, Singapore, Malaysia.

43. **Hoffman, S. L., V. Nussenzweig, J. C. Sadoff, and R. S. Nussenzweig.** 1991. Progress toward malaria pre-erythrocytic vaccines. *Science* **252:**520–521.

44. **Hoffman, S. L., C. N. Oster, C. V. Plowe, G. R. Wollett, J. C. Beier, J. D. Chulay, R. A. Wirtz, M. R. Hollingdale, and M. Mugambi.** 1987. Naturally acquired antibodies to sporozoites do not prevent malaria: vaccine development implications. *Science* **237:**639–642.

45. **Hopkins, D. R., E. Ruiz-Tiben, R. L. Kaiser, et al.** 1993. Dracunculiasis eradication: beginning of the end. *Am. J. Trop. Med. Hyg.* **49:**281–289.

46. **Howard, R. F., K. C. Jacobson, E. Rickel, and J. Thurman.** 1998. Analysis of inhibitory epitopes in the *Plasmodium falciparum* rhoptry protein RAP-1 including identification of a second inhibitory epitope. *Infect. Immun.* **66:**380–386.

47. **Hull, H. F., M. E. Birmingham, B. Melgaard, and J. W. Lee.** 1997. Progress toward global polio eradication. *J. Infect. Dis.* **175**(Suppl.):S4–S9.

48. **Jackobsen, P. H., M. M. Lemnge, Y. A. Abu-Zeid, H. A. Msangeni, F. M. Salum, J. I. Mhina, J. A. Akida, S. S. Ruta, A. M. Ronn, P. M. Heegaard, R. G. Ridley, and I. C. Bygbjerg.** 1996. Immunoglobulin G reactivities to rhoptry-associated protein-1 associated with decreased levels of *Plasmodium falciparum* parasitemia in Tanzanian children. *Am. J. Trop. Med. Hyg.* **55:**642–646.

49. **Jiang, J. B., G. Q. Li, X. B. Guo, Y. C. Kong, and K. Arnold.** 1982. Antimalarial activity of mefloquine and qinghaosu. *Lancet* **2:**285–288.

50. **Jones, T. R., and S. L. Hoffman.** 1994. Malaria vaccine development. *Clin. Microbiol. Rev.* **7:**303–310.

51. **Kaslow, D. C.** 1997. Transmission-blocking vaccines: uses and current status of development. *Intl. J. Parasitol.* **27:**183–189.

52. **Kondrashin, A. V., and W. Rooney.** 1992. Overview: epidemiology of malaria and its control in countries of the WHO South-East region. *Southeast Asian J. Trop. Med. Publ. Health* **23**(Suppl. 4):13–22.

53. **Krogstad, D. J.** 1991. Antiparasitic drugs: mechanisms of action, drug assays, pharmacokinetics and pharmacodynamics, p. 258–278. *In* V. Lorian (ed.), *Antibiotics and Laboratory Medicine, 3rd Edition.* Williams and Wilkins, Baltimore, Md.

53a.**Krogstad, D. J.** 1993. Blood and tissue protozoa, p. 597–615. *In* M. Schaechter, G. Medoff, and B. I. Eisenstein (ed.), *Mechanisms of Microbial Disease.* Williams & Wilkins, Baltimore, Md.

54. **Krogstad, D. J.** 1996. Malaria as a re-emerging disease. *Epidemiol. Rev.* **18:**77–89.

55. **Krogstad, D. J.** 1996. Malaria: the deteriorating situation, p. 6–10. *In* P. K. Russell and C. P. Howson (ed.), *Vaccines against Malaria: Hope in a Gathering Storm.* Institute of Medicine, National Academy Press, Washington, D.C.

56. **Krogstad, D. J., and D. De.** 1998. Chloroquine: modes of action and resistance and the activity of chloroquine analogs, p. 331–339. *In* I. W. Sherman (ed.), *Malaria: Parasite Biology, Pathogenesis, and Protection.* American Society for Microbiology, Washington, D.C.

57. **Krogstad, D. J., I. Y. Gluzman, B. L. Herwaldt, P. H. Schlesinger, and T. E. Wellems.** 1992. Energy-dependence of chloroquine accumulation and chloroquine efflux. *Biochem. Pharmacol.* **43:**57–62.

58. **Krogstad, D. J., I. Y. Gluzman, D. E. Kyle, S. K. Martin, W. K. Milhous, and P. H. Schlesinger.** 1987. Efflux of chloroquine from *Plasmodium falciparum*: mechanism of chloroquine resistance. *Science* **238:**1283–1285.

59. **Krotoski, W. A., D. M. Krotoski, P. C. C. Garnham, R. S. Bray, R. Killick-Kendrick, C. C. Draper, G. A. Targett, and M. W. Guy.** 1980. Relapses in primate malaria: discovery of two populations of exoerythrocytic stages: preliminary note. *Br. Med. J.* **280:**153–154.

60. **Lal, A. A., M. A. Hughes, D. A. Oliveira, C. Nelson, P. B. Bloland, A. J. Oloo, W. E. Hawley, A. W. Hightower, B. L. Nahlen, and V. Udhayakumar.** 1996. Identification of T-cell determinants

in natural immune responses to the *Plasmodium falciparum* apical membrane antigen (AMA-1) in an adult population exposed to malaria. *Infect. Immun.* **64:**1054–1059.

61. **Laughlin, L. W., and L. J. Legters.** 1993. Disease threats in Somalia. *Am. J. Trop. Med. Hyg.* **48:** vi–x.
62. **Lobel, H. O., and P. E. Kozarsky.** 1997. Update on prevention of malaria for travelers. *JAMA* **278:**1767–1771.
63. **Looareesuwan, S., T. Harinasuta, and T. Chongsuphajaisiddhi.** 1992. Drug resistant malaria, with special reference to Thailand. *Southeast Asian J. Trop. Med. Public Health* **23:**621–634.
64. **Lopez-Antunano, F. J.** 1992. Epidemiology and control of malaria and other arthropod-borne diseases. *Mem. Inst. Oswaldo Cruz* **87**(Suppl. 3):105–114.
65. **Luxemburger, C., K. L. Thwai, N. J. White, H. K. Webster, D. E. Kyle, L. Maelankirri, T. Chongsuphajaisiddhi, and F. Nosten.** 1996. The epidemiology of malaria in a Karen population on the western border of Thailand. *Trans. R. Soc. Trop. Med. Hyg.* **90:**105–111.
66. **Marsh, K., M. English, J. Crawley, and N. Peshu.** 1996. The pathogenesis of severe malaria in African children. *Ann. Trop. Med. Parasitol.* **90:**395–402.
67. **Marsh, K., D. Forster, C. Waruiru, I. Mwangi, M. Winstanley, V. Marsh, C. Newton, P. Winstanley, P. Warn, and N. Peshu, et al.** 1995. Indicators of life-threatening malaria in African children. *N. Engl. J. Med.* **332:**1399–1404.
68. **Marshall, V. M., L. Zhang, R. F. Anders, and R. L. Coppel.** 1996. Diversity of the vaccine candidate AMA-1 of *Plasmodium falciparum*. *Mol. Biochem. Parasitol.* **77:**109–113.
69. **Masinde, G. L., D. J. Krogstad, D. M. Gordon, and P. E. Duffy.** Immunization with SPf66 and subsequent infection with homologous and heterologous parasites. *Am. J. Trop. Med. Hyg.*, in press.
70. **Matola, Y. G., U. Mwita, and A. E. Mawsoud.** 1984. Malaria in the islands of Zanzibar and Pemba 11 years after the suspension of a malaria eradication programme. *Cent. Afr. J. Med.* **30:** 91–92.
71. **Mbogo, C. N., R. W. Snow, C. P. Khamala, E. W. Kabiru, J. H. Ouma, J. I. Githure, K. Marsh, and J. C. Beier.** 1995. Relationships between *Plasmodium falciparum* transmission by vector populations and the incidence of severe disease at nine sites on the Kenyan coast. *Am. J. Trop. Med. Hyg.* **52:**201–206.
72. **Meshnick, S. R., T. E. Taylor, and S. Kamchonwongpaisan.** 1996. Artemisinin and the antimalarial endoperoxides: from herbal remedy to targeted chemotherapy. *Microbiol. Rev.* **60:**301–315.
73. **Miller, L. H., M. F. Good, and G. Milon.** 1994. Malaria pathogenesis. *Science* **264:**1878–1883.
74. **Monath, T. P., and A. Nasidi.** 1993. Should yellow fever vaccine be included in the expanded program of immunization in Africa? a cost-effectiveness analysis for Nigeria. *Am. J. Trop. Med. Hyg.* **48:**274–299.
75. **Mons, B., J. J. Croon, W. van der Star, and H. J. van der Kaay.** 1988. Erythrocytic schizogony and invasion of *Plasmodium vivax in vitro*. *Intl. J. Parasitol.* **18:**307–311.
76. **Moore, D. V., and J. E. Lanier.** 1961. Observations on two *Plasmodium falciparum* infections with abnormal response to chloroquine. *Am. J. Trop. Med. Hyg.* **10:**5–9.
77. **Mouchet, J., S. Laventure, S. Blanchy, R. Fioramonti, A. Rakotonjanabelo, P. Rabarison, J. Sircoulon, and J. Roux.** 1997. The reconquest of the Madagascar highlands by malaria. *Bull. Soc. Pathol. Exot.* **90:**162–168.
78. **Nokes, D. J., and J. Swinton J.** 1997. Vaccination in pulses: a strategy for global eradication of measles and polio? *Trends Microbiol.* **5:**14–19.
79. **Nowak, R.** 1995. Malaria: how the parasite disguises itself. *Science* **269:**755.
80. **Nwanyanwu, O. C., C. Ziba, P. Kazembe, L. Chitsulo, J. J. Wirima, N. Kumwenda, and S. C. Redd.** 1996. Efficacy of sulphadoxine/pyrimethamine for *Plasmodium falciparum* malaria in Malawian children under five years of age. *Trop. Med. Int. Health* **21:**231–235.
81. **Okwo-Bele, J. M., A. Lobanov, R. J. Biellik, M. E. Birmingham, L. Pierre, O. Tomori, and D. Barakamfitiye.** 1997. Overview of poliomyelitis in the African region and current regional plan of action. *J. Infect. Dis.* **175**(Suppl.):S10–S15.
82. **Oplinger, M. L., S. Baqar, A. F. Trofa, J. D. Clements, P. Gibbs, G. Pazzaglia, A. L. Bourgeois, and D. A. Scott.** 1997. Safety and immunogenicity in volunteers of a new candidate oral mucosal

adjuvant, LT(R192G), abstr. G-10, p. 193. *In Abstracts of the 37th Interscience Conference on Antimicrobial Agents and Chemotherapy.* American Society for Microbiology, Washington, D.C.

83. **Packard, R. M.** 1997. Malaria dreams: postwar visions of health and development in the Third World. *Med. Anthropol.* **17:**279–296.

84. **Packard, R. M., and P. Gadehla.** 1997. A land filled with mosquitoes: Fred L. Soper, the Rockefeller Foundation and the *Anopheles gambiae* invasion of Brazil. *Med. Anthropol.* **17:**215–238.

85. **Patriarca, P. A, W. H. Foege, and T. A. Swartz.** 1993. Progress in polio eradication. *Lancet* **342:** 1461–1464.

86. **Paxton, L. A., L. Slutsker, L. J. Schultz, S. P. Luby, R. Meriwether, P. Matson, and A. J. Sulzer.** Imported malaria in Montagnard refugees settling in North Carolina: implications for prevention and control. *Am. J. Trop. Med. Hyg.* **54:**54–57.

87. **Payne, D.** 1987. Spread of chloroquine resistance in *Plasmodium falciparum. Parasitol. Today* **3:** 241–246.

88. **Payne, D.** 1988. Did medicated salt hasten the spread of chloroquine resistance in *Plasmodium falciparum? Parasitol. Today* **6:**112–115.

89. **Peragallo, M. S., G. Sabatinelli, G. Majori, G. Cali, and G. Sarnicola.** 1995. Prevention of malaria among Italian troops in Somalia and Mozambique (1993–1994). *Trans. R. Soc. Trop. Med. Hyg.* **89:**302.

90. **Peterson, D. S., W. K. Milhous, and T. E. Wellems.** 1990. Molecular basis of differential resistance to cycloguanil and pyrimethamine in *Plasmodium falciparum. Proc. Natl. Acad. Sci. USA* **87:**3018–3022.

91. **Plowe, C. V., and T. E. Wellems.** 1995. Molecular approaches to the spreading problem of drug resistant malaria. *Adv. Exp. Med. Biol.* **390:**197–209.

92. **Porignon, D., J. P. Noterman, P. Hennart, R. Tonglet, E. M. Soron'Gane, and T. E. Lokombe.** 1995. The role of the Zairian Health Services in the Rwandan refugee crisis. *Disasters* **19:**356–360.

93. **Riley, E. M., K. C. Williamson, B. M. Greenwood, and D. C. Kaslow.** 1995. Human immune recognition of recombinant proteins representing discrete domains of the *Plasmodium falciparum* gamete surface protein, Pfs230. *Parasite Immunol.* **17:**11–19.

94. **Robertson, S. E., B. P. Hull, O. Tomori, O. Bele, J. W. LeDuc, and K. Esteves.** 1996. Yellow fever: a decade of re-emergence. *JAMA* **176:**1157–1162.

95. **Sahkibaei, M., and U. Frevert.** 1996. Dual interaction of the malaria circumsporozoite protein with the low density lipoprotein receptor-related protein (LRP) and heparan sulfate proteoglycans. *J. Exp. Med.* **184:**1699–1711.

96. **Seebeck, T.** 1991. Molecular biology and parasites. *Experientia* **47:**163–166.

97. **Sharma, V. P.** 1996. Re-emergence of malaria in India. *Indian J. Med. Res.* **103:**26–45.

98. **Shortt, H. E., and P. C. C. Garnham.** 1948. Pre-erythrocytic stage in mammalian malaria parasites. *Nature* **161:**126.

99. **Silva, R. T.** 1994. Malaria eradication as a legacy of colonial discourse: the case of Sri Lanka. *Parassitologia* **36:**149–163.

100. **Slater, A. F.** 1993. Chloroquine: mechanism of drug action and resistance in *Plasmodium falciparum. Pharmacol. Ther.* **57:**203–235.

101. **Slater, A. F., and A. Cerami.** 1992. Inhibition by chloroquine of a novel haem polymerase enzyme activity in malaia trophozoites. *Nature* **355:**108–109.

102. **Soper, F. L.** 1949. Species sanitation and species eradication for the control of mosquito-borne diseases, p. 1167–1174. *In* M. F. Boyd (ed.), *Malariology: A Comprehensive Survey of All Aspects of This Group of Diseases from a Global Standpoint.* The W. B. Saunders Co., Philadelphia, Pa.

103. **Sowunmi, A., A. M. J. Oduola, O. A. Ogundahunsi, C. O. Falade, G. O. Gbotosho, and L. A. Salako.** 1997. Enhanced efficacy of chloroquine-chlorpheniramine combination in acute uncomplicated falciparum malaria in children. *Trans. R. Soc. Trop. Med. Hyg.* **91:**63–67.

104. **Spielman, A., U. Kitron, and R. J. Pollack.** 1993. Time limitation and the role of research in the worldwide attempt to eradicate malaria. *J. Med. Entomol.* **30:**6–19.

105. **Stoute, J. A., M. Slaoui, D. G. Heppner, P. Momin, K. E. Kester, P. Desmons, B. T. Wellde, N. Garcon, U. Krzych, and M. Marchand.** 1997. A preliminary evaluation of a recombinant

circumsporozoite protein vaccine against *Plasmodium falciparum* malaria: RTS,S Malaria Vaccine Evaluation Group. *N. Engl. J. Med.* **336:**86–91.

106. **Stowers, A., D. Tauylor, N. Prescott, Q. Cheng, J. Cooper, and A. Saul.** 1997. Assessment of the humoral immune response against *Plasmodium falciparum* rhoptry-associated proteins 1 and 2. *Infect. Immun.* **65:**2329–2338.

107. **Su, X. Z., V. M. Heatwole, S. P. Wertheimer, F. Guinet, J. A. Herrfeldt, D. S. Peterson, J. A. Ravetch, and T. E. Wellems.** 1995. The large diverse gene family *var* encodes proteins involved in cytoadherence and antigenic variation of *Plasmodium falciparum*-infected erythrocytes. *Cell* **82:** 89–100.

108. **Su, X.-Z., L. A. Kirkman, H. Fujioka, and T. E. Wellems.** 1997. Complex polymorphisms in a ~330 kDa protein are linked to chloroquine-resistant *Plasmodium falciparum* in Southeast Asia and Africa. *Cell* **91:**591–603.

109. **Sullivan, D. J. Jr., I. Y. Gluzman, D. G. Russell, and D. E. Goldberg.** 1996. On the molecular mechanism of chloroquine's antimalarial action. *Proc. Natl. Acad. Sci. USA* **93:**11865–11870.

110. **ter Kuile, F. O., G. Dolan, F. Nosten, et al.** 1993. Halofantrine versus mefloquine in treatment of multidrug-resistant falciparum malaria. *Lancet* **341:**1044–1049.

111. **Trager, W.** 1971. A new method for intraerythrocytic cultivation of malaria parasites (*Plasmodium coatneyi and P. falciparum*). *J. Protozool.* **18:**239–242.

112. **Trager, W. and J. B. Jensen.** 1976. Human malaria parasites in continuous culture. *Science* **193:** 673–675.

113. **Trenholme, G. M., R. L. Williams, R. E. Desjardins, et al.** 1975. Mefloquine (WR 142,490) in the treatment of human malaria. *Science* **190:**792–794.

114. **van der Hoek, W., D. A. Premasiri, and A. R. Wickremasinghe.** 1997. Early diagnosis and treatment of malaria in a refugee population in Sri Lanka. *Southeast Asian J. Trop. Med. Public Health* **28:**12–17.

115. **Vanham, G., and E. Bisalinkumi.** 1995. Immunology of human *Plasmodium falciparum* malaria. *Ann. Soc. Belge. Med. Trop.* **75:**159–178.

116. **van Hensbroek, M. B., E. Onyiorah, S. Jaffar, G. Schneider, A. Palmer, A. Nusmeijer, S. Bennett, B. M. Greenwood, and D. Kwiatkowski.** 1996. A trial of artemether or quinine in children with cerebral malaria. *N. Engl. J. Med.* **335:**69–75.

117. **Wallace, M. R., T. W. Sharp, B. Smoak, C. Iriye, P. Rozmajzl, S. A. Thornton, R. Batchelor, A. J. Magill, H. O. Lobel, C. F. Longer, and J. P. Burans.** 1996. Malaria among United States troops in Somalia. *Am. J. Med.* **100:**49–55.

118. **Wang, P., M. Read, P. F. Sims, and J. E. Hyde.** 1997. Sulfadoxine resistance in the human malaria parasite *Plasmodium falciparum* is determined by mutations in dihydropteroate synthase and an additional factor associated with folate utilization. *Mol. Microbiol.* **23:**979–986.

119. **Ward, S. A., P. G. Bray, M. Mungthin, and S. R. Hawley.** 1995. Current views on the mechanisms of resistance to quinoline-containing drugs in *Plasmodium falciparum. Ann. Trop. Med. Parasitol.* **89:**121–124.

120. **Warsame, M, W. H. Wernsdorfer, G. Huldt, and A. Bjorkman.** 1995. An epidemic of *Plasmodium falciparum* malaria in Balcad, Somalia, and its causation. *Trans. R. Soc. Trop. Med. Hyg.* **89:**142–145.

121. **Wickham, J. M., E. D. Dennis, and G. H. Mitchell.** 1980. Long term cultivation of a simian malaria parasite (*Plasmodium knowlesi*) in a semi-automated apparatus. *Trans. R. Soc. Trop. Med. Hyg.* **74:**789–792.

122. **Williamson, K. C., D. B. Keister, O. Muratova, and D. C. Kaslow.** 1995. Recombinant Pfs230, a *Plasmodium falciparum* gametocyte protein, induces antisera that reduce the infectivity of *Plasmodium falciparum* to mosquitoes. *Mol. Biochem. Parasitol.* **75:**33–42.

123. **Wongsrichanalai, C., H. K. Webster, and T. Wimonwattrawatee, et al.** 1992. Drug resistant malaria, with special reference to Thailand. *Southeast Asian J. Trop. Med. Public Health* **47:**112–116.

124. **World Health Organization.** 1997. World malaria situation in 1994, parts I–III. (*W. H. O.*) *Wkly. Epidemiol. Rec.* **72:**269–274, 277–283, 285–291.

*Emerging Infections 2*
Edited by W. M. Scheld, W. A. Craig, and J. M. Hughes
© 1998 ASM Press, Washington, D.C.

*Chapter 12*

# Immigrants, Imaging, and Immunoblots: the Emergence of Neurocysticercosis as a Significant Public Health Problem

*Peter M. Schantz, Patricia P. Wilkins, and Victor C. W. Tsang*

## INTRODUCTION AND HISTORICAL BACKGROUND

Taeniasis, or cysticercosis, caused by *Taenia solium* (often referred to as the pork tapeworm), is a classical zoonosis which has been recognized since antiquity. As a result of a variety of demographic, technologic, and political factors, it is emerging as an increasingly important condition in regions where it has long been endemic as well as regions into which it is imported or introduced. The two-host life cycle of the tapeworm involves humans as definitive hosts and swine as intermediate hosts (Fig. 1). Pigs are the source of human taeniasis, an intestinal tapeworm infection acquired by eating undercooked pork contaminated with cysticerci, the larval stage of the cestode. Cysticercosis, however, is acquired by ingesting *Taenia* eggs shed in the feces of a human tapeworm carrier and thus may occur in humans who neither eat pork nor share environments with pigs. Although cysticerci may localize throughout the body, most clinical manifestations result from their presence in the central nervous system (neurocysticercosis [NCC]), where they can cause seizures, hydrocephalus, and other neurologic dysfunctions (41).

Prominently visible in both its intestinal and tissue stages, the macroparasite *T. solium* has been known since the earliest times. Spontaneous elimination of individual tapeworm segments were alluded to by writers at the beginnings of recorded history (56). The ancient Greeks made reference to "measles" in pork which were the larval cysticerci; however, their significance was not understood. Aristotole compared their appearance to hailstones; he and others regarded them as wormlike animals. In the 16th century, European pathologists associated the condition with disease in humans and described cysticerci in the brains of epileptic persons. By the mid-19th century a number of investigators had demonstrated the link be-

*Peter M. Schantz, Patricia P. Wilkins, and Victor C. W. Tsang* • Division of Parasitic Diseases, National Center for Infectious Diseases, Centers for Disease Control and Prevention, Mailstop F22, 4770 Buford Highway, Atlanta, GA 30341.

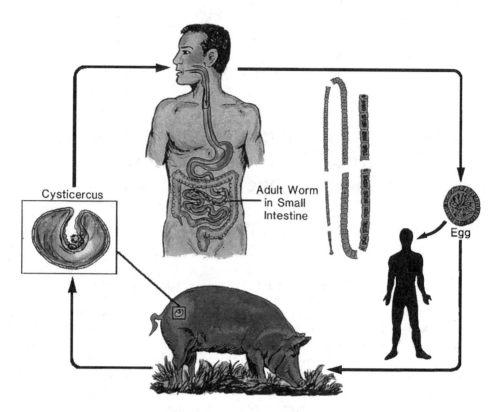

**Figure 1.** Life cycle of *T. solium.*

tween cystic and strobilar (intestinal) forms of several species of *Taenia* by showing that cystic worms metamorphosed into adult worms when ingested by suitable hosts. This relationship for *T. solium* was confirmed in 1855 by Kuchenmeister who administered cyst-infected pork to a condemned criminal and observed developing adult forms in the man's intestine after his execution (56). About the same time, van Beneden in Belgium demonstrated that he could produce cysticerci in the muscles of pigs by feeding them *T. solium* eggs obtained from tapeworm segments passed by infected humans. Further studies confirmed that humans alone were the definitive host of the worm and that pigs were the only significant intermediate host; thus, the reasons were now well understood for the well-recognized paucity of infection in persons of certain religions such as Muslims and Jews, who were forbidden to eat pork. Scattered reports suggest that the infection was prevalent in pigs and in humans in various parts of the world; however, the highest rates of transmission most likely occurred in populations with the poorest medical documentation. During the first half of the last century, approximately 2% of postmortem examinations of humans conducted in Berlin revealed cysticercosis. Details of the clinical and pathologic characteristics of NCC were extensively described in German medical literature by the turn of the 20th century (61). Although the infection has been virtually eliminated from Germany and most of the rest of Western Europe, similar or higher prevalence rates have been documented recently in parts of Africa, Asia, and Central and South America (9).

Improvements in diagnosis (neuroimaging methods and immunoblotting for immunodiagnosis) have revolutionized the antemortem recognition of this disease, thus improving our understanding of the nature of the disease and its true prevalence while large-scale immigration of populations in modern times have continued to expand its distribution.

## CLINICAL ASPECTS

### Neurocysticercosis

After ingestion, the eggs of *T. solium* hatch in the duodenum. The released embryos (oncospheres) penetrate the intestinal mucosa, gain access to the circulatory system, and are distributed to extraenteric sites, where they develop as larval cysticerci. The typical cysticercus is a tiny ellipsoid bladder (0.5 to 1.5 cm diameter) with a white translucent membrane that contains a single spherical, invaginated protoscolex bathed in a small amount of clear liquid. In pigs, the cysticerci of *T. solium* localize most frequently within the lymphatic capillaries of the skeletal muscles and in the brain. In humans, cysticerci often occur in skeletal muscles, but most important clinical manifestations emanate from cysticerci localized in the central nervous system (CNS). Within the CNS, 1 to more than 1,000 cysticerci may occur in the meninges, the ventricles, the subarachnoid space, or the brain parenchyma (Fig. 2). Less frequently, cysticerci may localize in the eyes, subcutaneous tissues, and heart. Pathogenesis is related to the number and sites of lo-

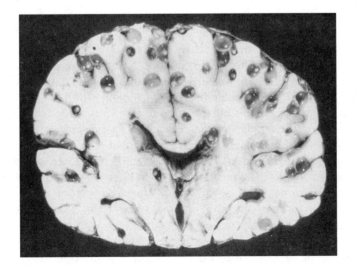

**Figure 2.** Multiple cysticerci in the brain of a 12-year-old girl at autopsy. (Courtesy of Ana Flisser.)

calization of cysticerci and to the host immune response; cysticerci in the CNS may be apparently tolerated and survive for years or may be overwhelmed within a few days by an intense inflammatory response (30). Consequently, NCC is characterized by extreme clinical polymorphism and variability in outcome, thus complicating prognostic evaluation and comparison of therapeutic regimens. Clinical NCC is diagnosed most frequently in adults; children account for fewer than 20% of clinical cases. The disease is most commonly heralded by new-onset generalized seizures. NCC has been shown to be the most common cause of late-onset seizures in Mexico and many other regions where *T. solium* is endemic, accounting for 30 to 50% of all cases; recently the International League Against Epilepsy called it the main cause of epilepsy worldwide (20). Cerebral imaging typically reveals a single "ring enhancing lesion" that may resolve spontaneously and disappear without clinical sequelae within 2 to 3 months. The minority of patients in whom the lesion persists as a calcified granuloma are more likely to have persistent seizures (72). Another common presentation is new-onset seizures in a person in whom cerebral imaging demonstrates single or multiple calcifications without evidence of viable cysticerci; in these patients the stages associated with invasion, development, and finally, destruction of parasites were presumably clinically silent. More complicated and severe clinical courses occur in patients with intraventricular and cisternal lesions. Another distinct clinical form is cysticercotic encephalitis. Typically seen in young female patients who present with acute onset of illness similar to viral encephalitis, this uncommon but often fatal form of NCC is associated with the early CNS-invasive stages; computed tomography (CT) or magnetic resonance (MR) imaging studies disclose severe and diffuse brain edema and (with contrast enhancement) multiple ring-enhancing "granulomas" (83).

## Taeniasis

Taeniasis, or intestinal infection by the adult-stage *T. solium*, is acquired by ingestion of cysticerci in raw or inadequately cooked pork and is characterized by the development of one or more chains of several hundreds of segments, or proglottids. The tapeworms, or strobila, grow to 1 to 3 m long and are attached to the wall of the small intestine by a pinhead-sized scolex that has four circular muscular suckers and is crowned by a double ring of 22 to 36 anterior movable hooks. Gravid proglottids, comprising the posterior portion of the worm, break off individually or in small clusters and are shed in the feces. Each segment carries an average of 60,000 eggs that are immediately infective if ingested by a susceptible intermediate host. The eggs are sticky and can be found attached to the perianal skin and even under the fingernails of tapeworm carriers. Internal autoinfection with cysticercosis can occur when, in the small bowel of the tapeworm carrier, the embryos of *T. solium* released from eggs can invade the bowel wall and disseminate hematogenously to muscle, subcutaneous tissues, the central nervous system (CNS), and other tissues. External autoinfection can also occur when tapeworm carriers ingest *T. solium* eggs that have adhered to the perianal skin. How frequently autoinfection occurs is not known; from 5% to 40% of patients diagnosed with cysticercosis have concurrent taeniasis (101). The fact that many *T. solium* tapeworm carriers develop antibodies to larval antigens suggests that "auto-exposure" to embryo antigens may be the norm (126a). Most cases of taeniasis are asymptomatic; the most commonly reported symptom is the observation of proglottids passed in stool.

## Treatment

### Neurocysticercosis

Current approaches to treatment of NCC have been reviewed recently by Sotelo et al. (112) and White (126). The initial focus of therapy for patients with symptomatic NCC is suppression of seizures or inflammation with anticonvulsants or corticosteroids, respectively. In certain circumstances, relief of increased intracranial pressure is achieved with shunting of cerebrospinal fluid (CSF). Surgical interventions are often necessary for cyst resection and alleviation of complications of the disease; however, surgical procedures are usually only palliative because of the multiple cysticerci that may be present. A major advance occurred in the 1980s when it was demonstrated that praziquantel and albendazole were effective for treating intracerebral cysticerci in patients (1, 11, 82, 110).

Anthelmintic drugs are now commonly used for management of NCC; however, the extreme variability of the clinical course of NCC and the high proportion of cases that tend to resolve spontaneously have hindered the interpretation of chemotherapy trials that lacked adequate comparison groups. This has prevented the development of clear guidelines for treatment. Although many patients continue to require anticonvulsive medication for control of seizures after anthelmintic treatment, recent studies concluded that a higher proportion of patients treated with anthelmintics become seizure-free than those not treated (31, 122). While some recent reports confirm the efficacy of anthelmintic treatment (24, 115), others question their efficacy (106) and point out inadequacies in prior studies (58, 65, 126). The outcome of a recently reported clinical trial in Ecuador in which patients were assigned randomly to treatment groups (albendazole or praziquantel) and that included a control group (15) may challenge some of the assumptions of those who routinely advocate the use of anthelmintic medication in NCC. In this study, 175 patients with active neurocysticercosis were randomly assigned to three treatment groups: (i) oral prednisolone alone (27), (ii) praziquantel (50 mg/kg for 15 days) with prednisolone (54), or (iii) albendazole (15 mg/kg) for 8 days with prednisolone (57). At 6 months and 1 year after treatment there were no significant differences in the three treatment groups in the proportion of patients free of cysts or the relative reduction of number of cysts. The efficacy of therapy was relatively low: only 20% to 41% of patients were totally free of cysts. At 2 years, there were no differences in the proportion who remained free of seizures; however, early and late sequelae (headaches, seizures, and hydrocephalus) occurred in a higher proportion of patients treated with anthelmintic drugs than in those receiving prednisolone alone. The authors concluded that the "improvement" attributed to either anthelmintic drug in prior studies may have been related to the lack of appropriate controls and is a reflection of the natural history of the condition. The results of this study suggest that we still lack reliable criteria to determine which patients require treatment with either praziquantel or albendazole.

## Taeniasis

Intestinal-stage *T. solium* infection is most effectively treated with praziquantel. A single dose of 10 mg per kg of body weight is >95% efficacious. Because this drug is well absorbed and active against larval stage *T. solium*, there is some risk of initiation or exacerbation of symptoms in persons with concomitant latent NCC (40). Niclosamide (adult dose, 2 g) is another drug with reported high efficacy against intestinal *Taenia* spp.; the fact that niclosamide is poorly absorbed from the intestine eliminates the possibility of provocation of symptoms incidental to destruction of intracerebral cysticerci.

## ROLE OF IMPROVED DIAGNOSIS

### Diagnosis of Neurocysticercosis

Clinical diagnosis of NCC is complicated by the wide spectrum of clinical presentations associated with the disease (126). Until recently, characterization of NCC was mainly based on clinical observations and findings at autopsy of deceased patients; antemortem diagnosis was limited by the inability to visualize the intracerebral lesions. Plain roentgenography was useful for visualization of calcified lesions only; invasive radiologic procedures such as pneumoencephalography were sometimes helpful for characterizing intraventricular and arachnoid forms. It was not until the advent of modern neuroimaging procedures that early, nonterminal clinical events could be characterized in patients.

### Neuroimaging Diagnosis

Contrasted CT and MR imaging of the brain have revolutionized the diagnosis of NCC by improving the discernment of intracerebral lesions (69, 114, 117) (Fig. 3). For many patients, information adequate for specific diagnosis is available from either CT or MR; however, studies comparing the two imaging procedures have concluded that the latter is more sensitive and specific for identifying most forms of NCC, with the exception of microcalcifications. MR shows clearly the degree of edema and inflammation as evidence of the host immune response. MR also discloses ocular, ventricular, and subarachnoid cysticerci better than CT and has a higher resolution for analysis of the fluid contents of the cyst, which in turn is an indication of the viability of the cysticercus (69, 114).

### Immunodiagnosis of Cysticercosis

The second major advance in diagnosis of cysticercosis was the development of sensitive and specific immunodiagnostic procedures. Immunologic methods have long been used for diagnosis of these conditions; however, until recently they involved a variety of quantitative methods using crude and poorly characterized antigens. Early experience at the Centers for Disease Control and Prevention (CDC) indicated considerable nonspecificity. When modern neuroimaging methods provided alternative methods for noninvasive diagnosis, results indicated that immunodiagnosis was seriously lacking in sensitivity (96, 100). Similar deficiencies in

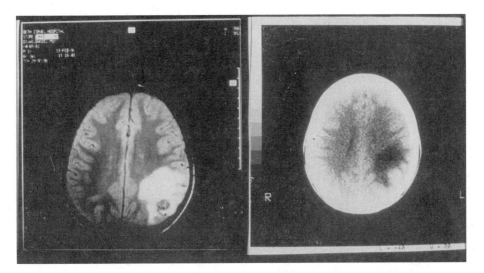

**Figure 3.** Radioimaging of neurocysticercosis. MR (left) and CT (right) images of the brain of a patient with a single cystic lesion are shown.

the value of immunodiagnosis were reported by others (53). In the mid-1980s, however, homologous species-specific antigenic components were demonstrated in crude *T. solium* larval materials, providing the basis for species-specific diagnosis (55). An improved immunoblot assay was developed by Tsang and others (119). This test has greatly impacted clinical diagnosis of NCC and, very importantly, provided a useful tool for surveillance and epidemiological studies. The immuno-blot assay (also known as enzyme-linked immunoelectrotransfer blot [EITB]) is based on serologic reactivity with purified *T. solium* glycoproteins. A soluble pro-tein fraction is prepared from cysticerci collected from infected pigs and further purified using lentil lectin affinity chromatography. The lectin-bound proteins are separated by sodium dodecyl sulfate-polyacrylamide gel electrophoresis (SDS-PAGE) and then transferred to nitrocellulose membranes. The immunoblot detects antibodies that are present in serum, plasma, or cerebrospinal fluid (CSF) to seven disease-specific glycoproteins. The diagnostic proteins are designated GP50, GP39-42, GP24, GP21, GP18, GP14, and GP13, based on relative molecular weight determinations by SDS-PAGE (Fig. 4). Immunoreactivity with any of the seven glycoproteins indicates present or prior disease.

Sera from infected individuals contain antibodies that typically react with more than one of the seven immunodiagnostic proteins (34, 44, 100). In a recent hospital-based study, about half of neurocysticercosis patients had serum antibodies that reacted to all seven diagnostic proteins (46). The proteins that are most frequently recognized are the GP42 complex and GP24 (119). The lower molecular weight proteins, GP14 and GP13, are the least often recognized, but antibodies to these proteins are present in 46 and 59% of sera, respectively. The test detects 98% of parasitologically proven cases with two or more cysts and is 100% specific (119).

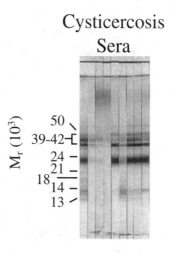

**Figure 4.** Immunoblot showing reactivity of sera from patients with cysticercosis. Individual sera from patients with cysticercosis were analyzed by the immunoblot assay. Cysticercosis-specific antibodies react with glycoproteins derived from *T. solium* cysts. The positions of the seven diagnostic glycoproteins are noted and designated according to their relative mobilities in SDS-PAGE.

In patients with a single parenchymal cyst, or microcalcifications, the test is less sensitive, between 60 and 80% (46, 48, 127), perhaps due to insufficient immune stimulation (100, 127). Antibodies present in CSF can also be detected by immunoblotting, but the test is more sensitive when serum or plasma samples are used. In fact, CSF testing has never detected a case of cysticercosis that was not detected using serum (119). Saliva has also been evaluated and was reported to detect only 70% of the cases (39).

A recent study examined the presence of anticysticercal antibodies in serum of neurocysticercosis patients following antiparasitic treatment (46). Approximately half of the patients in this study had anticysticercal antibodies that recognized all seven of the diagnostic proteins. Of these patients, those who were successfully treated had antibodies that reacted to all seven proteins 1 year after treatment. Of the patients with antibodies to fewer than 7 proteins, three patients (7%) were seronegative after 1 year, and 12% showed a decrease in the number of proteins recognized by immunoblot 1 year after treatment (46).

The immunoblot assay has also been used successfully to detect cysticercosis in pigs; the assay was 100% sensitive (53, 120) and is approximately two-fold more sensitive than tongue examination (120). Initial experiments in pigs suggested that detection of specific IgM antibody levels in comparison with those of IgG could differentiate between newly acquired or chronic infection (120); however, experiments to determine if these predictive criteria can be applied to human cysticercosis have not been performed.

Given the proven operational characteristics of the immunoblot assay, there is a need for a low-cost, field-applicable assay for detection of human and pig cysticercosis. Efforts center on the already proven glycoprotein antigens detected in the immunoblot assay. Preliminary experiments have demonstrated that the carbohydrate portions of the seven immunodiagnostic glycoproteins are not required for immunoreactivity. Furthermore, because several of these proteins are recognized by antibodies present in a high percentage of sera from patients with cysticercosis, these proteins have been targeted for further purification and molecular cloning. Although recombinant forms of any of these proteins may not be available for some time, a simple assay based on further purification of the lentil lectin bound fraction is currently being investigated. Some progress in this direction has recently been reported involving fractionation of the identified gp antigens (62, 78) although side-by-side comparisons await analysis; their use in immunoblot and ELISA formats showed expected high levels of sensitivity and specificity (62).

The immunoblot assay has proven utility for immunodiagnosis of *T. solium* cysticercosis in humans and swine and is the current test of choice for clinical and epidemiologic studies (34, 44, 53, 100); however, as with all antibody assays, the test has limitations, and interpretation of the results has to take into account that the presence of antibody may indicate only previous exposure or infection with the parasite and not necessarily current viable infection. Furthermore, clinical manifestations of NCC may remain long after the intracerebral cysticerci are dead and no longer producing antigenic stimuli; consequently, clinically symptomatic patients with long-dead parasites may be seronegative. Understanding these limitations provides a more realistic basis for utilization and interpretation of the test results.

## Diagnosis of Taeniasis

Diagnosis of adult taenia tapeworm infections is a critical element of any control and intervention study, but traditional methods lack sensitivity and specificity. Diagnosis of tapeworm carriers has long been limited to demonstration of ova and/or proglottids in direct examination of stool samples; however, recently developed immunologic methods promise increased sensitivity and wider applicability.

### Parasitology-Based Methods

Direct parasitologic examination of stool samples is the only method of diagnosis that is absolute. The diagnosis of taeniasis is made when eggs or gravid proglottids or both are present in the sample; however, due to the intermittent nature of excretion, prevalent infections are underdetected (59). The precise species of *Taenia* can be determined if gravid proglottids are present. Based on the number of uterine branches present in the proglottid, *T. solium* can be distinguished from *T. saginata*. Gravid proglottids from *T. solium* bear 10 or fewer uterine branches on each side of the central uterus; proglottids of *T. saginata* have 12 or more branches (80). In very rare cases, a scolex may be present in the sample. If so, then definitive species diagnosis of *T. solium* or *T. saginata* can be made by the presence of an armed (with hooks) or unarmed (without hooks) scolex, respectively (38). However, if ova alone are seen in the sample, the species of *Taenia* present cannot be determined. Both *T. solium* and *T. saginata* may be indigeneous to the same geographic area, making speciation particularly critical for intervention studies of cysticercosis. So, although microscopic-based parasitologic techniques are simple and relatively inexpensive, these techniques lack both sensitivity and specificity.

## Detection of Coproantigen

As an alternative to microscopic techniques for detection of taeniasis, Allan and colleagues have developed an assay that detects parasite antigens in stool samples (2). The coproantigen assay was developed as an antigen capture immunoassay with high sensitivity and specificity (2, 3). Originally the assay was developed in a microtiter plate format (2) and, more recently, has been simplified into a dipstick-based assay (4). The microtiter plate coproantigen assay is more sensitive (99% sensitive) and more specific than microscopic assays. The dipstick-based assay is less sensitive than the microtiter plate version of the assay, but was determined to be more sensitive than microscopy (3). The levels of coproantigen present in feces decline dramatically following elimination of the tapeworm, and the assay can be used for monitoring treatment success. One limitation of this assay is that it cannot distinguish between taeniasis caused by *T. solium* or *T. saginata*. Other limitations of the assay include problems associated with stool collection.

## Immunoblot for Detection of Taeniasis

In an effort to develop a serologic-based assay for detection of taeniasis carrier, an immunoblot assay using excretory/secretory (TS/ES) antigens of adult *T. solium* tapeworms has been developed (126a). The TS/ES proteins derived from in vitro culture of adult *T. solium* tapeworms were separated by SDS-PAGE and transferred onto nitrocellulose membranes. In an immunoblot assay, sera from parasite-confirmed *T. solium* carriers and sera from cysticercosis patients were incubated with the separated TS/ES proteins. A group of proteins that reacted with sera from adult worm carriers but not with sera from cysticercosis patients was identified. Antibodies in sera from persons with other helminthic infections (such as *Hymenelopis nana*, *Echinococcus* spp., *Ascaris*, *Trichinella*, and others) do not generate antibodies that react with the ES proteins, indicating that this assay is very specific. Furthermore, using sera from a limited number of parasitologically confirmed taeniasis cases, the immunoblot detects all cases of *T. solium* taeniasis and none of the *T. saginata* cases. These preliminary data suggest that the immunoblot assay may be a useful method for distinguishing *T. solium* from *T. saginata* tapeworm carriers. Although currently a complex assay format, when simplified, the assay may be an important tool for control and prevention strategies for cysticercosis.

## GEOGRAPHIC DISTRIBUTION AND PREVALENCE

### Geographic Distribution

*T. solium* infection is widely endemic in rural areas of developing countries in Central and South America, Asia, and Africa (Fig. 5 and 6).

Published reports document the occurrence of clinical NCC in most of the countries of the Americas (most notably Mexico, Guatemala, El Salvador, Honduras, Colombia, Ecuador, Peru, Bolivia, and Brazil). The infection was reported to be present in 18 countries of South and Central America whose combined populations

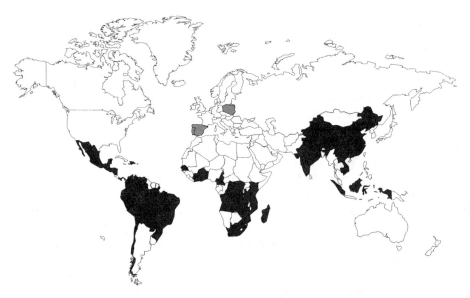

**Figure 5.** Approximate geographic distribution of *T. solium*. ■, high or moderate prevalence; ■, low or sporadic prevalence.

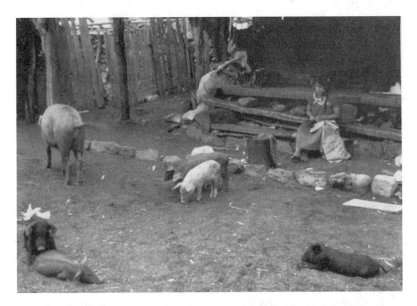

**Figure 6.** The outside commons area of a household in Mexico where *T. solium* infection is endemic. The unrestrained sow and piglets have access to human fecal wastes deposited on the open ground or in a shallow pit latrine.

represented 94% of the total 1980 population of the Latin American countries (103). Of the American countries, only Canada, the United States, and possibly Argentina and Uruguay appear to be free of transmission in the pig-to-human cycle. However, these latter countries are observing an increase in imported and introduced infections related to immigration of persons from neighboring countries where *T. solium* infection is endemic. No information is available concerning the occurrence or absence of infection in Guyana, Suriname, and French Guiana.

In Asia, almost all available data are from clinic-based populations and are biased in terms of the true geographic origin and epidemiologic factors associated with transmission. Transmission in much of Asia is strongly influenced by prevailing cultural practices and socioeconomic conditions. In India, for example, intestinal-stage *T. solium* infections occur mainly in pork-eating populations, particularly in rural populations and lower socioeconomic classes; 78% of children of pig farmers were reported to pass taeniid eggs (10, 108). Vegetarian populations are presumably exposed to cysticercosis through direct and indirect contact with *Taenia* carriers. The vast majority of clinical cases reported in India are of the single-lesion variety with relatively mild symptoms and benign outcomes; these are believed to be associated with exposure to eggs in contaminated foodstuffs or other indirect exposure to tapeworm carriers (118). Curiously, the greatest number of cases of the rare, massive, disseminated form of the disease has also been reported from India. The explanations for these extremes are unknown (125). As might be expected, there are no reports from the strictly Muslim countries of Iran, Pakistan, and Bangladesh. Human NCC is reported widely from China and parts of Korea. It is known to occur also, although few published data are available, in the Southeast Asian countries of Myanmar (Burma), Cambodia, Laos, Vietnam, and parts of the Philippines. In Indonesia, *T. solium* infection is endemic in parts of numerous islands including Sumatra, Bali, West Kalimantan, Sulawesi, Flores, East Timor, and Irian Jaya (107). The cestode was recently introduced into Irian Jaya when swine from Bali were translocated to (the former) West New Guinea (discussed below). Improvements in socioeconomic conditions were associated with reduction or disappearance of the conditions in Japan, Taiwan, Hong Kong, Singapore, and Thailand.

In Africa, *T. solium* is transmitted throughout most of the continent with the exception of the strictly Muslim areas of North and sub-Saharan Africa. Because of the limited development of medical and sanitary infrastructure, the impact of the disease is probably underestimated to a greater degree than in other regions (81). The general lack of sanitary services, especially adequate disposal of human excrement, and the widespread occurrence of free-roaming pigs permit transmission of *T. solium* in most of the regions. Controlled slaughter of swine is rarely practiced and consequently cysticerci-infected pork is generally consumed by humans who either ignore or are unaware of its significance. In South Africa, where medical services are more sophisticated, NCC has long been a subject of scientific reports (50, 68, 79, 87, 91); from other regions where *T. solium* infection is endemic; however, there are very limited data because of the lack of diagnostic capacity. NCC is reportedly a common clinical entity in many countries of West Africa (Senegal, Benin, Ivory Coast, Togo, and Ghana), central Africa (Zaire, Cameroon,

Burundi, and Rwanda), and southern Africa (Madagascar, Mozambique, South Africa, and Zimbabwe) (73, 81). Few reports of NCC in humans in East Africa have been documented; however, a recent report of *T. solium* cysticercosis in 13% of pigs slaughtered in three abattoirs in Tanzania suggests that the cestode occurs in at least some regions (11). NCC is an important cause of neurologic disability in the regions of Africa where it has been studied; epilepsy in several countries has been documented to be caused by *T. solium* infection in 30 to 51% of cases (81). In Africa, as in Asia, subcutaneous localization of cysticerci, concomitant with intracerebral infection, is common (>30%); this is in contrast to the infection in American countries where subcutaneous localization in patients with NCC is relatively rare (25).

Historically, *T. solium* occurred widely in European countries; indeed, many of the earliest recorded observations about the parasite and its life cycle were reported by European authors (56). In the mid-19th century, it was reported that cysticerci were observed in 2% of autopsied human cadavers in Germany and infections were commonly observed in swine at slaughter (56). The same was apparently true in many countries of the continent. Today, the infection has largely disappeared as a result of improvements in swine husbandry, sanitation, and hygiene. However, locally acquired infections are still occasionally reported from Spain (Castilla, Extremadura and Andalucia) (18), northern Portugal (89), southern Italy (90), and Poland (77a), indicating persisting foci of transmission in some regions.

## Prevalence

Until recently, the only available quantitative data on cysticercosis from any country were clinic-based statistics on the frequency of NCC among hospital patients or autopsied cadavers. In Mexico, for example, NCC has long been considered to have an important impact on health services expenditures. Through the 1980s, this diagnosis accounted for nearly 9% of admissions to neurology and neurosurgical services and was the final diagnosis in 11 to 25% of patients operated on for removal of brain tumors (96). NCC was found in 2.8 to 3.6% of all autopsies in Mexico City hospitals and was reported as the cause of death in 0.6 to 1.5% of hospitalized patients. Similar statistics documenting the frequency of clinical diagnoses of NCC have been reported from many other countries. Such statistics can be misleading, however, because differences in availability of medical services and lack of comprehensive and consistent reporting in most countries still confound attempts to compare incidence and prevalence among countries and (within a country) between rural and urban areas. For example, extensive documentation in the medical literature on the occurrence of NCC in Mexico over many years might have suggested that the disease was more prevalent there than in neighboring countries. However, surveys using comparable methods, although few in number, reveal that the prevalence of *T. solium* infection in neighboring countries exceeds rates in Mexico by considerable margins (Table 1).

In all countries, improved diagnostic technology, new options for treatment, and greater awareness of cysticercosis by the medical and public health communities have resulted in documentation of increased numbers of cases diagnosed in areas

**Table 1.** Prevalence estimates of *T. solium* cysticercosis and taeniasis in people and pigs in Latin American communities

| Country | Community | Sample size | Seroprevalence (%)[a] | Prevalence of taeniasis (%) | Prevalence in pigs (%) | Reference |
|---------|-----------|-------------|----------------------|-----------------------------|------------------------|-----------|
| Mexico | Angahuan | 1,552 | 10.8 | 0.3[b] | 4.0[c] | 94 |
| | Xoxocotla | 1,005 | 4.9 | 0.2[b] | 6.5[c] | 92 |
| Guatemala | Quesada | 862 | 11.0 | 1.0[b,d] | 4.0[c] | 6 |
| | El Jocote | 955 | 20.0 | 2.8[b,d] | 14.0[c] | 49 |
| Bolivia | "Rural community" | 159 | 22.6 | ND[e] | 38.9[f] | 121 |
| Ecuador | San Pablo del Lago | 118 | 10.4 | ND | 7.5[c] | 22 |
| Peru | Lima (urban) | 250 | 0 | ND | 0 | 121 |
| | Maceda | 371 | 8.0 | 0.3[b] | 43.0[f] | 33 |
| | Churusapa | 134 | 7.0 | ND | 49.0[f] | 45 |
| | Haparquilla | 108 | 13.0 | ND | 46.0[f] | 45 |
| | Monterredonda | 489 | 16.0 | ND | 13.0[f] | 45 |
| | Quilcas | | 18.0 | ND | 60–70[f] | 45 |
| | Saylla | 99 | 24.0 | ND | 36.0[f] | 45 |

[a]Determined by immunoblot assay.
[b]Prevalence of taeniasis measured by examination of fecal specimens for eggs.
[c]Prevalence of cysticercosis in pigs measured by visual examination and palpation of tongue.
[d]Prevalence of taeniasis measured by examination of fecal specimens for coproantigens.
[e]ND, not done.
[f]Prevalence of cysticercosis in pigs measured by detection of antibodies by immunoblot assay.

where the disease is traditionally endemic as well as new disclosures of active transmission from regions where the disease was previously unrecognized or not reported. Recent surveys and epidemiologic studies, using state-of-the-art diagnostic methods, have begun to better document the occurrence of the infection and its impact on affected populations. Table 1 compares recent prevalence estimates for *T. solium* cysticercosis and taeniasis in humans and cysticercosis in pigs in surveys of community-based population samples in Latin America in which comparable diagnostic methods were used. Prevalence varied among communities, but a consistent relative pattern of prevalence ratios of the different forms of infection has been observed. Prevalences of intestinal stage infection (taeniasis) are relatively low. However, relative rates of cysticercosis in humans and pigs are consistently related quantitatively to the rates of taeniasis. NCC is not usually specifically recognized by the population of affected communities as the cause of seizures and other neurologic disorders. However, use of new, improved serologic and imaging diagnostic technology has identified NCC as the most important contributor to the high rates of epilepsy and migraine headaches in many regions where *T. solium* infection is endemic.

In most studies in which clinical information has been collected, histories of seizures and some other disorders have been linked to NCC as evidenced by CT and serologic evidence. For example, in community-based studies from Mexico, Ecuador, and Peru, large proportions of persons with histories of seizures had serologic (21 to 34%) or neurologic imaging (54 to 70%) evidence of NCC, and these clinical findings were significantly more frequent than in persons without histories of seizures (22, 47, 100). It is important to note that the seizure episodes in these rural people had not previously been linked to NCC, and this type of active diagnostic intervention was needed to be able to demonstrate the impact of the disease on the health of these communities. Although there exist no data-based estimates of the worldwide prevalence of *T. solium* infection in humans, extrapolation from these limited serologic survey data suggests that 30 to 50 million persons may have been exposed to *T. solium* in Latin America alone (121).

In most countries where *T. solium* infection is endemic, community-based prevalence data are not yet available. There is a need for provision of diagnostic and therapeutic resources at the community level to determine the prevalence of infection and rates of associated morbidity. One useful approach to quantification of neurologic disorders at the community level is the World Health Organization protocol for epidemiologic evaluation of neurologic disorders in developing countries. This provides a standardized procedure for estimating the prevalence of major neurologic illnesses: epilepsy, migraine headaches, stroke, extrapyramidal disorders, and peripheral neuropathies. When complemented by cerebral imaging and serodiagnosis for *T. solium* infection, results can be used to characterize and quantify the contribution of NCC to the local prevalence of neurologic disorders (21, 22). Information provided by such studies serves to document the burdens of morbidity and disability imposed by NCC and may lead to implementation of cost-effective control interventions.

## PATTERNS OF TRANSMISSION

### Endemic Transmission

Throughout its worldwide distribution, *T. solium* is maintained by cyclic transmission in swine and human hosts. More than 35 years ago, *T. solium* infection was called a "testimony to under-development" (14), and that characterization remains true today. Transmission of *T. solium* requires that pigs have access to human feces and that humans ingest inadequately cooked meat of pigs. Such conditions are common in rural areas of many under-developed or unevenly developed countries characterized by poor hygiene, deficient sanitary facilities, and primitive swine husbandry practices that allow pigs to run loose all or part of the time. Such communities have not yet directly benefited from the achievements in sanitation and hygiene often referred to as the "first public health revolution." In situations where pigs are kept in enclosures or are restrained, they may be fed human feces purposefully (e.g., "pig-sty privies"). Such conditions may appear to be the endpoint of social neglect but usually represent an effective adaptation to poverty and circumstance whereby the pig is nourished adequately at virtually no cost to the owner and simultaneously serves as a community scavenger or "sanitary police." Through coprophagy, pigs readily become infected, often at high rates and very intense levels. Recent surveys in communities of Latin America where the disease is endemic have revealed infection rates in pigs from 5 to 50% (6, 7, 22, 27, 33, 45, 53, 91–95), and some pigs can have ~2,500 cysticerci per kg of meat (A. E. Gonzalez, cited in reference 33).

Although local persons are usually unaware of the threat to public health that this infection in pigs represents and do not relate the lesions in their animals to disease in humans, pig owners routinely check their live pigs for cysticercosis by direct examination of the tongue. This concern is motivated by the fact that cysticerci-infected meat will be rejected at slaughter (where control is practiced) or will bring a significantly reduced price. Consequently, infected pigs may be slaughtered and sold clandestinely or for consumption by the owner's family. In villages in central Peru, where infection rates in pigs varied from 14 to 25%, virtually none of the pigs were processed at the local slaughterhouse. Rather, pig owners and vendors purposefully bypassed formal slaughterhouses. The investigators estimated that 23% of total pork consumed in the community was derived from pigs infected with cysticerci (27). Studies in Mexico, Guatemala, and Peru have shown that the principal factors associated with the likelihood of infection in pigs include age (infection rates increase with age) and access to human feces. Confined pigs tend to be protected from infection but only if confinement is habitual and they are not deliberately fed feces (33, 92, 93).

Improved understanding of the epidemiology of *T. solium* transmission requires a better understanding of the risk factors for intestinal-stage infection and the modes of dispersal of infective eggs by human tapeworm carriers because taeniid eggs in feces or contamination of the hands of infected humans are the direct source of cysticercosis in pigs and humans. Some recent studies, utilizing improved diagnostic techniques, have begun to collect such information. Surveys in communities where the disease is endemic in Mexico, Guatemala, Peru, and Honduras have shown rates varying from 0.3 to 6.0% (5, 6, 28, 33, 91–94). Factors associated with taeniasis include age (rates of intestinal taeniid infections tend to peak in middle adulthood; although infections occur in all age groups) and frequency of pork consumption (6, 91, 92, 94). In some populations, taeniid infections are observed significantly more frequently in women than in men (6, 28, 49, 84). The presence of a tapeworm-infected individual within a household is an important risk factor for exposure to *T. solium* cysticercosis, and this risk may be increased if the tapeworm carrier is a woman engaged in food preparation and child care activities.

In Peruvian mountain villages, food handlers engaged in preparing and selling a traditional pork dish ("chicharrones") were shown to harbor intestinal taeniid infections at a significantly higher rate than other persons in the community (45). Serologic screening of humans from these villages using the same specific immunoblot assay documented levels of apparent exposure to cysticercosis varying from 5 to 24% (Table 1).

Higher levels of seropositivity in humans were associated with low levels of sanitary infrastructure (6) and personal hygiene (92), an age of over 20 years (33, 45, 47, 92, 94), and personal histories of taeniasis (33, 47, 92). The highest seropositivity rates were observed among persons with multiple factors (45), suggesting that these apparent risk factors and behaviors acted cumulatively. In some communities there was evidence of "clustering" of seropositive individuals in households of persons with histories of or current taeniasis (6, 22, 91, 92). In Guatemala, for example, one-third of all seropositive persons were clustered within the same households (6). These observations indicate the "focal" nature of transmission associated with the presence of a tapeworm carrier. There is a need for further studies in Latin America and in other areas where *T. solium* is currently transmitted to provide baseline epidemiologic data and suggest strategies for control.

## Imported and Introduced Disease

Imported cases of *T. solium* taeniasis/cysticercosis are those acquired in a foreign country. Onset of illness in NCC typically occurs a year or more after initial acquisition of the infection. Therefore, among internationally mobile persons exposed to infection it is not uncommon that development of the disease occurs in a different country than that in which the infection was acquired ("imported case"). Returning tourists or immigrants can also import intestinal-stage *T. solium* infections into the country. When the tapeworm carrier travels home or emigrates to a foreign country and inadvertently transmits the infection to another person (or to a pig) the infection has been "introduced" to the host country. More rarely, the infection can be introduced by international transport of infected pigs and subsequent consumption of their infected meat.

### Imported Disease

A unique historical epidemic of imported NCC occurred in British troops stationed in India. At least 450 soldiers or their family members developed symptoms from 1 to 30 years (average, 5 years) following their deployment in India (35). Approximately one-fourth of these patients reported a history of taeniasis, but little other information was reported on their possible sources of infection.

Smaller numbers of imported cases are currently diagnosed every year in many countries in immigrants or tourists returning from countries where *T. solium* infection is endemic. This phenomena is fed by the recent increases in international migrations as a result of tourist and business travel and emigration (the World Tourist Organization currently estimates that at least 400 million international border crossings occur each year). In recent years, series of imported cases of NCC have been reported from Australia (71, 76, 128), Norway (34a), Argentina (124), Denmark (60), and the United States (discussed below). The ratio of immigrants to tourists among these patients is about 10:1. Rarely was a specific source of infection identified for imported cases.

### Introduced Disease

On rare occasions *T. solium* has been introduced into a new area and spread epidemically. Such was the case in West Irian Jaya where the infection was introduced in swine brought from Bali and given to the Ekari people by the Indonesian government as part of an effort to induce them to accept Indonesian control. Unfortunately, these pigs turned out to be something of a "Trojan horse," because the swine were infected by cysticerci of *T. solium* and the human population also became infected, with disastrous consequences. Local cultural customs and pig husbandry practices facilitated the transmission and rapid spread of the cestode. The first indication of the problem was noted in 1971 when many of the people suffered seizures and burns caused by NCC (42). As a result of extensive migrations of people with their pigs, the infection has spread throughout the island, possibly including Papua New Guinea, and is now considered a serious emerging health problem there (107).

There are no other documented instances of foreign "introduction" and continued transmission of *T. solium* via infected pigs, yet imported cases of human taeniasis occasionally are linked epidemiologically to clusters of infected pigs in the United States (88, 101a). Such "outbreaks" have been identified by routine inspection of infected swine at slaughter and limited to the exposed cohorts of pigs.

## The U.S. Experience

By virtue of the number of immigrants entering the United States every year from countries where *T. solium* infection is endemic, more cases of imported NCC are diagnosed here every year than in all other countries combined. *T. solium* cysticercosis is (and apparently always has been) mostly an imported disease in the United States. Even 150 years ago, locally acquired cysticercosis was apparently rarely recognized or recorded although environmental and socioeconomic conditions were conducive to transmission in the pig-human cycle. "Thousands of swine" roamed the streets of New York City (and most other urban and rural communities) and were allowed to do so because they were efficient scavengers (85). The few cases of NCC recorded in those years were in German and other European immigrants (32). Of 42 cases recorded between 1857 and 1954, only three were "unequivocably" autochthonous (13). Of greater significance in recent decades is NCC's emergence as an important clinical entity in California and other southwestern states in immigrants from countries where *T. solium* infection is endemic. By 1980, NCC was recognized as the leading cause of nonalcoholic seizures in adults and a common cause of meningitis and intracranial masses (64). Review of published literature on more than 900 cases diagnosed through 1986 indicated that more than 90% of patients were born outside the country, most (80 to 90%) in Mexico (13, 16, 19, 36, 43, 64, 66, 70, 74, 102, 105, 116). Only 15 well-documented, locally acquired cases (e.g., patients born in the United States with no history of travel to a country where *T. solium* infection is endemic) had been reported in the published literature (36).

For some years beginning in the mid-1970s, we had been aware of increasing numbers of diagnosed cases of NCC in southern California and other southwestern states. This was apparent from the increase in numbers of serum specimens sent to CDC by physicians requiring confirmation of their presumptive diagnoses and by the increase of clinical reports that were published in American medical journals. To determine the nature of this phenomenon, we reviewed hospital records of four of the largest medical centers in Los Angeles County and obtained information on 447 cases diagnosed during the 11-year period from 1973 to 1983 (84). It was readily apparent that beginning the last few years of the 1970s, there was a significant increase in diagnoses of NCC. The number of cases diagnosed annually increased four-fold between 1977 and 1981. A number of factors may have been involved in this apparent emergence including an increase in the number of immigrants from areas where the disease is endemic and improved physician awareness of the disease. However, the major factor was the introduction and widespread utilization of CT scans, for example. This new technology had so enhanced the clinician's ability to identify and define the nature of intracerebral lesions that its introduction confounded other possible explanations. Ninety-five percent of the patients in the cases reported during this period were Hispanic. Hospital admission records did not record patients' country of origin. Three percent of patients had no history of travel to areas where the disease is endemic outside the United States; thus, their infections were presumably acquired locally.

Concerned about the implications of the findings of the hospital survey, the Los Angeles County Department of Health Services (LACDHS) took action to collect more information on the disease. An important step was to make cysticercosis a reportable disease and to conduct investigations of contacts of reported cases to look for factors associated with local transmission. In the first 3 years of reporting, 1988–1990, the LACDHS was notified of 138 cases (109). Although it was believed that many diagnosed cases were not reported, the overall rate per 100,000 population was 0.6; among the Hispanic population, however, it was 1.6 per 100,000. Mortality in this group of patients was 5.8 percent. Of 122 patients for whom detailed histories were available, most (85%) were foreign-born immigrants. Of 19 patients born in the United States, nine had traveled to Mexico or other countries where *T. solium* is endemic. The remaining 10 cases (7%) were presumably acquired locally from exposure to *T. solium* tapeworm carriers ("introduced cases"). Interestingly, the mean age of these patients was 14 years, considerably less than that of patients with imported disease (23 years). Routine follow-up investigations resulted in demonstration of active *Taenia* sp. infections among family contacts (the probable sources of the cysticercosis infections) in 22% of locally acquired cases and in 5% of imported cases (109). This demonstrated the value of such investigations for identifying potential sources of local transmission; treatment of these *Taenia* infections eliminates the potential for further transmission. Epidemiologic investigations of some cases acquired in California or other states have also identified household contact with persons who had imported tapeworm infections as probable sources of infection (16, 64, 67, 116). In 1989, cysticercosis was made a reportable disease in the state of California. During the following 12 months, 134 cases were reported. The characteristics of these patients were very similar to those described from Los Angeles County (37).

The continuing epidemic of imported disease has expanded to adjacent states and elsewhere in the country. Although cysticercosis is not a reportable disease in states other than California, extrapolation from the California surveillance data, the numbers of requests for immunodiagnosis, and the published case series from other states, it was estimated that >1,000 cases are currently diagnosed each year in the United States (106). In a single general hospital in Houston, Texas, 204 cases were identified by review of discharge diagnoses and neurology clinic records between 1994 and 1997 (29). More than 99% of the patients were Hispanic immigrants from Mexico and El Salvador; diagnoses of NCC accounted for 16% of seizure cases in Hispanics. These researchers estimated that >1,000 cases are diagnosed each year in the United States (106). In Chicago, two recent reports highlight the increasing frequency of NCC in children (86, 113). As in the past, most cases were diagnosed in persons of Hispanic origin (>90%), but increasing proportions of the patients (up to 42%) were persons born in the United States. Reported sources of possible exposure in these persons include recent travel to Mexico or Central America (50%) or visitors in the home from Latin America (20%) (86). From 6 to 28% lacked apparent risk factors, and one is left to speculate on their possible sources of infection. An ongoing multistate surveillance project of 11 university-affiliated hospital emergency departments (EDs) has preliminarily documented NCC as the apparent cause of approximately 2% of cases of seizures. Most cases were seen in the southwestern states (77). Patients with no travel history and in whom infections may have been locally acquired represented 8% of total.

Cases of NCC that were apparently acquired locally are being reported with increasing frequency and from regions of the country where there has been less local awareness on the part of physicians and public health authorities (8, 16, 86, 113). Direct or circumstantial evidence commonly links these cases to exposure to immigrants from Latin America, who are presumably carriers of *T. solium*. This was most dramatically shown in a cluster of cases in four unrelated families of an Orthodox Jewish community in New York City (97). The clue to the epidemiologic puzzle in these cases was the employment of live-in housekeepers in all of the homes. All of these women had recently emigrated from Latin American countries where *T. solium* is endemic and were considered the most likely source of infection for the members of these households. Examination of six housekeepers currently or previously employed in the four case households revealed an active *Taenia* sp. infection in one and a positive serologic test result in another. Employment of immigrants as domestic workers was very common in this community; a random telephone survey determined that 94% of the approximately 7,000 households in the community employed housekeepers, almost all of whom had recently emigrated from rural areas of Mexico or countries of Central America. Each household employed an average of three such women per year.

To further evaluate the extent of this problem, we conducted a serosurvey in the same community and sought to identify exposures and practices associated with acquisition of infection. Cysticercosis antibodies were detected by immunoblot assay (EITB) in 23 (1.3%) of 1,789 persons from 612 families (75). All 23 seropositive persons were asymptomatic, and no intracerebral lesions were found in the 21 seropositive persons who underwent brain imaging. Seropositivity was significantly associated ($P < 0.05$) with female sex, employment of a domestic worker for child care duties, and employment of persons from Central America.

Seropositivity in households in the Brooklyn community was associated with employment of housekeepers from Central America. This apparent link to the workers from Central America rather than Mexico is supported by the limited data on rates of *T. solium* infections. Pork tapeworm infection is endemic in many Latin American countries, but prevalence may be higher in rural Central America than in other areas (Table 1). A stool examination survey of migrant workers in North Carolina found taeniasis in Central American workers (4.4%), but none in those from Haiti or Mexico (26). Taeniasis prevalence among emigrant employees in surveyed households is unknown and may be difficult to determine; most employees live in the households, many are undocumented aliens, access to the population is limited, and confidentiality of test results is difficult to ensure. Widespread employment of domestic workers from regions where the disease is endemic and high employee turnover contribute to exposure risk. We have recommended that individuals at risk for *T. solium* who are to be employed as domestic workers or food handlers should be screened for tapeworm infection and treated if positive (75).

Of further concern are the numbers, possibly increasing, of cysticercosis cases in which inquiry and investigation fails to demonstrate a probable cause of cysticercosis (16, 86, 113). These patients are typically young, born in the United States, and without histories of foreign travel or employment of domestic workers in their households. In these cases one may presume that patients acquire their infection through ingestion of food, possibly served in a restaurant, accidentally contaminated with *T. solium* eggs by an infected food handler. It is important to note that the possibility of acquiring *T. solium* taeniasis by ingestion of pork in the U.S. is remote. Of more that 80 million swine slaughtered in the U.S. every year under government inspection, usually fewer than 10 carcasses with cysticercosis are recorded (88, 98).

Because immigration to the United States from countries where *T. solium* infection is endemic continues to rise, the numbers of imported cases of NCC as well as local transmission from imported tapeworm carriers are likely to increase. Immigration from Mexico and other countries has increased markedly in each of the last 3 decades. By the late 1980s the foreign-born population in the United States was estimated to be about 20 million; the numbers of immigrants born in Mexico alone doubled from 2.2 million to 4.3 million (124). Net legal and illegal immigration is currently estimated to surpass 1 million per year, and there is no immediate prospect that these numbers will decrease. However, these statistics are not fully indicative of the movement back and forth across the 2,000-mile border between the United States and Mexico. Many Mexican and Central American workers in the U.S. travel "home" to their villages or cities at least once a year (6, 29). It is estimated that movement in both directions across the U.S.-Mexico border exceeds 200 million persons per year. Thus opportunities for acquiring and transporting both intestinal- and tissue-stage *T. solium* infections are multiplied.

## CONTROL AND ERADICATION

The response in the United States to this emerging problem of cysticercosis has been to provide improved diagnostic tests, to increase physician awareness of the condition and its associated risk factors, and to look for opportunities to collect more accurate information about its epidemiology (84, 97, 109, 119). When high-risk communities or groups were identified, attempts were made to educate them about the disease and how to minimize chances for its transmission, e.g., by recommending that persons at high risk of having tapeworm infections be screened for intestinal parasites (and treated if infected) if they are to be employed as food handlers or housekeepers (97). The permanent solution to this public health problem, however, lies in controlling the infection in the hundreds or thousands of rural communities in Mexico and elsewhere in Latin America, where conditions exist to permit the life cycle of *T. solium* to be consummated.

In 1993, the International Task Force For Disease Eradication declared *Taenia solium* a potentially eradicable infection (17). The parasite has several characteristics that appear to make it vulnerable to eradication (99): (i) the life cycle requires humans as definitive hosts; (ii) tapeworm infections in humans are the only source of infection for pigs, the natural intermediate hosts; (iii) the life span of pigs rarely exceeds 1 year, and swine herds can be managed; (iv) no reservoirs for infection exist in wildlife; and (v) *T. solium* gradually disappeared from most European countries even without control measures targeted specifically at it. Factors credited with the elimination of *T. solium* include improvements in general sanitation and economic status, the introduction of indoor pig husbandry, and rigorous meat inspection.

Under the conditions that exist currently in countries where *T. solium* infection is endemic and given available resources, we do not yet know what is required to reduce and ultimately eliminate transmission. Although no intervention program specifically targeted against *T. solium* at the national or regional level has been implemented in recent times with proven success, several strategies for control have been proposed (8, 52, 99). They include the following measures.

## Comprehensive Programs of Long-Term Intervention

This involves appropriate legislation, health education, modernization of swine husbandry practices, more efficient and all-inclusive coverage of meat inspection, provision of adequate sanitary facilities, and measures to detect and treat human tapeworm carriers. Such comprehensive improvements, although not targeted at *T. solium*, are what incidentally reduced transmission in many European countries. Such programs are extremely desirable and represent the long-term goal of health development because they yield broad benefits at many levels of society. They are very expensive and require advanced levels of infrastructure development. Political and economic realities in many communities where *T. solium* is endemic today, however, provide little hope that all of these measures can be implemented in the near future. For example, the investment in water, sanitation, and health services needed to eliminate the risk of cholera throughout Latin America was estimated to exceed $200 billion over 12 years (57). It remains to be seen if resources of that magnitude can be mobilized for development in the face of a health threat.

## Short-Term, Targeted Intervention Programs

To achieve more rapid progress toward eradication and substantial reduction of sickness and death caused by neurocysticercosis, short-term intervention measures have been proposed and in some cases partially evaluated. These include the following measures.

### Mass or Selected Taeniacidal Treatment of Humans

This strategy is based on the identification of transmission foci and treatment of everyone or of all diagnosed or suspected cases of taeniosis in humans, with the goal of immediate interruption of transmission from humans to pigs and other humans. The feasibility of this strategy was shown in a trial in Ecuador in which approximately 15,000 persons in several communities were administered praziquantel (5 to 10 mg/kg); this intervention achieved at least a temporary reduction in the prevalence of cysticercosis in pigs (23). In a smaller trial in Mexico, however, this low dose of praziquantel appeared to have reactivated symptoms of neurocysticercosis in at least one case of previously undiagnosed NCC (41), thus revealing a potentially harmful reaction to this intervention. Niclosamide was used for mass treatment of populations in two villages in Guatemala; 10 months after treatment, significant reductions were noted in the prevalence of taeniasis in humans (3.5 to 1.0%) and cysticercosis in pigs (55 to 7%) (7). Niclosamide is not considered to be potentially harmful in patients with NCC and may be an effective alternative to praziquantel for mass administration. Further research on the costs, safety, and effectiveness of various taeniacidal drugs and strategies for their administration are necessary.

### Cysticercidal Treatment of Pigs

The recent demonstation of the 100% efficacy of the benzimidazole compound oxfendazole, given as a single dose, for destroying cysticerci while not damaging the animal or the meat product, introduces the possibility of treatment of pigs as a possible intervention (54). The pig is a good target for surveillance and intervention for many reasons, including its value to the owner, the local awareness that cysticercosis reduces market value (27), and the current availability of effective means of diagnosis and treatment. Intervention measures focused on pigs have not yet been evaluated on any scale. Cost, sustainability, and long-term effectiveness of these approaches need to be assessed.

### Vaccination of Pigs and/or Humans

Although the technology is not yet developed for *T. solium*, there is sound theoretical possibility that an effective vaccine to protect swine and human intermediate hosts could be developed. Such has already been demonstrated in the cases of the related taeniids *T. ovis* and *Echinococcus granulosus* for which cloned recombinant antigen vaccines have been produced (63). Although their production may be feasible, how vaccines could fit into the overall intervention strategy (i.e., their cost, effectiveness, and sustainability) would have to be demonstrated.

### Health Education

Experience with other zoonotic rural health problems, such as echinococcosis in New Zealand and Tasmania (Australia), indicated that educational interventions in the form of posters and pamphlets had no effect, by themselves, on transmission of the infection (51). They were believed, however, to have sensitized the population to accept the introduction of other interventions such as restrictions on home slaughter of livestock and diagnostic dosing of dogs; these latter actions have nearly eradicated infection from those island regions. The results of a recent field trial in Mexico of an educational intervention against *T. solium*, in which the educational strategy was based on careful ethnographic study and involved extensive community participation, suggested that education may succeed in changing knowledge and practices related to the infection. Within 6 months of completion of the educational intervention, rates of transmission had declined significantly as measured by infection prevalence in young pigs (95). Continued educational intervention, supported by legislation and active enforcement, may succeed in reducing and perhaps ultimately eliminating transmission of the cestode; however, further studies of the effectiveness of health education, with long-term followup, are needed. Health education, whether part of short-term or long-term programs, is a fundamental requirement to obtain local cooperation and sustainability of the intervention strategy. Experiences with other diseases indicate that to be maximally effective health education must be based on local perceptions, knowledge, and practices related to the disease and must involve participation of the community.

## Maintenance Activities

Fundamental to any strategy of intervention against *T. solium* is sustainability. Once substantial progress in reducing transmission of taeniasis/cysticercosis through targeted intervention has been achieved, means must be developed to sustain progress (9). One approach may be to integrate control activities into primary health care systems. Maintenance activities might include identification of new foci of transmission followed by targeted application of measures to eliminate infection. To be effective in the long term, control measures based on these short-term approaches have to be supported by aggressive educational campaigns and by significant improvements in personal hygiene and general sanitation within the area where the disease is endemic.

## Developing an Action Plan

As a first step toward achieving prevention and control of taeniasis and cysticercosis, it is necessary to implement national plans aimed at controlling this disease. A number of countries already have national action plans, yet few activities have been implemented. As a first step, it is necessary to identify regions where *T. solium* infection is endemic, to measure prevalence of taeniosis and cysticercosis in pigs and humans, and to evaluate the economic and social costs of the disease. There is a need for operational research aimed at verifying the effectiveness, costs, and benefits of alternative intervention strategies against *T. solium* in a variety of geographic and socioeconomic settings.

## CONCLUSIONS

*T. solium* infection is widely endemic in rural areas of developing countries where political, socioeconomic, and environmental conditions permit the tapeworm's life cycle in pigs and humans to be completed. Active intervention for control of *T. solium* infection is still at its infancy, and there are severe economic and social problems existing in most areas where the disease is endemic that hinder implementation of programs.

Special studies reveal that morbidity caused by NCC is measurable and severe in areas where NCC is endemic. Nevertheless, the nature of the disease and the lack of locally available diagnostic facilities make NCC an essentially silent and unrecognized disease of humans within most affected communities. These realities complicate attempts to motivate and empower the community to initiate measures to control the disease. Pig owners, however, easily recognize the infection in their animals; the fact that cysticercosis reduces the market value of infected pigs suggests a focus for education and prevention measures. In contrast, people rarely understand the relationship between cysticercosis in pigs and taeniosis or cysticercosis in humans and thus lack knowledge and incentive to change behavior that fosters transmission. In many, if not most, communities where *T. solium* infection is endemic there is an absence of piped water, sanitary infrastructure, waste disposal, and other basic services. Consequently, to be effective in the short term, intervention measures must be designed to circumvent these deficiencies to the extent possible. Primary health care facilities are also often lacking or inadequate. Since the disease is generally related to poverty and all its associated manifestations, all strategies to control the disease must consider costs and locally available resources (9, 52, 99). Nevertheless, the many recent advances in diagnosis and treatment of the disease and the new knowledge of the impact of the zoonotic disease on local health and the economy, provide incentives and improved means to undertake these tasks.

## REFERENCES

1. **Alarcon, F., G. Duenas, L. Escalante, M. Montalvo, and M. Roman.** 1989. Neurocysticercosis. Short course of treatment with albendazole. *Arch. Neurol.* **46:**1231–1236.
2. **Allan, J. C., G. Avila, A. Flisser, J. Garcia-Noval, and P. S. Craig.** 1990. Immunodiagnosis of taeniasis by coproantigen detection. *Parasitology* **101:**473–477.
3. **Allan, J. C., P. S. Craig, J. Garcia-Noval, D. Lui, F. Mencos, M. Rogan, R. Stringer, Y. Wang, H. Wen, E. Zeyhle, and P. Zhou.** 1992. Coproantigen detection for the immunodiagnosis of echinococcus and taeniasis in dogs and humans. *Parasitology* **104:**347–355.
4. **Allan, J. C., A. Flisser, J. Garcia-Noval, F. Mencos, and E. Sarti.** 1993. Dipstick dot ELISA for detection of *Taenia* coproantigens in humans. *Parasitology* **107:**79–85.
5. **Allan, J. C., J. Garcia-Noval, R. Torres-Alvarez, M. Velasquez-Tohom, and P. Yurrita.** 1996. Field trial of diagnosis of *Taenia solium* taeniasis by coproantigen enzyme-linked immunosorbent assay. *Am. J. Trop. Med. Hyg.* **54:** 352–356.
6. **Allan, J. C., H. Soto de Alfaro, R. Torres-Alvarez, P. S. Craig, C. Fletes, J. Garcia-Noval, F. de Mata, R. M. Velasquez-Tohom, and P. Yurrita.** 1996. Epidemiology of intestinal taeniasis in four rural Guatemalan communities. *Ann. Trop. Med. Parasitol.* **90:**157–165.
7. **Allan, J. C., C. Fletes, M. Velasquez-Tohom, et al.** 1997. Mass chemotherapy for intestinal *Taenia Solium* infection: effect on prevalence in humans and pigs. *Trans. R. Soc. Trop. Med. Hyg.* **91:**595–598.
8. **Anonymous.** 1990. Cysticercosis in California. *California Morbidity* (Biweekly reports 23 and 24.) Infectious Disease Branch, Department of Health Services, State of California, Berkeley.
9. **Anonymous** 1997. *PAHO/WHO Informal Consultation on the Taeniasis/Cysticercosis Complex.* p. 1–20. Pan American Health Organization Series HCT/AIEPI-5. Pan American Health Organization, Washington, D.C.
10. **Banerjee, P. S., B. B. Bhatia, and B. A. Pandit.** 1994. *Sarcocystis suihominis* infection in human beings in India. *J. Vet. Parasitol.* **8:**57–58.
11. **Boa, M. E., H. O. Bogh, A. A. Kassuku, and P. Nansen.** 1995. The prevalence of *Taenia solium* metacestodes in pigs in northern Tanzania. *J. Helm.* **69:**113–117.
12. **Camacho, S. P. D., R. Lozano, M. F. Medina, V. S. Peraza, M. L. Z. Ramos, A. C. Ruiz, and K. Willms.** 1991. Epidemiologic study and control of *Taenia solium* infections with praziquantel in a rural village of Mexico. *Am. J. Trop. Med. Hyg.* **145:**522–531.
13. **Campagna, M., and C. Schwartzwelder.** 1954. Human cysticerosis in the United States. *J. Parasitol.* **40**(Suppl.):46.
14. **Canelas, H. M.** 1962. Neurocisticercose: incidencia diagnostico y formas. *Arg. Neuropsiquiatr.* **20:** 1–15.
15. **Carpio, A., C. Flores, P. Leon, F. Santillan, and W. A. Hauser.** 1995. Is the course of neurocysticercosis modified by treatment with antihelminthic agents? *Arch. Intern. Med.* **155:**1982–1995.

16. **Centers for Disease Control and Prevention.** 1992. Locally-acquired neurocysticercosis—North Carolina, Massachusetts, and South Carolina. *Morbid. Mortal. Weekly Rep.* **41:**1–4.

17. **Centers for Disease Control and Prevention.** 1993. Recommendation of the International Task Force for Disease Eradication. *Morbid. Mortal. Weekly Rep.* **42**(RR-16):1–27.

18. **Chinchilla, N., D. De Andres, and S. Gimenez-Roldan.** 1989. Neurocysticercosis in the urban area of Madrid. *Arch. Neurobiol.* **52**(6):287–294.

19. **Cohen, B.** 1962. Cysticercosis cerebri: a case report. *South. Med. J.* **55:**48–55.

20. **Communicable Tropical Diseases, International League Against Epilepsy.** 1994. Relationship between epilepsy and tropical diseases. *Epilepsia* **35:**89–93.

21. **Cruz, M. E., I. Cruz, M. Dumas, P. M. Preux, and P. Schantz.** 1994b. Headache and cysticercosis in Ecuador, South America. *Headache* **35:**93–97.

22. **Cruz, M. E., P. M. Schantz, I. Cruz, et al.** 1998. Epilepsy and neurocysticercosis in an Andean community. Submitted for publication.

23. **Cruz, M., A. Davis, H. Dixon, and Z. S. Pawlowski.** 1989. Operational studies on the control of *Taenia solium* taeniasis/cysticercosis in Ecuador. *Bull. W. H. O.* **67:**563–566.

24. **Cruz, M., I. Cruz, and J. Horton.** 1991. Albendazole versus praziquantel in the treatment of cerebral cysticercosis: clinical evaluation. *Trans. R. Soc. Trop. Med. Hyg.* **85:**244–247.

25. **Cruz, M., I. Cruz, P. M. Schantz, and W. Teran.** 1994. Human subcutaneous *Taenia solium* cysticercosis in an Andean population with neurocysticercosis. *Am. J. Trop. Med. Hyg.* **51:**405–407.

26. **Csiesielski, S. D., J. Metts, J. C. Ortiz, and J. R. Seed.** 1991. Parasites among North Carolina migrant farm workers. *Am. J. Public Health* **82:**1258–1262.

27. **Cysticercosis Working Group in Peru.** 1993. The marketing of cysticercotic pigs in the Sierra of Peru. *Bull. W. H. O.* **71:**223–228.

28. **de Kaminsky, R. G.** 1991. Taeniasis-cysticercosis in Honduras. *Trans. R. Soc. Trop. Med. Hyg.* **85:**531–534.

29. **De La Garza, Y., E. Graviss, W. Shandera, R. Armstrong, P. Schantz, and A. C. White.** Epidemiology of neurocysticercosis in Houston, Texas, abstr. P-28.2, p. 148. *In International Conference on Emerging Infectious Diseases Program & Abstracts Book.*

30. **Del Brutto, O. H., and J. Sotelo.** 1988. Neurocysticercosis: an update. *Rev. Infect. Dis.* **6:**1075–1087.

31. **Del Brutto, O. H., C. A. Boboa, and R. Santibanez.** 1992. Epilepsy due to neurocysticercosis. Analysis of 203 patients. *Neurology* **42:**389–392.

32. **Diamond, I. B.** 1899. Cysticercus of brain and spinal cord. *JAMA* **32:**1365–1369.

33. **Diaz, J. F., H. H. Garcia, R. H. Gilman, A. E. Gonzales, M. Castro, V. C. Tsang, J. B. Pilcher, L. E. Vasquez, M. Lescano, C. Carcamo, G. Madico, E. Miranda, and the Cysticercosis Working Group in Peru.** 1992. Epidemiology of taeniasis and cysticercosis in a Peruvian village. *Am. J. Epidemiol.* **185:**875–882.

34. **Diaz, J. F., M. Verastegui, R. H. Gilman, V. C. Tsang, J. B. Pilcher, C. Gallo, H. H. Garcia, P. Torres, T. Montenegro, E. Miranda, and the Cysticercosis Working Group in Peru.** 1992. Immunodiagnosis of human cysticercosis: A field comparison of an antibody enzyme-linked immunosorbent assay (ELISA), and an enzyme-linked immunoelectro transfer blot (EITB) assay in Peru. *Am. J. Trop. Med. Hyg.* **46:**610–615. .

34a. **Dietrichs, E., N. O. Aanonsen, S. J. Bakke, K. Skullerud, and T. Tyssvang.** 1994. Tapeworms in the brain—current problem in Norway. *J. Norw. Med. Assoc.* **114:**3089–3092.

35. **Dixon, H. B. F., F. M. Lipscomb, and W. H. Hargreaves.** 1961. Cysticercosis: An analysis and follow-up of 450 cases. Privy Council. *Med. Res. Spec. Rep. Ser.* **229:**1–58.

36. **Earnest, M. P., C. M. Filley, and L. B. Reller.** 1987. Neurocysticercosis in the United States: 35 cases and a review. *Rev. Infect. Dis.* **9:**961–979.

37. **Ehnert, K. L, L. Barrett, R. R. Roberto, G. W. Rutherford, and F. J. Sorvillo.** 1992. Cysticercosis: first 12 months of reporting in California. *Bull. Pan. Am. Health Organ.* **26:**165–169.

38. **Eldson-Dew, R., and E. M. Proctor.** 1965. Distinction between *Taeniarhynchus saginata* and *Taenia solium. S. Afr. J. Sci.* **61:**215–217.

39. **Feldman, M., A. Plancarte, M. Sandoval, and A. Flisser.** 1990. Comparison of two assays (EIA and EITB) and two samples (saliva and serum) for the diagnosis of neurocysticercosis. *Trans. R. Soc. Trop. Med. Hyg.* **84:**559–562.

40. **Flisser, A., J. Allan, P. Craig, I. Madrazo, A. Plancarte, E. Sarti, and P. Schantz.** 1993. Neurological symptoms in occult neurocysticercosis after single taeniacidal dose of praziquantel. *Lancet* **342:**748.

41. **Flisser, A.** 1994. Taeniasis and cysticercosis due to *Taenia solium. Prog. Clin. Parasitol.* **4:**77–115.

42. **Gadjusek, D. C.** 1978. Introduction of *Taenia solium* into West New Guinea with a note on an epidemic of burns from cysticercus epilepsy in the Ekari people of the Wissel Lake area. *Papua New Guinea Med. J.* **21:**329–342.

43. **Garbutt, G. D., and C. B. Courville.** 1967. Cysticercosis cerebri. A retrospective study including 14 new cases personally investigated. *Bull. Los Angel. Neurol. Soc.* **32:**6–16.

44. **Garcia, H. H., E. J. Candy, J. F. Diaz, R. H. Gilman, G. Herrera, E. Miranda, J. Naranjo, V. C. W. Tsang, and the Cysticercosis Working Group.** 1994. Discrepancies between cerebral computed tomography and western blot in the diagnosis of neurocysticercosis. *Am. J. Trop. Med. Hyg.* **50:**152–157.

45. **Garcia, H. H., R. H. Gilman, A. E. Gonzales, and the Cysticercosis Working Group.** 1996. Epidemiología de la cisticercosis en el Peru, p. 313–326. *In* H. H. Garcia and S. M. Martinez (ed.), *Taeniasis/Cisticercosis por* T. Solium. Editorial Universo S. A., Lima, Peru.

46. **Garcia, H. H., M. Catacora, R. H. Gilman, A. Gonzalez, V. C. W. Tsang, M. Verastegui, and the Cysticercosis Working Group.** 1997. Serologic evaluation of neurocysticercosis patients after antiparasitic therapy. *J. Infect. Dis.* **175:**486–489.

47. **Garcia-Noval, J., J. C. Allan, P. S. Craig, C. Fletes, H. Higueros, F. de Mata, F. Mencos, E. Moreno, H. Soto, R. Torres, and P. Yurrita.** 1996. Epidemiology of *Taenia solium* taeniasis and cysticercosis in two rural Guatemalan communities. *Am. J. Trop. Med. Hyg.* **55:**282–289.

48. **Garcia, H. H., R. H. Gilman, V. C. W. Tsang, et al.** 1997. Clinical significance of neurocysticercosis in endemic villages. *Trans. R. Soc. Trop. Med. Hyg.* **91:**176–178.

49. **Garcia, H. H., M. Alvarado, F. Diaz, C. Gallo, R. Gilman, G. Herrera, M. Martinez, E. Miranda, J. Naranjo, J. B. Pilcher, M. Porras, V. C. W. Tsang, M. Verastegui, and the Cysticercosis Working Group in Peru.** 1991. Diagnosis of cysticercosis in endemic regions. *Lancet* **338:**549–551.

50. **Gelfand, M., and C. Jeffrey.** 1973. Cerebral cysticercosis in Rhodesia. *J. Trop. Med. Hyg.* **76:**87–89.

51. **Gemmel, M. A., and P. M. Schantz.** 1997. Formulating policies for control of *Echinococus granuloses*: an overview of planning, implementation, and evaluation, p. 329–345. *In* F. L. Andersen, M. Kachari, and H. Ouhelli (ed.), *Compendium on Cystic Echinococosis.* Brigham Young University Print Services, Provo, Utah.

52. **Gilman, R. H., M. Dunleavy, C. A. W. Evans, H. Garcia, A. E. Gonzalez, M. Verastegui, and the Cysticercosis Working Group in Peru.** 1996. Methods for the control of taeniasis-cysticercosis, p. 327–340. *In* H. H. Garcia and M. Martinez (ed.), *Taeniasis/Cisticercosis por* T. solium. Editorial Universo S. A., Lima, Peru.

53. **Gonzalez, A. E., H. Balazar, V. Cama, M. Castro, A. Chavera, R. H. Gilman, E. Miranda, T. Montenegro, J. B. Pilcher, V. C. W. Tsang, and M. Verastegui.** 1990. Prevalence and comparison of serologic assays, necropsy, and tongue examination for the diagnosis of porcine cysticercosis in Peru. *Am. J. Trop. Med. Hyg.* **43:**194–199.

54. **Gonzalez, A. E., H. H. Garcia, R. H. Gilman, C. M. Gavidia, V. C. W. Tsang, T. Bernal, N. Falcon, M. Romero, and M. T. Lopez-Urbina.** 1996. Effective single dose treatment of porcine cysticercosis with oxfendazole. *Am. J. Trop. Med. Hyg.* **54:**391–394.

55. **Gottstein, B., P. M. Schantz, and V. C. W. Tsang.** 1985. Demonstration of species-specific and cross-reactive components of *Taenia solium* mestacestode antigens. *Am. J. Trop. Med. Hyg.* **35:**308–18.

56. **Grove, D. I.** 1990. *Taenia Solium* and *Taeniasis Solium* and cysticercosis, p. 335–383. *In A History of Human Helminthology.* CAB International, Oxford, United Kingdom.

57. **Guerra de Macedo, C.** 1991. Proposal for investment in health. *Bull. Pan Am. Health Organ.* **25:**i.

58. **Hachinski, V. C.** 1995. Controversies in neurology. *Neurology* **52:**104.

59. **Hall, A., D. W. T. Crompton, M. C. Latham, and L. S. Stephenson.** 1981. *Taenia saginata* (cestoda) in western Kenya: the reliability of faecal examination in diagnosis. *Parasitology* **83**:91–101.

60. **Hansen, N. J. D., T. Christensen, and L. H. Hagelskjaer.** 1992. Neurocysticercosis: a short review and presentation of a Scandinavian case. *Scand. J. Infect. Dis.* **24**:255–262.

61. **Henneberg, R.** 1912. The animal parasites of the central nervous system. *Handb. Neurol.* **3**:642–683. (In German.).

62. **Ito, A., A. Plancarte, L. Ma, et al.** Novel antigens for neurocysticercosis: Simple method for preparation and evaluation for serodiagnosis. *Am. J. Trop. Med. Hyg.*, in press.

63. **Johnson, K. S., G. B. L. Harrison, and M. W. Lightowlers.** 1989. Vaccination against ovine cysticervosis using a defined recombinant antigen. *Nature* **338**:585–587.

64. **Kean, J. R.** 1980. Cysticercosis acquired in the United States. *Ann. Neurol.* **8**:643.

65. **Kramer, L. D.** 1994. Medical treatment of cysticercosis: Ineffective. *Arch. Neurol.* **52**:101–102.

66. **Loo, L., and A. Braude.** 1982. Cerebral cysticercosis in San Diego: a report of 23 cases and a review of literature. *Medicine* (Baltimore) **61**:341–359.

67. **Los Angeles County Department of Health Services.** 1982. Cysticercosis acquired in Los Angeles County. *Public Health Lett.* **4**:34–35.

68. **Mafojane, N. A.** 1994. The Neurocysticercosis Project in Atteridgeville-Mamelodi townships. *S. Afr. Med. J.* **84(4)**:208–211.

69. **Martinez, H. R., G. Elizondo, R. Rangel-Guerra.** 1989. MR imaging in neurocysticercosis. *Am J. Neuroradiol.* **10**:1011–1019.

70. **McCormick, G. F.** 1985. Cysticercosis—Review of 230 patients. *Bull. Clin. Neurosci.* **13**:76–101.

71. **McDowell, D., and C. G. Harper.** 1990. Neurocysticercosis—two Australian cases. *Med. J. Aust.* **152**:217–218.

72. **Medina, M. T., E. Rosas, F. Rubio-Donnadieve, and J. Sotelo.** 1990. Neurocysticercosis as the main cause of late-onset epilepsy in Mexico. *Arch. Intern. Med.* **150**:325–327.

73. **Michel, P., P. Callies, C. Genin, H. Raharison, and J. Roux.** 1992. Cysticercosis in Madagascar: diagnostic and therapeutic improvement. *Dakar Med.* **37**:191–197.

74. **Mitchell, W. G., and T. O. Crawford.** 1988. Intraparenchymal cerebral cysticercosis in children: diagnosis and treatment. *Pediatrics* **82**:76–82.

75. **Moore, A. C., E. I. M. Abter, R. Antar, R. L. Barbour, E. K. Chapnick, J. A. Fried, J. R. Grossman, X. Haichou, A. Hakim, A. W. Hightower, S. S. Hyon, L. I. Lutwick, J. B. Pilcher, P. M. Schantz, D. A. Ware, and M. Wilson.** 1995. Seroprevalence of cysticercosis in an Orthodox Jewish community. *Am. J. Trop. Med. Hyg.* **53(5)**:439–442.

76. **Oman, K. M., M. L. Grayson, and P. Kempster.** 1994. Neurocysticercosis and new-onset seizures in short term travellers to Bali. *Med. J. Aust.* **161**:399.

77. **Ong, S., G. J. Moran, D. A. Talan, et al.** 1998. Radiographically-imaged seizures and neurocysticercosis. p. 28.4, 149. *In Program Abstract, International Conference on Emerging Infectious Diseases, Atlanta, Ga, March 8–11, 1998.*

77a. **Pawlowski, Z., and A. Ramisz.** 1997. Personal communication.

78. **Plancarte, A., M. Fexas, and A. Flisser.** 1994. Reactivity in ELISA and dot blot of purified GP24, an immunodominant antigen of *Taenia solium* for the diagnosis of human neurocysticercosis. *Int. J. Parasitol.* **24**:733–738.

79. **Powell, S. J., I. N. MacLend, E. M. Proctor, and A. J. Wilmot.** 1966. Cysticercosis and epilepsy in Africans: a clincial and serological study. *Am. Trop. Med. Parasitol.* **60**:152–158.

80. **Proctor, E. M.** 1972. Identification of tapeworms. *S. Afr. Med. J.* **46**:234.

81. **Preux, P. M., G. Avode, B. Bouteille, M. Cruz, M. Dumas, M. Druet-Cabanac, E. K. Grunitzky, and Z. Melaku.** 1996. Cysticercosis and neurocysticercosis in Africa: current status. *Neurol. Infect. Epidemiol.* **1**:63–68.

82. **Quintero-Rodriquez, E.** 1989. Praziquantel vs. albendazole for cysticercosis. *Neurosurgery* **23**:128.

83. **Rangel, R., O. Del Brutto, J. Sotelo, and B. Torres.** 1987. Cysticercotic encephalitis: a severe form in young females. *Am. J. Trop. Med. Hyg.* **36**:387–392.

84. **Richards, F. R., E. Ruiz-Tiben, P. M. Schantz, and F. J. Sorvillo.** 1985. Cysticercosis in Los Angeles County. *JAMA* **254**:3444–3448.

85. **Rosenberg, C. E.** 1987. *The Cholera Years.* p. 17, 103, 113, 144. University of Chicago Press, Chicago, Ill.

86. **Rosenfeld, E. A., S. E. Byrd, and S. T. Shulman.** 1996. Neurocysticercosis among children in Chicago. *Clin. Infect. Dis.* **23:**262–268.

87. **Sachs, L. V., and I. Berkowitz.** 1991. Cysticercosis in an urban black South African community: prevalence and risk factors. *Trop. Gastro-enterol.* **11:**30–33.

88. **Saini, P. R., P. C. McCaskey, and D. W. Webert.** 1997. Food safety and regulatory aspects of cattle and swine cysticercosis. *J. Food Prot.* **59:**447–453.

89. **Santos Meneses Monteiro, L. A.** 1995. Neurocisticercose no norte de Portugal, p. 247. Doctoral dissertation. Instituto de Ciencias Biomedicas A. Salazar, Lisbon, Portugal.

90. **Saporiti, A., A. Brocchieri, and G. Grignani.** 1994. Neurocysticercosis as a cause of epilepsy. A case report. *Minerva Med.* **85:**403–407.

91. **Sarti, E. J., P. M. Schantz, R. Lara, H. Gomez, and A. Flisser.** 1988. *Taenia solium* taeniasis and cysticercosis in a Mexican village. *Trop. Med. Parasitol.* **39:**194–198.

92. **Sarti, E., A. Flisser, I. O. Guiterrez, A. S. Lopez, A. Plancarte, J. Roberts, P. M. Schantz, and M. Wilson.** 1992. Prevalence and risk factors for *Taenia solium* taeniasis and cysticercosis in humans and pigs in a village in Morelos, Mexico. *Am. J. Trop. Med. Hyg.* **46:**677–685.

93. **Sarti, E., J. Aguilera, A. Lopez, and P. M. Schantz.** 1992. Epidemiologic observations on porcine cysticercosis in a rural community of Michoacan State, Mexico. *Vet. Parasitol.* **41:**195–201.

94. **Sarti, E., A. Plancarte, P. M. Schantz, H. Gomez, and A. Flisser.** 1994. Epidemiological investigation of *Taenia solium* taeniasis and cysticercosis in a rural village of Michoacan state, Mexico. *Trans. R. Soc. Trop. Med. Hyg.* **88:**49–52.

95. **Sarti, E., A. Flisser, P. M. Schantz, M. Gleizer, M. Loya, A. Plancarte, G. Avila, J. Allan, P. Craig, M. Bronfman, and P. Wijeyaratne.** 1997. Development and evaluation of a health education intervention against *Taenia solium* in a rural community in Mexico. *Am. J. Trop. Med. Hyg.* **56:**127–132.

96. **Schantz, P. M., and E. Sarti.** 1989. Diagnostic methods and epidemiological surveillance of *Taenia solium* infection. *Acta Leiden.* **57:**153–163.

97. **Schantz, P. M, A. M. Aron, A. Flisser, B. J. Hartman, A. C. Moore, J. L. Munoz, D. Persaud, E. Sarti, J. A. Schaefer, E. Sarti, and M. Wilson.** 1992. Neurocysticercosis in an orthodox Jewish community in New York City. *N. Engl. J. Med.* **327:**692–695.

98. **Schantz, P. M., and J. McCauley.** 1991. Current status of foodborne parasitic zoonoses in the United States. *Southeast Asian J. Trop. Med. Public Health* **22:**65–71.

99. **Schantz, P. M., M. Cruz, Z. Pawlowski, and E. Sarti.** 1993. Potential eradicability of taeniasis and cysticercosis. *Bull. Pan Am. Health Organ.* **27:**397–403.

100. **Schantz, P. M., J. L. Criales, A. Flisser, A. Plancarte, J. Roberts, E. Sarti, A. Plancarte, and M. Wilson.** 1994. Community-based epidemiological investigations of cysticercosis due to *Taenia solium*: comparison of serological screening tests and clinical findings in two populations in Mexico. *Clin. Infect. Dis.* **18:**879–885.

101. **Schantz, P. M., and M. H. J. Kramer.** 1995. Larval cestode infections: cysticercosis and echinococcosis. *Curr. Opin. Infect. Dis.* **8:**342–350.

101a.**Schantz, P. M.** Unpublished data.

102. **Scharf, D.** 1988. Neurocysticercosis. *Arch. Neurol.* **45:**777–780.

103. **Schenone, H., R. Ramirez, A. Rojas, and F. Villarroel.** 1982. Epidemiology of human cysticercosis in Latin America, p. 25–38. *In* A. Flisser, K. Willms, J. P. Laclette, C. Larralde, C. Ridaura, and F. Beltran (ed.), *Cysticercosis: Present State of Knowledge and Perspectives.* Academic Press, New York, N.Y.

104. **Schultz, T. S., and G. F. Ascherl, Jr.** 1978. Cerebral cysticercosis: occurrence in the immigrant population. *Neurosurgery* **3:**164–169.

105. **Shanley, J. D., and M. C. Jordan.** 1980. Clinical aspects of CNS cysticercosis. *Arch. Int. Med.* **140:**1309–1313.

106. **Shandera, W. X., R. Armstrong, J. Chen, P. Diaz, and A. C. J. White.** 1994. Cysticercosis in Houston, Texas: a report of 112 cases. *Medicine* (Baltimore) **73:**37–52.

107. **Simanjuntak, G. M., S. S. Margono, M. Okamoto, and A. Ito.** 1997. Taeniasis/cysticercosis in Indonesia as an emerging disease. *Parasitol. Today* **13:**321–322.

108. **Singh, S., N. Singh, R. Pandav, C. S. Pandav, and M. G. Karmarker.** 1994. *Toxoplasma gondii* infection and its association with iodine deficiency in a residential school in a tribal area of Maharashtra. *Indian Journal of Medical Research* **99:**27–31.

109. **Sorvillo, F. J., F. O. Richards, P. M. Schantz, and S. H. Waterman.** 1992. Cysticercosis surveillance: locally acquired and travel-related infections and detection of intestinal tapeworm carriers in Los Angeles County. *Am. J. Trop. Med. Hyg.* **47:**365–371.

110. **Sotelo, J., F. Escobedo, J. and Rodriguez-Carbajal.** 1984. Therapy of parenchymal brain cysticercosis with praziquantel. *N. Engl. J. Med.* **310:**1001–1007.

111. **Sotelo, J., F. Escobedo, and P. Penagos.** 1988. Albendazole vs praziquantel for therapy for neurocysticercosis: a controlled trial. *Arch. Neurol.* **45:**532–534.

112. **Sotelo, J., O. H. Del Brutto, and G. C. Roman.** 1996. *Cysticercosis*, p. 240–259. In J. S. Remington and M. N. Swartz (ed.), *Current Clinical Topics in Infectious Diseases*. Blackwell Science, Boston, Mass.

113. **Stamos, J. K., E. G. Chadwick, Y. S. Hahn, A. H. Rowley, P. M. Schantz, and M. Wilson.** The changing epidemiology of neurocysticercosis: Report of unusual pediatric cases. Submitted for publication.

114. **Suss, R. A., K. R. Maravilla, and J. Thompson.** 1986. MR imaging of intracranial cysticercosis with CT and anatomopathologic features. *Am. J. Neuroradiol.* **7:**235–242.

115. **Takayanugui, O. M., and E. Jardin.** 1992. Therapy for neurocysticercosis. Comparison between albendazole and praziquantel. *Arch. Neurol.* **49:**290–294.

116. **Tasker, W. G., and S. A. Plotkin.** 1979. Cerebral cysticercosis. *Pediatrics* **63:**761–763.

117. **Teitelbaum, G. P., R. J. Otto, and M. Lin.** 1989. MR imaging of neurocysticercosis. *Am. J. Roentgenol.* **153:**857–866.

118. **Thakur, L. C., and K. S. Anand.** 1991. Childhood neurocysticercosis in South India. *Indian J. Pediatr.* **58:**815–819.

119. **Tsang, V. C. W., A. E. Boyer, and J. A. Brand.** 1989. An enzyme-linked immunotransfer blot assay and glycoprotein antigens for diagnosing human cysticercosis (*Taenia solium*). *J. Infect. Dis.* **159:**50–59.

120. **Tsang, V. C. W., A. E. Boyer, R. H. Gilman, E. I. Kamango-Sollo, K. D. Murrell, J. A. Pilcher, M. L. Rhoads, P. M. Schantz, and W. Zhou.** 1991. Efficacy of the immunoblot assay for cysticercosis in pigs and modulated expression of distinct IgM/IgG activities to *Taenia solium* antigens in experimental infections. *Vet. Immunol. Immunopathol.* **29:**69–78.

121. **Tsang, V. C. W., and M. Wilson.** 1995. *Taenia solium*: an under recognized but serious public health problem. *Parasitol. Today* **11:**124–126.

122. **Vazquez, V., and J. Sotelo.** 1992. The course of seizures after treatment for cerebral cysticercosis. *N. Engl. J. Med.* **327:**696–701.

123. **Vernez, G., and Ronfeldt, D.** 1991. The current situation in Mexican immigration. *Science* **251:**1189–1193.

124. **Villa, A. M., D. A. Monteverde, and W. Rodriguez.** 1993. Neurocisticercosis en un hospital de la ciudad de Buenos Aires: estudio de once casos. *Arg. Neuropsiquiatr.* **51:**333–336.

125. **Wadia, N. H., S. B. Desai, and M. B. Bhett.** 1988. Disseminated cysticercosis—new observations including CT scan findings and experience with treatment by praziquantel. *Brain* **11:**597–614.

126. **White, A. C.** 1997. Neurocysticercosis: a major cause of neurological disease worldwide. *Clin. Infect. Dis.* **24:**101–115.

126a.**Wilkins, P., and V. C. W. Tsang.** 1998. Unpublished data.

127. **Wilson, M., R. T. Bryan, J. A. Fried, D. A Ware, P. M. Schantz, J. B. Pilcher, and V. C. W. Tsang.** 1991. Clinical evaluation of the cysticercosis enzyme-linked immunoelectrotransfer blot in patients with neurocysticercosis. *J. Infect. Dis.* **164:**1007–1009.

128. **Yong, J. L. C., and B. A. Warren.** 1994. Neurocysticercosis: a report of four cases. *Pathology* **26:**244–249.

*Emerging Infections 2*
Edited by W. M. Scheld, W. A. Craig, and J. M. Hughes
© 1998 ASM Press, Washington, D.C.

*Chapter 13*

# The North American Liver Fluke, *Metorchis conjunctus*

## J. Dick MacLean

In the past 25 years parasitic infections have contributed to the growing number of emerging infections in North America. There have been a number of reasons for this growth, which has been almost entirely due to protozoa (1). The increased number of severely immunocompromised individuals in North America has been a major factor in the emergence of two new opportunistic protozoa, *Cryptosporidium parvum* and *Enterocytozoon bieneusi*, and one "old" protozoan, *Toxoplasma gondii*. Public health failures in water sanitation have led to epidemics of *C. parvum* in Milwaukee, Wis., and toxoplasmosis in British Columbia, Canada. The increasing globalization of food supplies, which reflects improving food processing and transportation technologies, has supplied us with outbreaks of *Cyclospora cayetanensis*, associated with fresh berry importations from Central America.

Protozoa have contributed the most important emerging parasite examples to date; the helminths have played a far smaller role. In this era of immunodeficiency, *Strongyloides stercoralis* (the classic opportunistic helminth) has fortunately not "emerged" (for reasons that remain unclear).

However, there is a slowly emerging helminth problem, an increasing frequency of helminth infections due to the consumption of raw or undercooked fish. Both total fish consumption and the percentage that is purchased (fresh or frozen) have increased by 50% and 100%, respectively, in the past 35 years (Fig. 1). These consumption patterns reflect a number of influences. There have been improvements in the preservation and transportation of fish and an increase in public awareness of the nutritional benefits of a fish diet. A spread of ethnic cuisines has been stimulated by a continuing multicultural immigration, travel, and television. Finally, an increase in per capita disposable income has also had an influence. Fresh fish sales have risen, but the amount consumed raw is difficult to ascertain. If the number of sushi bars is any measure, there has been a significant increase.

*J. Dick MacLean* • McGill University Centre for Tropical Disease, Montreal General Hospital, 1650 Cedar Ave., Room D7-153, Montreal, Quebec, Canada H3G 1A4.

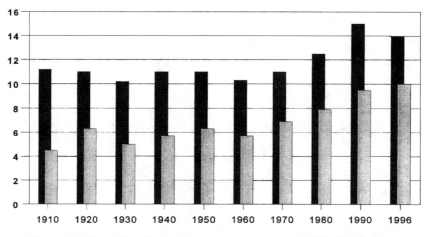

**Figure 1.** Total and fresh/frozen fish consumption (pounds of edible fish) in North America. Solid columns represent total; shaded columns represent fresh/frozen. (Source: Personal communication from the National Marine Fisheries Service, Fisheries Statistics and Economics Division.)

The following is a description of an outbreak of a new clinical disease, acute metorchiasis, following the consumption of sashimi (raw fish) prepared from freshly caught white sucker, *Catastomus commersoni*.

## THE OUTBREAK

Twenty-seven individuals attended one or both of two picnics north of Montreal, Canada, on 16 and 23 May 1993. Sashimi (pieces of raw fish) prepared from freshwater fish caught locally the same day was one of the principal foods served at the picnic. In the days following the picnic 19 individuals developed an illness with clinical pathology and/or laboratory abnormalities. These were defined as cases for the purpose of the outbreak investigation (22).

### Index Case

The index patient, a 50-year-old male, is presented because the progression of his illness was typical of the cases as a whole. A day after the first picnic, where he had eaten a number of pieces of sashimi, he developed steady upper abdominal pain, nausea, anorexia, feverishness, fatigue, a slight cough, and muscle aches and pains. The symptoms persisted at roughly the same intensity for 10 days, when he presented at a hospital emergency department and was noted to have a temperature of 38.3°C and epigastric tenderness. His hematological parameters were normal, and he was sent home. His symptoms persisted for another 3 days. On return to the emergency department, he had a raised eosinophil count of $1.8 \times 10^9$/liter (normal, $\leq .45 \times 10^9$/liter). Over the following week, his eosinophil counts continued to rise, and he developed liver enzyme elevations with an obstructive pattern

**Table 1.** Laboratory results of index case

| Parameter[a] | Normal value | 28 May | 31 May | 1 June | 9 June | 7 July |
|---|---|---|---|---|---|---|
| Leukocytes | $4.8 \times 10^9$–$10.8 \times 10^9$/liter | 12.4 | 12.4 | 12.0 | 21.1 | 5.4 |
| Eosinophils | $<0.45 \times 10^9$/liter | 0.3 | 1.8 | 2.7 | 15.2 | 0.4 |
| ALT | 10–40 U/liter | 25 | 157 | 142 | 76 | 29 |
| GGT | 11–50 U/liter | 10 | 416 | 406 | 304 | 179 |
| AP | 37–117 U/liter | | 425 | 466 | 300 | 125 |
| Amylase | 0–160 U/liter | | | 61 | 91 | |
| Stool ova | Negative | | | Positive | Positive | Negative |

[a]ALT, alanine aminotransferase; GGT, γ-glutamyl transferase; AP, alkaline phosphatase.

(Table 1). Opisthorchid eggs were found in his stool on day 15 of his illness (Fig. 2).

The clinical features of the cases as a whole resembled the index case (Table 2). Of note, however, were two patients who developed laboratory abnormalities without clinical symptomatology. Both persons had eaten only a small quantity of sashimi (two or three pieces). A number of other clinical parameters revealed a clear association between quantity of sashimi eaten and the subsequent clinical illness (Table 3). The ova found in the stools of patients measured 28.5 ± 2.1 by 15.6 ± 1.6 μm in size and could not be distinguished by light microscopy from *Opisthorchis viverrini*. Treatment with praziquantel (60 mg/kg for 1 day) was initiated from 19 to 25 days after the illness had begun. In those who were still sick, resolution of all symptoms occurred within 48 hours of treatment. Eosinophil counts returned to normal within 31 days of treatment with praziquantel.

Six gutted fish, caught but not consumed on the picnic days, had been kept frozen and were available for examination. These were identified by J. R. Arthur

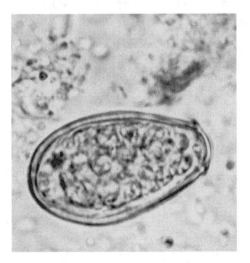

**Figure 2.** Egg of *M. conjunctus* from golden hamsters (average size 28.5 by 15.6 μm).

**Table 2.** Clinical and laboratory features in 19 cases

| Parameter | Value |
|---|---|
| Clinical | |
| Fatigue | 79% |
| Fever | 63% |
| Abdominal pain | 63% |
| Headache | 63% |
| Weight loss | 58% |
| Anorexia | 53% |
| Nausea | 32% |
| Diarrhea | 26% |
| Ate sashimi | 100% |
| Sashimi eaten (mean) | 30 g |
| Laboratory | |
| Leukocytes ($10^9$/liter; mean)[a] | 11,716 |
| Eosinophils ($10^9$/liter, mean)[a] | 4,114 |
| Eosinophils ($>0.45 \times 10^9$/liter, mean)[a] | 79% |
| Elevated liver enzymes | 58% |
| Opisthorchid eggs in stool | 57% |

[a]Mean of highest values durng illness of each case.

(Maurice Lamontagne Institute, Fisheries and Oceans Canada) as *C. commersoni*, the common (white) sucker. To determine whether these fish were infected, they were processed with a pepsin-HCl digestion and forced through a 500–$\mu$m pore screen. Examination revealed an average per fish of 7.2 (range: 0.1 to 18.9) metacercaria/g of flesh (Fig. 3). These were tentatively identified as the metacercaria of *Metorchis conjunctus*; further identification was difficult because of the immature nature of this stage of the parasite. To make a definitive identification of the parasite, a further lot of fish was caught 3 weeks later from the same small river, and live (unfrozen) metacercaria were recovered. Mark Curtis of the Institute of Parasitology, Macdonald Campus, McGill University, fed 20 metacercaria to each of two golden hamsters (*Cricetus auratus*). The hamsters were found to have operculated eggs in their stools by day 12 of the infection, and these were identical to the eggs found in the human cases. The two animals were examined on days 16

**Table 3.** Course of illness related to quantity of fish (sashimi) eaten[a]

| Parameter | Value relative to no. of sashimi pieces eaten | |
|---|---|---|
| | ≤5 | ≥10 |
| No. of cases | 7 | 10 |
| Incubation period (days) | 9 | 4 |
| Fever | 3 | 10 |
| Raised liver enzyme levels | 0 | 10 |
| Emergency department visit | 1 | 6 |
| Opisthorchid eggs in stool | 3 | 7 |
| Symptoms resolved before treatment | 5 | 3 |

[a]Each piece weighed ~2 g.

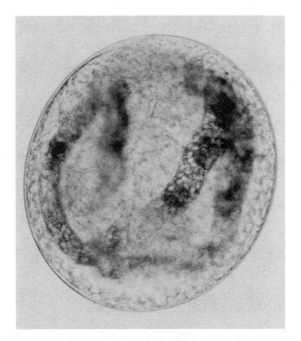

**Figure 3.** Metacercaria (0.27 mm by 0.29 mm) of *M. conjunctus* recovered from the flesh of *C. commersoni*. (Reproduced from reference 22 with permission of the publisher.)

and 23 postinfection; 11 and 7 adult flukes, respectively, were found distributed throughout the extra- and intrahepatic bile ducts and gallbladder. These flukes were identified as *M. conjunctus* on the basis of comparisons with published morphological descriptions by Cameron, Skrjabin, and Watson (6, 36, 38) (Fig. 4).

A crude antigen was prepared from adult flukes harvested from the golden hamsters and the metacercaria from *C. commersoni*. Antibodies directed against the adult antigens were measured with an enzyme-linked immunosorbent assay (ELISA) and were found in all patients who had eaten more than three pieces of sashimi and none of the picnickers who did not eat sashimi. The ELISA using metacercarial antigen was less sensitive (Fig. 5).

## THE PARASITE

*M. conjunctus* is a fluke in the family Opisthorchiidae. Like other flukes in this family, it lives within the biliary tree of the definitive host (Fig. 6) (6, 17). The adult fluke produces eggs which pass down the common bile duct to the intestine and are excreted via feces into fresh water where they are ingested by and hatch within specific snails. Within the snail, the first intermediate host, they subsequently metamorphose through several generations of rediae and are then released as free-swimming cercaria that can penetrate the skin and encyst in the flesh of fish, the second intermediate host. These small oval (0.26 × 0.33 mm) metacercariae in the

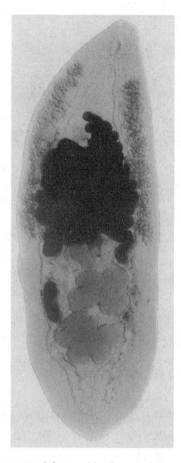

**Figure 4.** Adult fluke removed from golden hamster biliary tree (size range, 3.56 to 3.90 by 1.16 mm). (Reproduced from reference 22 with permission of the publisher.)

fish flesh excyst in the intestine of the definitive host when the fish is eaten raw. The larvae mature to adults in 2 to 3 days and migrate through the sphincter of Oddi and up the biliary tree where they become lodged within the intrahepatic bile ducts and survive for an unknown length of time (38).

The first intermediate host of *M. conjunctus* is the aquatic snail *Amnicola limosa limosa*. It is widely distributed in North America, from Labrador in the north to Florida in the south, and from the Atlantic seaboard in the east to Utah in the west (4, 8). The second intermediate hosts include several freshwater fish species; the most important is the white sucker. It has a geographic range that also covers much of central and eastern Canada and the United States (Fig. 7) (21, 35).

The definitive hosts of *M. conjunctus* are a wide range of North American carnivores, including bears, wolves, foxes, coyotes, raccoons, muskrats, mink, fishers, dogs, and cats, and occasionally humans. Infected animals have been found from

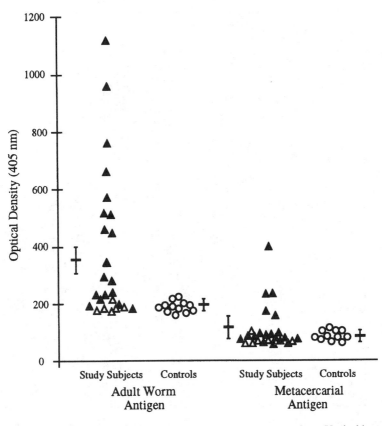

**Figure 5.** Results of ELISA for antibodies to *M. conjunctus* serology. Vertical bars are standard error of the mean. (Reproduced from reference 22 with permission of the publisher.)

the Atlantic coast to the western prairies and from South Carolina to Great Slave Lake in the Northwest Territories of Canada (Fig. 7) (5, 7, 12, 15, 41). *M. conjunctus* has been the cause of death of sufficient numbers of working sled dogs in central Canada to have merited several investigations by the government (1, 25). Necropsies of the dogs have indicated the cause of death to be liver damage associated with *M. conjunctus* infection. Similar pathology has been reproduced in a number of laboratory animal models (e.g., cat, dog, ferret, fox, racoon, mink, hamster, rat, mouse) (38).

Asymptomatic human infection with *M. conjunctus* has been seen occasionally during stool parasite surveys in aboriginal populations in Canada (Fig. 7) (39). In some small isolated communities prevalence levels have reached 20%. Symptomatic infections have never been described in humans. The duration of the asymptomatic carrier state is not known.

*M. conjunctus* belongs to the family Opisthorchidae, in which human infections with the closely related *O. viverrini*, *O. felineus*, and *Clonorchis sinensis* have been extensively investigated. Chronic infection with *O. viverrini* results in reactive in-

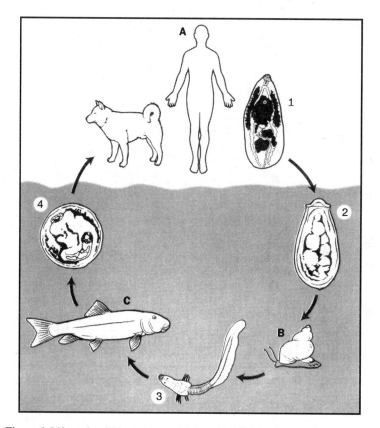

**Figure 6.** Life cycle of *M. conjunctus*. Hosts: (A) definitive human, dog, etc.); (B) first intermediate (snail [*A. limosa limosa*]; (C) second intermediate (fish [*C. commersoni*]). Stages: (1) adult fluke, (2) egg, (3) cercaria, (4) metacercaria. (Reproduced from reference 22 with permission of the publisher.)

flammation of the biliary tree epithelium with subsequent metaplasia, periductal inflammation, and fibrosis leading to obstruction, bacterial superinfection and (at times) cholangiocarcinoma (17, 30, 37). There have been only rare descriptions of an acute illness associated with these related species, but similarities to the present outbreak have been remarkable (20, 42). The most recent reports have come from the former Soviet Union (3, 24).

## CONTEXT

Although fish have not been implicated to date in human protozoan infections, they are the source of more than 50 different human helminth infections (32). The helminths include trematodes (e.g., the Oriental liver fluke, *C. sinensis*); cestodes (e.g., the fish tapeworm, *Diphyllobothrium latum*) and nematodes (e.g., the cod-worm, *Anisakis simplex*). A number of these parasites are important causes of morbidity and mortality in parts of the world such as Southeast Asia where raw

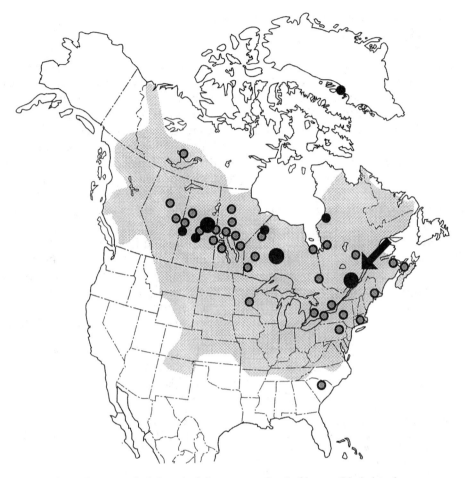

**Figure 7.** Range (shaded area) of *C. commersoni* and of human (black dots; larger dots represent larger outbreaks) and animal (shaded dots) infection with *M. conjunctus*. The arrow indicates the present outbreak. (Reproduced from reference 22 with permission of the publisher.)

fish and fish products are a substantial source of nutrition. The morbidity associated with fish parasites varies from asymptomatic to serious and is based on the parasite itself, the parasite load, and host response. At one extreme, in northern Thailand, cholangiocarcinoma is associated with chronic infections with the liver fluke *O. viverrini* (16).

North American fish can be as infected with helminths as fish on other continents. Raw fish consumption has been a tradition in several North American communities in the past. The Inuit and a number of other aboriginal societies have a long tradition of raw fish consumption, either as a matter of choice because of taste or at times of necessity. Some *Diphyllobothrium* species have been found only in Alaska and northern Canada, suggesting their indigenous origins. In fact, it is in these northern communities where the greatest range of fish parasites have been described in the human population (9, 32) (Table 4).

Reports in the literature have described many different helminth species that have infected humans subsequent to the consumption of raw fish indigenous to North America (32). Many of these case reports are individual case descriptions; infections have been acquired through the consumption of uncommon fish species. The university students' goldfish swallowing contest is an example. The vast majority of North American reports of indigenous fish parasites in humans are caused by five helminths. These are the cestodes *Diphyllobothrium spp.*, the trematodes *Metorchis* and *Nanophyetus*, and the nematodes *Anisakis* and *Pseudoterranova* (Table 5). Except for *Nanophyetus* (limited in distribution to the West Coast) and *Metorchis* (excluded from the West Coast), the other three species are widely distributed. *Metorchis* is limited to one important freshwater fish species, *Anisakis* and *Pseudoterranova* are limited to salt water fish, and *Diphyllobothrium* and *Nanophyetus* are limited to salt water fish and fish that live in both fresh and salt water (e.g., the Salmonidae). The fish tapeworms *Diphyllobothrium* spp. (of which there are three and possibly more species described in North America) (Table 4) are the most frequently described human helminths of fish origin on the continent. Aboriginal communities consuming raw fish, Jewish women who prepare gefilte fish, and recently West Coast salmon sashimi/sushi eaters are notable for higher-than-

**Table 4.** Fish parasites infecting persons in the United States and Canada

| Parasite | Fish host(s) | Reference(s) |
|---|---|---|
| Cestodes | | |
| *Diphyllobothrium latum* | Salmonids, pike, perch, burbot | 2 |
| *Diphyllobothrium dendriticum*[a] | Salmonids | 2 |
| *Diphyllobothrium ursi*[a] | Salmonids | 23, 28 |
| *Diphyllobothrium* spp.[a,b] | Salmonids | 2, 28 |
| *Schistocephalus solidus*[a] | Sticklebacks | 28 |
| Trematodes | | |
| *Nanophyetus salmincola* | Salmonids | 11 |
| *Metorchis conjunctus* | White sucker | 22 |
| *Cryptocotyle lingua* | Flounder | 28 |
| *Amphimerus pseudofelineus* | Freshwater fish | 32 |
| Nematodes | | |
| *Anisakis simplex* | Salmonids, tuna, herring, mackerel, squid | 9, 10 |
| *Pseudoterranova decipiens* | Cod, pollack, haddock | 19 |
| *Eustrongyloides* spp. | Killifish, estuarine species | 40 |
| *Dioctophema renale* | Freshwater fish, estuarine species | 14 |
| Acanthocephelans | | |
| *Corynostoma strumnosum* | Salmon? | 34 |
| *Acanthocephalus rauschi* | Salmon? | 13 |

[a]Found primarily in Alaska and northern Canada.
[b]The taxonomy of a number of North American *Diphyllobothrium* spp. that have been reported as infecting humans remains unclear (e.g., *D. ursi*, *D. lanceolatum*, *D. alascense*, and *D. dalliae*) (2).

**Table 5.** Features of most frequent parasite infections acquired from North American parasites acquired from raw fish

| Parasite | Size of infective stage in fish | Geographic range | Clinical presentation |
|---|---|---|---|
| *Diphyllobothrium* spp. | 1–20 cm × 1 mm | Whole continent | Adult worm in stool |
| *Anisakis simplex* | 2 cm × 1 mm | Atlantic and Pacific coasts | Abdominal pain, eosinophilia |
| *Pseudoterranova decipiens* | 2–5 cm | Atlantic and Pacific coasts | Vomited worm |
| *Metorchis conjunctus* | 0.33 × 0.26 mm | East and central continent | Abdominal pain, eosinophilia |
| *Nanophyetus salmincola* | 0.1 × 0.33 mm | Pacific coast | Abdominal pain, diarrhea, eosinophilia |

average rates of *Diphyllobothrium* infection (31). Although these parasitic infections have received little clinical study in North America, they appear to cause little to no pathology. Vitamin $B_{12}$ deficiency, which has been described to occur in infected individuals in Finland, has not been seen in North America. Diagnosis is made by finding the proglottids or eggs in stool specimens.

*Nanophyetus salmincola* has been recently described as a human infection along the Pacific coast of North America. It has been well described along the Pacific coast of Siberia where it is a common problem in raw salmon eaters (11). The small, 1-mm-long intestinal flukes become deeply embedded in the mucosa of the small intestine. In heavy infections (>500 flukes), they produce abdominal pain, diarrhea, and peripheral eosinophilia. Diagnosis is made by finding the eggs in stool specimens.

The helminths that have received the greatest attention have been the anisakids, *A. simplex* and *Pseudoterranova decipiens*. After ingestion, the 2 to 3 cm larvae of *A. simplex* become embedded in the stomach or the wall of the small intestine and produce a vigorous inflammatory response. The clinical presentation is abdominal pain, peripheral eosinophilia, and at times diarrhea. As these worms do not reach maturity in the human host, no eggs are passed in the stool. The diagnosis is made by a direct visualization of the worm by upper intestine endoscopy. *P. decipiens* appears to be less capable of penetrating the intestinal mucosa than *A. simplex* and presents frequently as a worm that has been vomited or coughed up.

In Japan, cases of anisakiasis have occurred at a frequency of more than 1000 per year (10). In the Netherlands, anisakiasis became a major problem in the 1960s when pickled herring became a source of infection. The Netherlands government legislated that fish must be frozen for a set period before it can be sold to be eaten uncooked.

Deardorff and Overstreet described an increase in anisakid infections acquired in the United States and reported in the literature during the period from 1951 to 1988 (9). Both increasing availability of upper-intestine endoscopy and the increase in raw fish consumption during the period are certain to have increased the reporting of these infections (27, 33). This legislation had an important positive impact on the *Anisakis* problem and was undoubtedly an important precedent for the U.S. Food and Drug Administration (FDA) (18, 29). In 1987 the FDA issued recommendations that fisheries products not cooked throughout to 140°F (60°C) or above, must before service or sale in ready-to-eat form be blast frozen to −31°F (−35°C) or below for 15 hours, or be frozen by regular means to −10°F (−23°C) or below for 168 hours (7 days). Neither the United States nor Canada requires that infections with parasites from fish be reported. It will be difficult to ascertain the impact of these recommendations.

## CONCLUSIONS

The present outbreak and the prevalence of the fluke *M. conjunctus* place this parasite among the more common fish-borne helminths that infect humans in North America. Important questions regarding the duration of the asymptomatic phase of this infection and its oncogenic potential remain unanswered.

**Acknowledgements.** The collaboration of J. Richard Arthur, Brian J. Ward, Theresa W. Gyorkos, Mark A. Curtis, and Evelyne Kokoskin in the research related to the outbreak is acknowledged with thanks.

### REFERENCES

1. **Allen, J. A., and R. A. Wardle.** 1934. Fluke disease in northern Manitoba sledge dogs. *Can. J. Res. (Sect. D)* **10**:404–408.
2. **Anderson, K., H. I. Ching, and R. Vik.** 1987. A review of freshwater species of *Diphyllobothrium* with redescriptions of *D. dendriticum* (Nitzsch, 1824) and *D. ditremum* (Creplin, 1825) from North America. *Can. J. Zool.* **65**:2216–2228.
3. **Bronshtein, A. M., and N. N. Ozeretskovskaya.** 1985. First trials of Praziquantel for the treatment of patients with acute or chronic *Opisthorchis felineus* infections. *Med. Parazitol.* (Moscow). **5**:31–34.
4. **Burch, J. B.** 1982. *Freshwater snails (Mollusca: Gastropoda) of North America.* Contract No 68-03-1280. U.S. Environmental Protection Agency, Cincinnati, Ohio.
5. **Cameron, T. W. M., I. W. Parnell, and L. L. Lyster.** 1940. The helminth parasites of sledge-dogs in northern Canada and Newfoundland. *Can. J. Res. (Sect. D)* **18**:325–332.
6. **Cameron, T. W. M.** 1944. The morphology, taxonomy, and life history of *Metorchis conjunctus* (Cobbold, 1860). *Can. J. Res. (Sect. D)* **22**:6–16.
7. **Cameron, T. W. M.** 1945. Fish-carried parasites in Canada. (1) Parasites carried by fresh-water fish. *Can. J. Comp. Med.* **9**:302–311.
8. **Clarke, A. H.** 1981. *The Freshwater Molluscs of Canada.* National Museum of Science, National Museum of Canada, Ottawa, Ontario, Canada.
9. **Deardorff, T. L., and R. M. Overstreet.** 1990. Seafood-transmitted zoonoses in the United States. The fishes, the dishes, and the worms, p. 211–265. *In* D. R. Ward and C. Hackney (ed.), *Microbiology of Marine Food Products.* Van Nostrand Reinhold, New York, N.Y.
10. **Deardorff, T. L., S. G. Kayes, and T. Fukumura.** 1991. Human anisakiasis transmitted by marine food products. *Hawaii Med. J.* **50**:9–16.
11. **Eastburne, R. L., T. R. Fritsche, and C. A. Terhune.** 1987. Human intestinal infection with *Nanophyetus salmincola* from Salmonid fishes. *Am. J. Trop. Med. Hyg.* **36**:586–591.
12. **Evans, W. S.** 1963. Fish-carried liver trematodes of Manitoba mammals. M.Sc. thesis. University of Manitoba, Winnipeg, Manitoba, Canada.
13. **Golvan, Y. J.** 1969. Systématique des acanthocéphales (Acanthocephala Rudolphi 1801) Prèmiere partie. L'ordre des Palaeacanthocephala Meyer 1931. Premier fascicule. La super-famille des Echinorhynchoidea (Cobbold 1876) Golvan et Houin 1963. *Mem. Mus. Natl. Hist. Natur.* **47**:1–373.
14. **Gutierrez, Y., M. Cohen, and C. N. Machicao.** 1989. *Dioctophyma* larva in the subcutaneous tissues of a woman in Ohio. *Am. J. Surg. Path.* **13**:800–802.

15. **Harkema, R., and G. C. Miller.** 1964. Helminth parasites of the raccoon, *Procyon lotor* in the southeastern United States. *J. Parasitol.* **50:**60–66.

16. **Haswell-Elkins, M. R., S. Satarug, and D. B. Elkins.** 1992. *Opisthorchis viverrini* infection in Northeast Thailand and its relationship to cholangiocarcinoma. *J. Gastroenterol. Hepatol.* **7:**538–548.

17. **Haswell-Elkins, M. R., and D. B. Elkins.** 1992. Food-borne trematodes. p. 1457. *In* C. C. Cook (ed.), *Manson's Tropical Medicine*, 20th ed.The W. B. Saunders Co., London, England.

18. **Jackson, G. J., J. W. Bier, and T. L. Schwartz.** 1990. More on making sushi safe. *N. Engl. J. Med.* **322:**1011.

19. **Kates, S., K. A. Wright, and R. Wright.** 1973. A case of human infection with the cod nematode *Phocanema* sp. *Am. J. Trop. Med. Hyg.* **22:**606–608.

20. **Koenigstein, R. P.** 1949. Observations on the epidemiology of infections with *Clonorchis inensis*. *Trans. R. Soc. Trop. Med. Hyg.* **42:**503–506.

21. **Lee, D. S., C. R. Gilbert, C. H. Hocutt, R. E. Jenkins, D. E. McAllister, and J. R. Stauffer.** 1980. *Atlas of North American Freshwater Fishes*. North Carolina Biological Survey, Raleigh.

22. **MacLean, J. D., J. R. Arthur, B. J. Ward, T. W. Gyorkos, M. A. Curtis, and E. Kokoskin.** 1996. Common-source outbreak of acute infection due to the North American liver fluke *Metorchis conjunctus*. *Lancet* **347:**154–158.

23. **Margolis, L., R. L. Rausch, and E. Robertson.** 1973. *Diphyllobothrium ursi* from man in British Columbia—first report of this tapeworm in Canada. *Can. J. Public Health* **64:**588–589.

24. **Mel'nikov, V. I., and N. I. Skarednov.** 1979. The clinical picture of acute opisthorchiasis in the immigrant population of the northern Ob' region. *Med. Parazitol.* (Moscow) **48:**12–16.

25. **Mongeau, N.** 1961. Hepatic distomatosis and infectious canine hepatitis in northern Manitoba. *Can. Vet. J.* **2:**33–38.

26. **Morse, S. S.** 1995. Factors in the emergence of infectious diseases. *Emerg. Infect. Dis.* **1:**7–15.

27. **Oshima, T.** 1987. Anisakiasis: is the sushi bar guilty? *Parasitol. Today* **3:**44–48.

28. **Rausch, R. L., E. M. Scott, and V. R. Rausch.** 1967. Helminths in Eskimos in western Alaska, with particular reference to *Diphyllobothrium* infection and anaemia. *Trans. R. Soc. Trop. Med. Hyg.* **61:**351–357.

29. **Retail Food Protection Branch, Food and Drug Administration.** 1987. Food Preparation: raw, marinated or partially cooked fishery products. Program Information Manual, Code Interpretation 2-403. Food and Drug Administration, Washington, D.C.

30. **Rim, H-J.** 1986. The current pathobiology and chemotherapy of clonorchiasis. *Korean J. Parasitol.* **24**(Suppl.):1–141.

31. **Ruttenber, A. J., B. G. Weniger, F. Sorvillo, R. A. Murray, and S. L. Ford.** 1984. Diphyllobothriasis associated with salmon consumption in Pacific coast states. *Am. J. Trop. Med. Hyg.* **33:**455–459.

32. **Sakanari, J. A., M. Moser, and T. L. Deardorff.** 1995. *Fish Parasites and Human Health*. Report T-CSGCP-034. California Sea Grant College, University of California, La Jolla.

33. **Schantz, P. M.** 1989. The dangers of eating raw fish. *N. Engl. J. Med.* **320:**1143–1145.

34. **Schmidt, G. D.** 1971. Acanthocephalan infections of man, with two new records. *J. Parasitol.* **57:**582–584.

35. **Scott, W. B., and E. J. Crossman.** 1973. *Freshwater Fishes of Canada*. Fish Research Board Canada, Ottawa, Canada.

36. **Skrjabin, K. I.** 1950. *Trematodes of Animals and Man. Essentials of Trematodology*, vol. 4. Izdat. Akad. Nauk. S. S. S. R., Moscow, Russia.

37. **World Health Organization.** 1995. *Control of Foodborne Trematode Infections*. World Health Organization, Geneva, Switzerland.

38. **Watson, T. G.** 1979. Aspects of the biology of *Metorchis conjunctus* in laboratory and field hosts. Ph.D. thesis. McGill University, Montreal, Canada.

39. **Watson, T. G., R. S. Freeman, and M. Staszak.** 1979. Parasites in native people of the Sioux Lookout zone, northwestern Ontario. *Can. J. Public Health.* **70:**179–182.

40. **Wittner, M., J. W. Turner, G. Jacquette, L. A. Ash, M. P. Salgo, and H. B. Tanowitz.** 1989. Eustrongylidiasis—A parasitic infection acquired by eating sushi. *N. Engl. J. Med.* **320:**1124–1189.

41. **Wobeser, G., W. Runge, and R. R. Stewart.** 1983. *Metorchis conjunctus* (Cobbold, 1860) infection in wolves (*Canis lupus*), with pancreatic involvement in two animals. *J. Wildl. Dis.* **19:**353–356.
42. **Xu, Z., H. Zhong, and W. Cho.** 1979. Acute clonorchiasis. *Chin. Med. J.* **93:**423–426.

*Emerging Infections 2*
Edited by W. M. Scheld, W. A. Craig, and J. M. Hughes
© 1998 ASM Press, Washington, D.C.

*Chapter 14*

# Opportunistic Infections (OIs) as Emerging Infectious Diseases: Challenges Posed by OIs in the 1990s and Beyond

*Jonathan E. Kaplan, Debra L. Hanson, Jeffrey L. Jones,*
*Charles B. Beard, Dennis D. Juranek, and Clare A. Dykewicz*

Opportunistic infections (OIs) have been defined as infections that occur with increased frequency and/or severity because of immunosuppression (18). That is, the microbial pathogen avails itself of the "opportunity" to multiply and cause disease in a host with diminished immune response. The concept of OIs is not new; OIs have been described for decades in children with congenital immunodeficiency syndromes and in both children and adults with a variety of conditions, such as hematopoietic malignancies, diabetes, and chronic pulmonary disease. However, in the context of emerging infectious diseases, OIs have assumed importance because of immunocompromised populations that are either new or have increased over the past two decades. Such populations may be immunocompromised as the result of a pathologic process, such as occurs in human immunodeficiency virus (HIV) infection, or because of medical treatments that induce immunosuppression, such as radiation or chemotherapy for cancer or immunosuppressive therapy for organ transplantation.

## OPPORTUNISTIC INFECTIONS ASSOCIATED WITH HIV/AIDS

The most visible emergence of OIs in the past two decades (and probably the greatest source of OIs in terms of numbers of cases of human disease) has been

*Jonathan E. Kaplan, Debra L. Hanson, and Jeffrey L. Jones* • Division of HIV/AIDS Prevention, National Center for HIV, SID, and TB Prevention, Centers for Disease Control and Prevention, Atlanta, GA 30333.    *Charles B. Beard and Dennis D. Juranek* • Division of Parasitic Diseases, National Center for Infectious Diseases, Centers for Disease Control and Prevention, Atlanta, GA 30333.    *Clare A. Dykewicz* • Division of AIDS, STD, and TB Laboratory Research, National Center for Infectious Diseases, Centers for Disease Control and Prevention, Atlanta, GA 30333.

in association with the HIV/AIDS pandemic. HIV is currently estimated to infect approximately 750,000 persons in the United States and more than 30 million persons globally (20, 46). HIV infection is characterized by a gradual loss of $CD4^+$ T lymphocytes; when the $CD4^+$ count falls below 200 cells/$\mu$l, the infection is associated with a wide variety of opportunistic infections. An estimated 200,000 to 250,000 persons in the United States have $CD4^+$ counts below 200 cells/$\mu$l (8).

A review in 1995 yielded a list of more than 100 microorganisms, ranging from viruses to arthropods, that have been associated with OIs in HIV-infected persons (18); all of these OIs could be considered emerging infectious diseases. Fortunately, only a minority of these diseases cause most of the morbidity in HIV-infected persons; these diseases are included in the Centers for Disease Control and Prevention (CDC) surveillance case definition of AIDS (5). Table 1 indicates the prevalence of various AIDS-defining conditions among adults and adolescents reported with AIDS in the United States in 1996; all of those listed except HIV wasting syndrome are associated with a known (or highly suspected) infectious etiology (7).

Because more than half of U.S. AIDS cases are currently reported based on the patient's having a $CD4^+$ T-lymphocyte count of <200 cells/$\mu$l and may not have OIs reported and because national surveillance data generally reflect only initial and not follow-up AIDS conditions, these data do not accurately reflect the burden of OIs in the HIV-infected population. A more accurate depiction is provided by the Adult and Adolescent Spectrum of Disease (ASD) Project, a medical record review study that has been conducted since 1990 in 11 U.S. cities (14). In this study, HIV-infected persons ≥13 years of age are enrolled at their first visit to an ASD facility. Their records are reviewed for demographic information and history of AIDS-defining illnesses; information on other illnesses, laboratory tests, and prescribed medications are collected for the 1-year period prior to enrollment. Subsequently, records are reviewed every 6 months until the patient is lost to follow-

**Table 1.** Prevalence of AIDS indicator conditions among adults and adolescents reported with an AIDS illness, United States, 1996[a]

| Condition | Prevalence (%) |
| --- | --- |
| *Pneumocystis carinii* pnemonia | 38.9 |
| HIV wasting syndrome | 19.1 |
| Candidiasis | 17.0 |
| Kaposi's sarcoma | 8.3 |
| Tuberculosis | 7.1 |
| *Mycobacterium avium* complex disease | 6.0 |
| Herpes simplex virus disease | 5.7 |
| Pneumonia, recurrent | 5.6 |
| Cryptococcosis | 5.0 |
| Toxoplasmosis of brain | 4.7 |
| Cytomegalovirus (CMV) disease other than retinitis | 4.7 |
| CMV retinitis | 4.2 |

[a]Of the 68,473 cases of AIDS reported in 1996, 59,284 were reported with severe immunosuppression ($CD4^+$ T-lymphocyte count of <200 cells/$\mu$l or $CD4^+$ percentage of ≤14), 29,227 were reported with an AIDS indicator condition, and 20,038 were reported with both. Source: CDC surveillance data (7).

up or dies. Enrollment is diverse with respect to race, ethnicity, gender, and HIV risk mode. It includes more than 40,000 persons as of July 1997.

Figure 1 indicates the incidence of various OIs among adults and adolescents in the ASD project who had CD4$^+$ T-lymphocyte counts of <200 cells/$\mu$l in 1992 to 1996. Although in the past 2 years the availability of potent antiretroviral drugs has resulted in dramatic declines in the incidence of OIs in some populations (32, 34), these data indicate that on average the incidence of OIs in this population of severely immunocompromised persons is high. These illnesses and their associated hospitalizations impact the cost of the U.S. HIV epidemic, which was estimated at $15.2 billion in 1995 (15).

The challenges posed by OIs in HIV-infected persons are numerous and go beyond simple measurements of incidence of disease and costs of medical care. They are perhaps best illustrated by a discussion of two OIs that present a different array of challenges—*Pneumocystis carinii* pneumonia (PCP) and cryptosporidiosis.

## *Pneumocystis carinii* Pneumonia

In the United States, PCP continues to be the most common serious OI in HIV-infected adults and adolescents (Table 1; Figure 1) and in children (data not shown), despite the availability of effective chemoprophylaxis. Such prophylaxis was recommended for HIV-infected adults and adolescents as early as 1989 (3) and for HIV-exposed/infected children in 1991 (4). PCP is characterized by shortness of breath, fever, dry cough, and bilateral infiltrates on chest X-ray; despite the availability of effective therapy, mortality remains about 8% in adults (19) and over 30% in children (42). Because the causative organism is thought to be ubiquitous in the environment, prevention of exposure is unlikely to be a realistic mode of disease prevention.

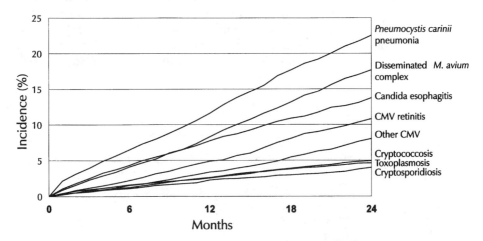

**Figure 1.** Incidence of opportunistic infections in HIV-infected persons following their first CD4$^+$ T-lymphocyte count of <200 cells/$\mu$l. Data are from the CDC's Adult and Adolescent Spectrum of Disease Project, averaged for the period 1992 to 1996.

Chemoprophylaxis against the first episode of PCP is recommended for any HIV-infected adolescent or adult with a CD4$^+$ T-lymphocyte count of <200 cells/$\mu$l or a history of oral candidiasis (thrush) or unexplained fever with a $\geq$2-week duration (8). The drug of choice is trimethoprim-sulfamethoxazole (TMP/SMX); dapsone or aerosolized pentamidine are alternatives for persons who cannot tolerate sulfa-containing drugs (8). Chemoprophylaxis is also recommended for all HIV-exposed children during their first year of life or until HIV infection is excluded; recommendations for older HIV-infected children are based on age-specific CD4$^+$ count thresholds (6). The drug of choice for children is also TMP/SMX.

The reasons that HIV-infected adults and adolescents continue to develop PCP were investigated recently by using data from CDC's ASD Project. To ascertain the factors leading to the development of PCP, a case of PCP (including cases definitively or presumptively diagnosed) in a person not in medical care was defined as one in which no positive HIV test result or CD4$^+$ T-lymphocyte count had been recorded before PCP diagnosis, or if no other AIDS illness (which would have brought the person into care) had been diagnosed. Persons who were in care but who had not been prescribed prophylaxis prior to illness were defined as those who had been enrolled in ASD and had at least one CD4$^+$ T-lymphocyte count recorded but who had not been prescribed TMP/SMX, dapsone, or aerosolized pentamidine prior to illness. These persons were in turn categorized as having met the criteria for PCP prophylaxis (CD4$^+$ count of <200 cells/$\mu$l or history of thrush or unexplained fever), and they should have been prescribed prophylaxis or categorized as not having met these criteria and therefore might not be expected to have had prophylaxis prescribed. Finally, persons with PCP were deemed to have "broken through" prophylaxis if any of the three drugs mentioned above had been prescribed before diagnosis.

The results of this analysis of causes of PCP are shown in Fig. 2. As of July 1997, more than 9,000 cases of PCP had been included in this analysis. More than half (54%) of cases occurred in persons who met our definition of "not in care." This suggests that failure to have had HIV infection diagnosed or to access medical care is responsible for a majority of cases of PCP in this study. Similar results have been obtained in other U.S. studies (40, 41). As the average interval between HIV

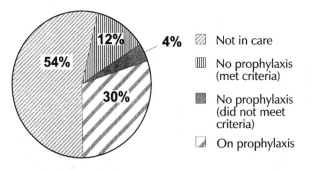

**Figure 2.** Reasons for development of PCP among 9,079 persons with PCP enrolled in the CDC ASD Project through July 1997.

infection and development of AIDS has been estimated at 10 years (33), the implications of these observations are obvious in terms of lost opportunities for prevention of illness as well as for prevention of transmission of HIV to others.

Approximately 12% of PCP cases occurred in persons who were in care and who satisfied the criteria for PCP prophylaxis but had not been prescribed prophylaxis. Some of these cases may have occurred in persons who did not return for follow-up and thus could not have prophylaxis prescribed, and some may have occurred in persons who were offered but refused prophylaxis. Nevertheless, these data suggest that adherence to this preventive measure on the part of health care providers is incomplete and could be improved.

Approximately 4% of cases occurred in persons in care who were not offered prophylaxis because they did not satisfy current criteria for PCP prophylaxis, i.e, a CD4$^+$ count of >200 cells/$\mu$l and no history of thrush or unexplained fever. Although this observation suggests that current criteria for prophylaxis could be improved to prevent such cases, it is noteworthy that this category accounted for only a small proportion of PCP cases in this study.

Approximately 30% of PCP cases occurred in persons who had been prescribed prophylaxis. Almost certainly, many of these cases occurred in persons who failed to adhere to their prophylaxis regimen, although this proportion cannot be assessed from these data. Some may have occurred because of incomplete efficacy of prophylaxis, i.e, prophylaxis may be less effective in those persons with the lowest CD4$^+$ counts (39). Finally, it is possible that some cases of PCP may occur because of antimicrobial resistance.

Because *P. carinii* cannot be cultivated in vitro, antimicrobial resistance cannot be measured directly. However, Meshnick and colleagues have reported data suggesting the possibility of the emergence of *P. carinii* resistance to sulfa drugs (21, 26). By sequencing the dihydropteroate synthase (DHPS) gene (mutant sequences of which have been associated with sulfa resistance in other diseases [e.g., malaria]), they found a statistically significant association between breakthrough on sulfa prophylaxis and the presence of mutant DHPS sequences. This is an intriguing finding, given the small numbers of subjects in their analysis (21) (Table 2). Although information regarding clinical response to TMP/SMX was not available, these data suggest the possiblity of drug resistance and highlight the need for further work in this area.

In addition to the challenges posed by PCP in HIV-infected adults and adolescents illustrated above, another is diagnostics. Diagnosis of PCP currently requires

**Table 2.** Occurrence of mutant DHPS gene in *Pneumocystis carinii* from persons with breakthrough PCP[a]

| Prophylaxis | No. of isolates with indicated form of DHPS gene | |
| --- | --- | --- |
| | Mutant | Wild type |
| Sulfa drug | 5 | 2 |
| No sulfa drug | 2 | 11 |

[a]Source: reference 21. $P = 0.02$ for difference in prevalence of mutant DHPS gene in persons receiving sulfa prophylaxis versus that in persons receiving nonsulfa prophylaxis.

bronchoscopy, although induced sputum examination has been sensitive in some studies (25). These procedures are obviously difficult to perform in children; whether more sensitive PCR assays (47) will allow testing of sputum or possibly gastric aspirates and whether serologic assays (44) will prove valuable in the diagnosis of PCP are the subjects of ongoing investigations.

## Cryptosporidiosis

Cryptosporidiosis, caused by the protozoan parasite *Cryptosporidium parvum*, is a diarrheal disease that can be severe and debilitating and can cause death in severely immunocompromised persons. Its incidence in AIDS patients has been reported to be as high as 5 to 10% per year (17, 43), and no treatment or chemoprophylaxis has been proven to be consistently effective. This disease poses quite different challenges from those for PCP, as sources of this organism in the environment are largely known and prevention thus involves avoidance of these exposures. Known modes of exposure include person-to-person, animal-to-person, consumption of contaminated tap and recreational water, consumption of contaminated food, and possibly fomite transmission (17, 30, 36) (Table 3).

The exposure mode that has drawn most attention in recent years has been consumption of municipal water. Several waterborne outbreaks of cryptosporidiosis have been documented in the past 15 years (Table 4). The most noteworthy of these was the outbreak in Milwaukee, Wis., in 1993 that sickened more than 400,000 persons and was associated with premature deaths in immunocompromised persons (16, 29). Of note is that nearly all these waterborne outbreaks occurred in the setting of adequately chlorinated water systems, which is not surprising, as chlorination is known to be ineffective against this parasite (24). Outbreaks also occurred in sev-

**Table 3.** Modes of transmission of cryptosporidiosis

Person to person
    Sexual contact (oral-anal sex)
    Day care center attendees and workers
    Health care workers, home care givers

Animal to person
    Farm animals (calves, lambs)
    Pets (puppies, kittens)[a]

Water
    Drinking and recreational

Food
    Apple cider, potato salad

Environment
    Fomite transmission[a]

[a]Transmission has not been demonstrated epidemiologically but potentially exists because of the presence of *C. parvum* oocysts in the environment.

**Table 4.** Outbreaks of cryptosporidiosis in the United States (drinking water)

| Year | Location | No. of persons ill | Water | | | Coliforms in treated water |
|------|----------|--------------------|-------|------|-----------|---------------------------|
| | | | Source | Filtered | Chlorinated | |
| 1984 | Texas | 2,000 | Artesian well | No | Yes | No |
| 1987 | Georgia | 13,000 | River | Yes | Yes | No |
| 1991 | Pennsylvania | 500 | Noncommunity well | No | Yes | No |
| 1992 | Oregon | 3,000 | Spring | No | Yes | No |
| 1992 | Oregon | | River | Yes | Yes | No |
| 1993 | Wisconsin | >400,000 | Lake | Yes | Yes | No |
| 1994 | Nevada | Unknown | Lake | Yes | Yes | No |
| 1994 | Washington | 113 | Well | No | No | Yes |

eral communities, including Milwaukee, with filtered municipal drinking water; these water treatment plants were also in compliance with Environmental Protection Agency standards regarding filtration.

The occurrence of these outbreaks has raised questions about the safety of municipal tap water for immunocompromised persons in the absence of a recognized outbreak. Data collected by LeChevallier and others indicated that *Cryptosporidium* oocysts can be found in virtually all surface water supplies (rivers and lakes) and in approximately one-half of "finished" water supplies (i.e., water processed for consumption by both chlorination and filtration) (27, 28). Oocysts in finished water are generally present in small numbers. Whether they all represent *C. parvum* or other, nonpathogenic species, whether they are viable and infective, and the dose required to produce illness in immunocompromised persons are unknown. Hence, the magnitude of risk to immunocompromised persons is also unknown.

The proportions of cryptosporidiosis illnesses in HIV-infected persons associated with the various modes of transmission, including consumption of municipal tap water, are unknown. However, a higher incidence in men who have sex with men than in other HIV risk groups suggests that sexual exposures are important (9). To investigate the feasibility of studying this issue further, Davis et al. collected information concerning the frequency of these various exposures in HIV-infected persons attending an outpatient facility in New York City in 1994 (11). More than three-fourths of these patients reported at least one risk factor (other than consumption of municipal tap water) known to be associated with cryptosporidiosis transmission. Approximately one-fourth of subjects reported trying to avoid municipal tap water by boiling water, using point-of-use water filters, or using bottled water. However, virtually all persons were exposed to at least some municipal drinking water through ice, teeth brushing, or occasional drinks of water while away from home (11). The data indicate some heterogeneity in this population regarding exposure to municipal tap water, and it is hoped that future studies will allow the delineation of the proportion of cryptosporidiosis illness associated with consumption of tap water, as well as with other environmental exposures.

A recent discovery that may prove useful in delineating environmental sources of cryptosporidial infections is a genotypic heterogeneity in isolates of *C. parvum*

(Fig. 3). Sequencing of *C. parvum* in the TRAP-C2 region of the genome suggests two genotypes: one appears to be of human and the other of animal origin (35). These sequencing differences are supported by biologic differences in these isolates; genotype 1 isolates do not appear to be infective to laboratory animals or calves, while genotype 2 isolates can readily infect calves and mice as well as humans (35). The ability to identify two types of *C. parvum* may prove useful in delineating the source of *C. parvum* infections and in guiding prevention strategies. For example, the finding that the Milwaukee isolates from 1993 are genotype 1 suggests a human origin of the outbreak. It further suggests that greater attention should be given to human sewage effluent as a significant contributor of *Cryptosporidium* oocysts in rivers and lakes serving as community water sources.

Other challenges posed by cryptosporidiosis in HIV-infected persons include development of assays to quantitate and determine viability of *C. parvum* oocysts in drinking water, more effective methods of removing such oocysts from water, and improved labeling of bottled water products to assist consumers in identifying products that have undergone treatments that kill or remove oocysts.

A summary of the major challenges posed by OIs in HIV-infected persons, many of which have been alluded to in the examples above, is given in Table 5. Noteworthy additions are the challenges posed by adverse consequences of chemoprophylaxis, which may diminish the advisability of offering prophylaxis that has been shown to be effective, such as chemoprophylaxis against cytomegalovirus (CMV) and deep fungal diseases. Vaccinations pose challenges in terms of efficacy in immunocompromised persons and possible stimulation of HIV replication and acceleration of HIV disease. Finally, in the developing world, many OIs that are

| Position: | 15 | 42 | 64 | 111 | 244 | |
|---|---|---|---|---|---|---|
| Isolate: | | | | | | |
| Milwaukee 93 /1 | G | C | T | C | T | |
| Milwaukee 93 /2 | G | C | T | C | T | |
| Milwaukee 93 /3 | G | C | T | C | T | |
| Milwaukee 96 | G | C | T | C | T | |
| Georgia-DC 95 | G | C | T | C | T | |
| Georgia-WP 95 /1 | G | C | T | C | T | |
| Georgia-WP 95 /2 | G | C | T | C | T | **Genotype 1** |
| Florida 95 /1 | G | C | T | C | T | |
| Florida 95 /2 | G | C | T | C | T | |
| Florida 95 /3 | G | C | T | C | T | |
| Florida 95 /4 | G | C | T | C | T | |
| Florida 95 /5 | G | C | T | C | C | |
| Texas 96 | G | C | T | C | C | |
| Maine Cider 93 | A | T | G | T | C | |
| B.C. Canada 96 | A | T | G | T | C | |
| Pennsylvania 97 (H) | A | T | G | T | C | **Genotype 2** |
| Pennsylvania 97 (C) | A | T | G | T | C | |
| Iowa calf (CDC) | A | T | G | T | C | |
| Published calf | A | T | G | T | C | |
| Other bovine (n=21) | A | T | G | T | C | |

Human Isolates (Milwaukee 93/1 through Texas 96); Calf Isolates (Maine Cider 93 through Other bovine)

**Figure 3.** Alignment of TRAP-C2 sequences from *Cryptosporidium parvum* isolates. Source: reference 35.

**Table 5.** Challenges posed by opportunistic infections in HIV-infected persons

Testing for HIV/access to care
Environmental sources of pathogens/methods to reduce exposure
Chemoprophylaxis: efficacy, toxicities, drug interactions, potential for antimicrobial resistance, cost
Vaccinations
Diagnostics
Better therapies
OIs of international importance

uncommon in the United States pose unique challenges in specific geographic areas. These include *Penicillium marneffei* infection in Southeast Asia (45), *Trypanosoma cruzi* in South America (12), and leishmanial infections in southern Europe (31) and probably in other areas where leishmaniasis is endemic.

## OPPORTUNISTIC INFECTIONS ASSOCIATED WITH OTHER DISEASES

A variety of other conditions are associated with immunosuppression and increased susceptibility to OIs (Table 6). Because denominators for these populations are often elusive, it is unclear whether such populations are increasing and therefore relevant to the concept of emerging infectious diseases. However, some of these populations are known to be increasing and hence are highly relevant in this regard.

## BONE MARROW AND SOLID ORGAN TRANSPLANTATION

Transplantation of hematopoietic stem cells, generally referred to as bone marrow transplantation (BMT), was initially used only as treatment for hematopoietic neoplasms (such as leukemia and lymphoma) and involved tissue from living related donors. Such transplantation from one person to another is referred to as allogeneic BMT. However, BMT is now used for treatment of many other, non-hematopoietic disorders. In these situations, the primary condition is treated with aggressive, marrow-ablative chemotherapy and radiation therapy, and the patient is

**Table 6.** Non-HIV-infected populations with impaired immunity

Children with congenital immunodeficiencies
Bone marrow and solid organ transplant recipients
Cancer patients receiving radiation and/or chemotherapy
Patients receiving chronic corticosteroid therapy
Patients with diabetes, chronic renal or pulmonary disease, sickle-cell anemia, asplenia
Patients with indwelling catheters
Burn and trauma victims
Premature newborns (<32 weeks of gestation)
Elderly persons

"rescued" by infusion of his or her own hematopoietic stem cells. This procedure is referred to as autologous transplantation and is used for an increasing variety of neoplasms, including solid tumors such as breast cancer (37). Because of the expanding uses and increasing survival of BMT patients (1), the numbers of BMT performed annually have increased dramatically in the past decade (Fig. 4). These increases are particularly noteworthy in that the International Bone Marrow Transplant Registry (IBMTR) and the Autologous Blood and Marrow Transplant Registry (ABMTR) estimate that only about 40% of allogeneic BMTs and about 50% of autologous BMTs are reported to their registries; hence, it is likely that more than 12,000 BMTs are performed in the United States yearly. In addition to the increased frequency of these procedures, a variety of stem cell preparations are being used, including not only bone marrow but also peripheral and umbilical blood stem cells. Concomitantly, a variety of preparative regimens are being employed. BMTs are also being performed in outpatient as well as inpatient settings. Therefore, these procedures pose increasing challenges in terms of the spectrum and incidence of OIs that may be anticipated and the surveillance systems required to monitor them.

BMT patients are at a unique time-dependent risk for OIs, depending on the stage of immunosuppression following BMT (Fig. 5). These stages include (i) the pre-engraftment phase (<30 days after BMT), when patients are at high risk for infections associated with neutropenia, such as bacteremias, herpes simplex virus disease, candidiasis, and aspergillosis; (ii) the early post-engraftment phase (the 2nd and 3rd months post-BMT) when depression of cell-mediated immunity is profound and the risks of CMV and aspergillosis are high; and (iii) the late post-engraftment phase (>100 days post-BMT) when patients are at increased risk of varicella-zoster virus infection as well as infection with encapsulated gram-positive bacteria (Fig. 5). Although no systematic surveillance is conducted for these

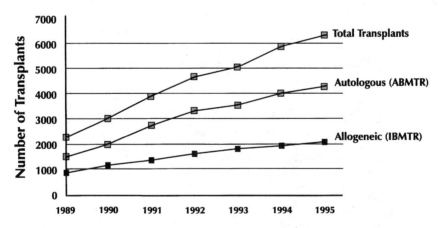

**Figure 4.** Number of reported bone marrow transplants, United States, 1989 to 1995. Data are from the Statistical Center of the International Bone Marrow Transplant Registry and the Autologous Blood and Marrow Transplant Registry.

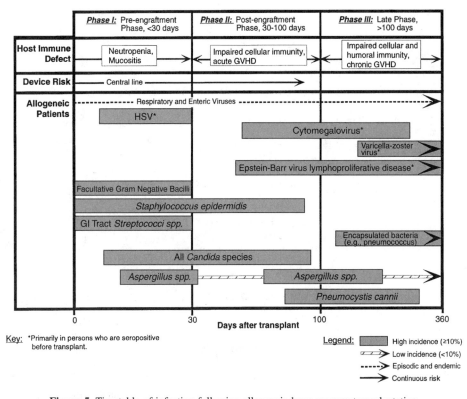

**Figure 5.** Timetable of infection following allogeneic bone marrow transplantation. The figure indicates disease in the absence of opportunistic infection chemoprophylaxis, which can reduce the incidence of herpes simplex virus (HSV) and cytomegalovirus (CMV) disease, candidiasis, and *Pneumocystis carinii* pneumonia.

infections, reports from large volume BMT centers suggest appreciable incidence rates of these infections, particularly in allogeneic versus autologous transplant patients and in the setting of acute or chronic graft versus host disease. For example, without prophylaxis, rates of invasive candidiasis, aspergillosis, and CMV disease in allogeneic transplant recipients can be as high as 25, 11, and 38%, respectively (2, 48, 50); however, rates of candidiasis and CMV disease can be reduced by chemoprophylaxis (2, 51).

## SOLID ORGAN TRANSPLANTS

The number of solid organ transplants (SOTs) has also been increasing in the past decade (Fig. 6). Although the time-dependent relationship between SOT and OIs is not as pronounced as for BMT, patients are at highest risk for OI in the first year following SOT. Again, systematic surveillance for these OIs is not performed, but data from large volume SOT centers indicate that infection is the leading cause of death in SOT patients; of these, CMV disease is the most important (38). SOTs

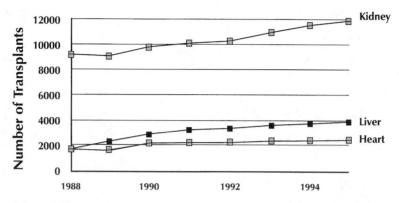

**Figure 6.** Number of solid organ transplants performed in the United States, 1988–1995. Data for kidney, liver, and heart transplants are shown; those for pancreas and lung (which are also increasing but totaled fewer than 2000 in 1995) are omitted. Data are from the United Network for Organ Sharing.

are also unique in that the transplanted organ may be the most frequent site of infection, particularly within 3 months of SOT surgery (13).

## THE ELDERLY

The elderly, here defined as persons ≥65 years of age, constitute an ever-increasing proportion of the U.S. population (Fig. 7) as well as of the population worldwide (49). Elderly persons are at increased risk for a variety of infections (10) (Table 7). Most of the conditions in Table 7 may be classified as OIs if the definition of immune impairment is expanded beyond defects of humoral and cel-

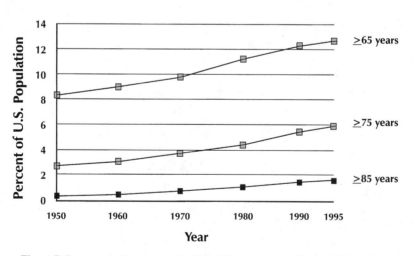

**Figure 7.** Percentage of persons in the United States who are elderly, 1950 to 1995. Data are from the U.S. Bureau of the Census.

**Table 7.** Opportunistic infections in the elderly[a]

rinary tract infections
Pneumonia
Tuberculosis
Pressure sores and skin infections
Bacteremia
Infective endocarditis
Infectious diarrhea
Meningitis
Septic arthritis

[a]Adapted from reference 10.

lular immunity to include defects in the cough reflex, defects in the integrity of the skin and mucous membranes, decreased gastric acidity, breaching of barriers by catheters and other indwelling devices, and anatomical defects in the urinary tract. In addition to these conditions, others associated with immunosuppression, such as diabetes and cancer, increase with age and therefore can be expected to increase as the U.S. population ages (22, 23).

## CONCLUSIONS

OIs pose significant challenges as emerging infectious diseases in increasing populations of immunocompromised persons, including persons with HIV infection, persons receiving bone marrow or solid organ transplants, and the elderly. Challenges include defining and quantitating the populations at risk, conducting surveillance for and determining risk factors for OIs among these populations, developing better diagnostic techniques and therapies, and developing strategies for disease prevention.

**Acknowledgments.** We thank Esther Benenson, Raleigh Bowden, Lawrence Davis, Edward Gregory, Altaf Lal, Steven Meshnick, Thomas Navin, Melodee Nugent, Michael Osterholm, Rosemary Ramsey, Philip Rowlings, Robert Rubin, Rosemary Soave, and John Wingard for sharing data and reviewing the manuscript and Sharon Cox, Claire Kiernan, Renee Maciejewski, Robin Moseley, and Patricia Tyson for graphics, secretarial, and editorial assistance.

## REFERENCES

1. **Antman, K. H., P. A. Rowlings, W. P. Vaughan, J. W. Fay, K. K. Fields, C. O. Freytes, R. P. Gale, B. E. Hillner, H. K. Holland, M. J. Kennedy, J. P. Klein, H. M. Lazarus, P. L. McCarthy, C. J. Pelz, R. Saez, G. Spitzer, E. A. Stadtmauer, S. F. Williams, S. Wolff, K. A. Sobocinski, J. O. Armitage, and M. M. Horowitz,** 1997. High-dose chemotherapy with autologous hematopoietic stem cell support for breast cancer in North America. *J. Clin. Oncol.* **15:**1870–1879.
2. **Boeckh, M., and R. Bowden.** 1995. Cytomegalovirus infection in marrow transplantation, p. 97–136. *In* C. D. Buckner (ed.), *Technical and Biological Components of Bone Marrow Transplantation.* Kluwer Academic Publishers, Boston, Mass.
3. **Centers for Disease Control.** 1989. Guidelines for prophylaxis against *Pneumocystis carinii* pneumonia for persons infected with human immunodeficiency virus. *Morbid. Mortal. Weekly Rep.* **38**(S-5):1–9.

4. **Centers for Disease Control.** 1991. Guidelines for prophylaxis against *Pneumocystis carinii* pneumonia for children infected with human immunodeficiency virus. *Morbid. Mortal. Weekly Rep.* **40**(RR-2):1–13.

5. **Centers for Disease Control and Prevention.** 1992. 1993 revised classification system for HIV infection and expanded surveillance case definition for AIDS among adolescents and adults. *Morbid. Mortal. Weekly Rep.* **41**:608–610.

6. **Centers for Disease Control and Prevention.** 1995. 1995 revised guidelines for prophylaxis against *Pneumocystis carinii* pneumonia for children infected with or perinatally exposed to human immunodeficiency virus. *Morbid. Mortal. Weekly Rep.* **44**(RR-4):1–11.

7. **Centers for Disease Control and Prevention.** 1996. *HIV/AIDS Surveillance Rep.* **8**(2):18.

8. **Centers for Disease Control and Prevention.** 1997. 1997 USPHS/IDSA guidelines for the prevention of opportunistic infections in persons infected with human immunodeficiency virus. *Morbid. Mortal. Weekly Rep.* **46**(RR-12):1–46.

9. **Ciesielski, C., J. Kaplan, M. Mays, J. Ward, and D. Juranek.** 1995. Cryptosporidiosis in AIDS patients in the United States—relationship to municipal water supplies, abstr. 308. *In Program and Abstracts of the 2nd National Conference on Human Retroviruses and Related Infections.*

10. **Crossley, K. B., and P. K. Peterson.** 1995. Infections in the Elderly. p. 2737–2742. *In* Mandell, G. L., J. E. Bennett, and R. Dolin (ed.), Principles and Practice of Infectious Diseases. Churchill Livingstone, Inc., New York, N.Y.

11. **Davis, L. J., H. L. Roberts, D. D. Juranek, S. R. Framm, and R. Soave.** Survey of risk factors for cryptosporidiosis: drinking water and other exposures. *Am. J. Prev. Med.*, in press.

12. **Del Castillo, M., G. Mendoza, J. Oviedo, R. P. Perez Bianco, A. E. Anselmo, and M. Silva.** 1990. AIDS and Chagas' disease with central nervous system tumor-like lesion. *Am. J. Med.* **88**: 693–694.

13. **Dummer, J. S., M. Ho, and R. L. Simmons.** 1995. Infections in Solid Organ Transplant Recipients. p. 2722–2732. *In* G. L. Mandell, J. E. Bennett, amd R. Dolin, (ed.), *Principles and Practice of Infectious Diseases.* Churchill Livingstone, Inc., New York, N.Y.

14. **Farizo, K. M., J. W. Buehler, M. E. Chamberland, B. M. Whyte, E. S. Froelicher, S. G. Hopkins, C. M. Reed, E. D. Mokotoff, D. L. Cohn, S. Troxler, A. F. Phelps, and R. L. Berkelman.** 1992. Spectrum of disease in persons with human immunodeficiency virus infection in the United States. *JAMA* **267**:1798–1805.

15. **Hellinger, F. J.** 1992. Forecasts of the costs of medical care for persons with HIV: 1992–1995. *Inquiry* **29**:356–365.

16. **Hoxie, N. J., J. P. Davis, J. M. Vergeront, R. D. Nashold, K. A. Blair, and W. R. MacKenzie.** 1997. Cryptosporidiosis-associated mortality following a massive waterborne outbreak in Milwaukee, Wisconsin. *Am. J. Public Health* **7**:2032–2035.

17. **Juranek, D. D.** 1995. Cryptosporidiosis: sources of infection and guidelines for prevention. *Clin. Infect. Dis.* **21**(Suppl. 1):S57–61.

18. **Kaplan, J. E., H. Masur, K. K. Holmes, M. M. McNeil, L. B. Schonberger, T. R. Navin, D. L. Hanson, P. A. Gross, H. W. Jaffe, and the USPHS/IDSA Prevention of Opportunistic Infections Working Group.** 1995. USPHS/IDSA guidelines for the prevention of opportunistic infections in persons infected with human immunodeficiency virus: introduction. *Clin. Infect. Dis.* **21**(Suppl. 1): S1–11.

19. **Kaplan, J. E., J. L. Jones, D. L. Hanson, and J. W. Ward.** 1996. Risk factors for death from *Pneumocystis carinii* pneumonia in the United States, abstr. Tu. B. 2300. *In Program and Abstracts of the XI International Conference on AIDS. Vancouver, Canada, July 7–12, 1996.*

20. **Karon, J. M., P. S. Rosenberg, G. McQuillan, M. Khare, M. Gwinn, and L. R. Petersen.** 1996. Prevalence of HIV infection in the United States, 1984 to 1992. *JAMA* **276**:126–131.

21. **Kazanjian, P., A. B. Locke, P. A. Hossler, B. R. Lane, M. S. Bartlett, J. W. Smith, M. Cannon, and S. R. Meshnick.** 1998. *Pneumocystis carinii* mutations associated with sulfa prophylaxis failures in AIDS patients. *AIDS* **12**:873–878.

22. **Kennedy, B. J., S. A. Bushhouse, and A. P. Bender.** 1994. Minnesota population cancer risk. *Cancer* **73**:724–729.

23. **Kenny, S.J., R. E. Aubert, and L. S. Geiss.** 1995. Prevalence and incidence of non-insulin dependent diabetes. p. 47–67. *In* M. I. Harris, C. C. Cowie, M. P. Stern, E. J. Boyko, G. E. Reiber, and

P. H. Bennett (ed.), *Diabetes in America*, 2nd ed. DHHS publication (NIH)95-1468. U.S. Department of Health and Human Services, Public Health Service, Washington, D.C.

24. **Korich, D. G., J. R. Mead, M. S. Madore, N. A. Sinclair, and C. R. Sterling.** 1990. Effects of ozone, chlorine dioxide, chlorine, and monochloramine on *Cryptosporidium parvum* oocyst viability. *Appl. Environ. Microbiol.* **56:**1423–1428.

25. **Kovacs, J. A., V. L. Ng, H. Masur, G. Leoung, K. Hadley, G. Evans, C. Lane, F. P. Ognibene, J. Shelhamer, J. E. Parrillo, and V. J. Gill.** 1988. Diagnosis of *Pneumocystis carinii* pneumonia. Improved detection in sputum with monoclonal antibodies. *N. Engl. J. Med.* **318:**589–593.

26. **Lane B. R., J. C. Ast, P. A. Hossler, D. P. Mindell, M. S. Bartlett, J. W. Smith, and S. R. Meshnick.** 1997. Dihydropteroate synthase polymorphisms in *Pneumocystis carinii. J. Infect. Dis.* **175:**482–485.

27. **LeChevallier, M. W., W. D. Norton, and R. G. Lee.** 1991. Occurrence of *Giardia* and *Cryptosporidium spp.* in surface water supplies. *Appl. Environ. Microbiol.* **57:**2610–2616.

28. **LeChevallier, M. W., W. D. Norton, and R. G. Lee.** 1991. *Giardia* and *Cryptosporidium spp.* in filtered drinking water supplies. *Appl. Environ. Microbiol.* **57:**2617–2621.

29. **MacKenzie, W. R., N. J. Hoxie, M. E. Proctor, M. S. Gradus, K. A. Blair, D. E. Peterson, J. J. Kazmierczak, D. G. Addiss, K. R. Fox, J. B. Rose, and J. P. Davis.** 1994. A massive outbreak in Milwaukee of *Cryptosporidium* infection transmitted through the public water supply. *N. Engl. J. Med.* **331:**161–167.

30. **Martino, P., G. Gentile, A. Caprioli, L. Baldassarri, G. Donelli, W. Arcese, S. Fenu, A. Micozzi, M. Venditti, and F. Mandelli.** 1988. Hospital acquired cryptosporidiosis in a bone marrow transplantation unit. *J. Infect. Dis.* **158:**647–648.

31. **Montalban, C., J. L. Calleja, A. Erice, F. Laguna, B. Clotet, D. Podzamczer, J. Cobo, J. Mallolas, M. Yebra, A. Gallego, and the Cooperative Group for the Study of Leishmaniasis in AIDS.** 1990. Visceral leishmaniasis in patients infected with human immunodeficiency virus. *J. Infect. Dis.* **21:**261–270.

32. **Moore, R. D., J. C. Keruly, and R. E. Chaisson.** 1997. The effectiveness of combination antiretroviral therapy in clinical practice, abstr. 213. *In Program and Abstracts of the 35th Annual Meeting of the Infectious Diseases Society of America.*

33. **Munoz, A., M.-C. Wang, S. Bass, J. M. G. Taylor, L. A. Kingsley, J. S. Chmiel, B. F. Polk, and the Multicenter AIDS Cohort Study Group.** 1989. Acquired immunodeficiency syndrome (AIDS)-free time after human immunodeficiency virus type 1 (HIV-1) seroconversion in homosexual men. *Am. J. Epidemiol.* **130:**530–539.

34. **Palella, F., A. Moorman, K. Delaney, M. Loveless, J. Fuhrer, D. Aschmand, S. Holmberg, and the HIV Outpatient Study (HOPS) Group.** 1997. Dramatically declining morbidity and mortality in ambulatory HIV-infected patients, abstr. 478. *In* Program and Abstr. 35th Ann. Meet. Infect. Dis. Soc. of Am.

35. **Peng, M., L. Xiao, A. R. Freeman, M. J. Arrowood, A. A. Escalante, A. C. Weltman, C. S. L. Ong, W. R. MacKenzie, A. A. Lal, and C. B. Beard.** 1997. Genetic polymorphism among *Cryptosporidium parvum* isolates: evidence of two distinct human transmission cycles. *Emerg. Infect. Dis.* **3:**567–573.

36. **Roncoroni, A. J., M. A. Gomez, J. Mera, P. Cagnoni, and M. D. Michel.** 1989. *Cryptosporidium* infection in renal transplant patients. *J. Infect. Dis.* **160:**559.

37. **Rowlings, P. A., J. R. Passweg, J. O. Armitage, R. P. Gale, K. A. Sobocinski, J. P. Klein, M. J. Zhang, and M. H. Horowitz.** 1995. Report from the International Bone Marrow Transplant Registry and the Autologous Blood and Marrow Transplant Registry—North America, p. 87–98. *In* P. I. Terasaki and J. M. Checka (ed.), *Clinical Transplants 1994.* UCLA Tissue Typing Laboratory, Los Angeles, Calif.

38. **Rubin, R. H.** 1994. Infection in the organ transplant recipient. p. 629–705. *In* R. H. Rubin, L. S. Young (ed.), *Clinical Approach to Infection in the Compromised Host*, 3rd ed. Plenum Medical Book Company, New York, N.Y.

39. **Saah, A. J., D. R. Hoover, Y. Peng, J. P. Phair, B. Visscher, L. A. Kingsley, L. K. Schrager, and the Multicenter AIDS Cohort Study Group.** 1995. Predictors for failure of *Pneumocystis carinii* pneumonia prophylaxis. *JAMA* **273:**1197–1202.

40. **Schwarcz, S. K., M. H. Katz, A. Hirozawa, J. Gurley, and G. F. Lemp.** 1997. Prevention of *Pneumocystis carinii* pneumonia: who are we missing? *AIDS* **11:**1263–1268.

41. **Shapiro, J., and P. Simon.** 1996. Late HIV diagnosis and failure to receive chemprophylaxis against *Pneumocystis carinii* pneumonia, abstr. I93. *In Abstracts of the 36th Interscience Conference on Antimicrobial Agents and Chemotherapy.* American Society for Microbiology, Washington, D.C.

42. **Simonds, R. J., M. L. Lindegren, P. Thomas, D. Hanson, B. Caldwell, G. Scott, M. Rogers, and the *Pneumocystis carinii* Pneumonia Prophylaxis Evaluation Working Group.** 1995. Prophylaxis against *Pneumocystis carinii* pneumonia among children with perinatally acquired human immunodeficiency virus infection in the United States. *N. Engl. J. Med.* **332:**786–790.

43. **Smith, P. D.** 1992. Gastrointestinal infections in AIDS. *Ann. Intern. Med.* **116:**63–77.

44. **Smulian, A. G., and P. D. Walzer.** 1994. Serologic studies of *Pneumocystis carinii* infection, p. 141–151. *In* P. D. Walzer (ed.), Pneumocystis carinii *Pneumonia.* Marcel Dekker, New York, N.Y.

45. **Supparatpinyo, K., S. Chiewchanvit, P. Hirunsri, C. Uthammachai, K. E. Nelson, and T. Sirisanthana.** 1992. *Penicillium marneffei* infection in patients infected with human immunodeficiency virus. *Clin. Infect. Dis.* **14:**871–874.

46. **United Nations Joint Programme on HIV/AIDS and World Health Organization.** 1997. *Report on the Global HIV/AIDS Epidemic.* United Nations Joint Programme on HIV/AIDS and World Health Organization, Geneva, Switzerland.

47. **Wakefield, A. E., R. F. Miller, L. A. Guiver, and J. M. Hopkin.** 1993. Oropharyngeal samples for detection of *Pneumocystis carinii* by DNA amplification. *Q. J. Med.* **86:**401–406.

48. **Wald, A., W. Leisenring, J. A. van Burik, and R. A. Bowden.** 1997. Epidemiology of *Aspergillus* infections in a large cohort of patients undergoing bone marrow transplantation. *J. Infect. Dis.* **175:** 1459–1466.

49. **Weiss, R., and K. Kasmauski.** 1997. Aging: new answers to old questions. *Natl. Geogr. Mag.* **192**(5):2–31.

50. **Wheat, L. J.** 1994. Fungal infections in the immunocompromised host, p. 211–237. *In* R. H. Rubin and L. S. Young (ed.), *Clinical Approach to Infection in the Compromised Host,* 3rd ed. Plenum Medical Book Company, New York, N.Y.

51. **Wingard, J. R., W. G. Merz, M. G. Rinaldi, T. R. Johnson, J. E. Karp, and R. Saral.** 1991. Increase in *Candida krusei* infection among patients with bone marrow transplantation and neutropenia treated prophylactically with fluconazole. *N. Engl. J. Med.* **325:**1274–1277.

*Emerging Infections 2*
Edited by W. M. Scheld, W. A. Craig, and J. M. Hughes
© 1998 ASM Press, Washington, D.C.

*Chapter 15*

# Food-Borne Diseases in the Global Village: What's on the Plate for the 21st Century

*David L. Swerdlow and Sean F. Altekruse*

At the beginning of this century, food-borne diseases were a common cause of illness because of poor sanitation, inadequate refrigeration and canning practices, and because diseased animals were killed under unsanitary conditions. Improvements in hygiene, availability of refrigeration, educational efforts, and industry regulations have improved many of these conditions; however, food-borne diseases remain a major public health problem. The yearly incidence of food-borne illness in the United States is estimated at between 6 and 80 million illnesses resulting in approximately 500 to 9,000 deaths (15, 40, 111). (Table 1). The annual economic burden is estimated at 5 billion U.S. dollars (7). New food safety concerns include new and emerging pathogens, changes in the food industry including globalization of the food supply, and changing populations with increased numbers of persons more susceptible to food-borne pathogens.

It is now recognized that food-borne pathogens do not just cause diarrhea; complications of infection can be severe. For example, infection with *Listeria monocytogenes* can cause meningitis or sepsis in neonates and immunosuppressed patients and miscarriage in pregnant women (86). Salmonellosis may also result in sepsis (64). Infection with some food-borne pathogens can be followed by chronic sequelae or disability. Toxoplasmosis is an important cause of congenital malformation (58). *Escherichia coli* O157:H7 is a leading cause of hemolytic uremic syndrome, the most common cause of acute kidney failure in children (48). Nontyphoidal *Salmonella* or *Yersinia enterocolitica* infection can cause reactive arthritis (19, 99), and campylobacteriosis can cause Guillain-Barré syndrome, one of the most common causes of flaccid paralysis in the United States since the control of poliomyelitis (72). In this review we present examples of new and emerging food-borne pathogens followed by examples of how changes in the food industry and

*David L. Swerdlow and Sean F. Altekruse* • Foodborne and Diarrheal Diseases Branch, Division of Bacterial and Mycotic Diseases, National Center for Infectious Diseases, Centers for Disease Control and Prevention, Atlanta, GA 30333.

**Table 1.** Estimated illnesses and deaths per year caused by selected food-borne pathogens in the United States and commonly implicated foods[a]

| Food-borne pathogen | Estimated cases | Estimated deaths | Commonly implicated foods |
|---|---|---|---|
| *Campylobacter jejuni* | 4,000,000 | 200–1,000 | Poultry, raw milk, untreated water |
| *Salmonella* (nontyphoid) | 2,000,000 | 500–2,000 | Eggs, poultry, meat, other raw foods |
| *Escherichia coli* O157:H7 | 20,000 | 100–200 | Ground beef, fresh produce, raw milk, untreated water, unpasteurized fruit juice |
| *Listeria monocytogenes* | 1,500 | 250–500 | Ready-to-eat foods (e.g., soft cheese, deli foods, pâté) |
| *Vibrio* species | 10,000 | 50–100 | Seafood (e.g., molluscan and crustacean shellfish, finfish) |

[a]Sources: reference 7, 15, and 40.

in the population affect the safety of our food supply. Finally we discuss approaches that may help to prevent and control emerging food-borne hazards.

## EMERGING FOOD-BORNE PATHOGENS

Emerging food-borne pathogens include new or newly recognized pathogens such as *Campylobacter jejuni*, *E. coli* O157:H7, *Vibrio vulnificus*, and *Cyclospora cayetanensis*; previously recognized pathogens that have emerged because of new modes of transmission such as *Salmonella* serotype Enteritidis transmitted by shell eggs; pathogens recently recognized to be transmitted by food-borne routes such as *L. monocytogenes*; and pathogens that have selectively adapted to environmental conditions such as antimicrobial-resistant *Salmonella* Typhimurium DT104.

### C. jejuni

*C. jejuni* is a food-borne pathogen that was not recognized as a cause of human illness until the late 1970s but has since emerged as the leading cause of food-borne bacterial infection (101). The estimated *C. jejuni* infection rate for the United States is more than two million cases per year (approximately 1% of the United States population) (101). The Guillain-Barré syndrome, which causes severe neurologic manifestations, can result from *Campylobacter* infections (72). In a multicenter study of 118 patients in the United States with Guillain-Barré syndrome, 36% had serologic evidence of *C. jejuni* infection during the weeks before onset of neurologic symptoms (72).

Outbreaks and sporadic illnesses caused by *C. jejuni* have different epidemiologic characteristics. The seasonality for common-source outbreaks is bimodal, with peaks in May and October and a low point in summer. The number of *Campylobacter* isolates reported to the Centers for Disease Control and Prevention (CDC), which largely represent sporadic illnesses, peaks in the summer months. These observations suggest that the circumstances that lead to outbreaks and sporadic illnesses are different. Epidemiologic studies indicate that outbreaks are frequently linked to consumption of contaminated raw milk or water, while sporadic illnesses are frequently associated with handling and consumption of undercooked poultry (101).

The use of unchlorinated drinking water in the production of food animals may be an important risk factor for the spread of *C. jejuni* in the farm environment (57, 77). Chlorination of drinking water used in food animal production may be a practical method to reduce contamination of raw meat and poultry with *C. jejuni*. The effectiveness of this inexpensive technology should be explored.

### *Escherichia coli* O157:H7

*E. coli* O157:H7 was first recognized to be a human pathogen in 1982, when two outbreaks in the United States were associated with eating undercooked hamburgers from a fast-food restaurant chain (81). Since then, this food-borne pathogen has emerged as a major cause of bloody and nonbloody diarrhea, causing up to 20,000 cases and up to 250 deaths per year in the United States (48). Outbreaks of infection have also been reported in Canada, Japan, Africa, the United Kingdom, Germany, and other countries (48). In addition to causing bloody diarrhea, *E. coli* O157:H7 infection is the most common cause of hemolytic uremic syndrome (HUS), the leading cause of kidney failure among children in the United States. HUS is associated with significant long-term complications. Between 3% and 5% of patients who develop HUS die, and approximately 12% are left with significant sequelae including end-stage renal disease, hypertension, and neurologic injury (87). Consumption of ground beef, lettuce, unpasteurized cider or milk, and untreated water have been associated with outbreaks, and person-to-person transmission is well documented (48).

Tracing *E. coli* O157:H7-contaminated ground beef to the farm of origin is a challenge because meat from a variety of sources may be combined to make ground beef. Trimmings from 100 or more carcasses may be combined in 2,000-pound lots of ground beef. When a shipment of ground beef is contaminated, it can lead to widespread illness, such as occurred in a well-publicized outbreak in the western United States in 1993 associated with consumption of hamburgers from a single restaurant chain. In Washington State alone, over 500 illnesses, 151 hospitalizations, and 3 deaths were attributed to this outbreak (13). Monitoring the microbial quality of ground beef to trace the source of contaminated beef is problematic because herds may have intermittent or low-prevalence infections and the pathogen may be difficult to detect in ground beef if it is present in low concentration (13).

### *V. vulnificus*

In the United States, the emergence of *V. vulnificus* was first reported in 1979 (20). *V. vulnificus* illnesses from eating shellfish have a summer seasonality, and most tracebacks have implicated consumption of raw oysters from the Gulf of Mexico (29). Although the annual oyster harvest from the U.S. Gulf of Mexico has not significantly changed since the 1930s, the percentage of oysters harvested during summer months increased from 8% of annual harvest in 1970 to 30% in 1994 (74). This change in practice is temporally associated with the decline of a competing oyster industry in the Chesapeake due to parasitism, pollution, and other processes (32). Thus, the emergence of *V. vulnificus* infections associated with consumption of Gulf Coast oysters may be a consequence of market forces brought about by the decline of summer harvesting by the nearest competing oyster industry.

*V. vulnificus* infections from shellfish can result in primary septicemia, a syndrome that generally affects persons with underlying illnesses characterized by iron overload (e.g., liver disease) (54). The clinical presentation may include shock, the appearance of bullous lesions on the skin, and swift progression to death. More than 55% of reported shellfish-associated *V. vulnificus* infections in Florida are fatal (54).

## C. cayetanensis

The initial report of human *Cyclospora* infection came from Papua New Guinea in 1979 (8). The first *C. cayetanensis* outbreak in the United States occurred in 1990 in a hospital dormitory in Chicago and was linked to drinking tap water from open storage tanks on the dormitory roof (55). The symptoms of infection with this parasite include prolonged, sometimes cyclical or relapsing watery diarrhea, profound fatigue, weight loss, and vomiting. Although the illness is self-limited, it may last for weeks, and progressive anorexia, fatigue, and weight loss may overshadow the presenting diarrheal symptoms (90). Before 1996, most documented cases of cyclosporiasis in North America were in overseas travelers. In 1996, a large outbreak occurred in North America; overall 1,465 cases were reported from 20 states, the District of Columbia, and two Canadian provinces (52). Raspberries imported from Guatemala were epidemiologically implicated as the vehicle of infection. The source of contamination of the berries was not determined, but a suggested hypothesis was that water contaminated with *C. cayetanensis* was used to spray insecticide on the raspberry plants (52). No animals have yet been identified as reservoirs of infection for *C. cayetanensis* isolates that infect humans; however, recent evidence suggests that *Eimeria*, a recognized coccidian parasite in birds, may be very similar to *C. cayetanensis* (79).

## Salmonella Serotype Enteritidis

An example of an emerging food-borne infection of global significance is *Salmonella* serotype Enteritidis (SE). In the late 20th century, isolation rates for SE increased worldwide (82). In the United States, the proportion of *Salmonella* isolates reported to CDC that were SE increased from 6% in 1980 to 25% in 1996 (Fig. 1) (30a). Between 1985 and 1991 in the United States, grade A shell eggs were implicated in 82% of outbreaks with information on the specific food vehicle (73).

The emergence of SE is related to the ability of the organism to infect the ovaries of egg-laying hens (89), resulting in contamination of the internal contents of intact shell eggs (92). SE can be transmitted vertically from breeding flocks to egg-laying hens, which then produce contaminated eggs. Once present in a flock, the infection is difficult to eliminate because transmission is sustained through environmental sources, including rodents, feed, and other hens.

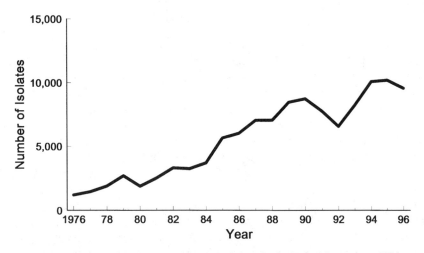

**Figure 1.** *Salmonella* serotype Enteritidis isolations in the United States from 1976 to 1996. Source: CDC, National Center for Infectious Diseases, Division of Bacterial and Mycotic Diseases.

The control of SE is complicated by economic pressures that emphasize egg production over infection control (14). In 1945 a typical henhouse contained 500 birds. By 1995, many houses contained 100,000 hens and multiple houses were linked by common machinery (14), resulting in large flocks with common risk profiles. Large-scale distribution of shell eggs from infected flocks has caused outbreaks in which contaminated eggs were disseminated across many states over a long period (73).

The practice of combining contents of several eggs together, called egg pooling, has caused many outbreaks. A small inoculum of *Salmonella* from a single egg may contaminate the entire batch and, if allowed to incubate, can cause illness in many people. SE outbreaks associated with pooled eggs have been particularly severe in nursing homes. In such outbreaks reported to CDC between 1975 and 1987, 9.7% of patients were hospitalized, and 6.8% died (63).

The predominant SE phage types (PT) reported from outbreak and sporadic illnesses in the United States between 1979 and 1984 were types 8, 13a, non-typeable, 14b, 9a, and 13 (37a). During the 1980s SE PT 4 was rarely reported in the United States (83), but it had emerged as the predominant phage type in both humans and poultry in Europe and Mexico, virtually replacing other phage types. Marked increases in reported human infections with SE have consistently accompanied the spread of SE PT 4. In the 1990s, SE PT 4 emerged in Southern California, resulting in a fivefold increase in reported SE infections (76). In 1995, similar increases in SE infection due to PT 4 were also reported in Utah (91). Surveillance to monitor regional trends in the prevalence of SE in the United States, including the prevalence of SE PT 4, is important to determine if the epidemic is spreading and to focus control measures.

## *L. monocytogenes*

Food-borne transmission has recently been recognized as a major source of human listeriosis (86). Listeriosis can cause meningitis or sepsis in neonates and immunocompromised hosts and fetal loss in pregnant women. Sporadic listeriosis is associated with a case-fatality rate of approximately 20% (46). Food-borne outbreaks of invasive listeriosis have been associated with cole slaw, pasteurized milk, pâté, pork tongue in jelly, and soft cheeses made with inadequately pasteurized milk (86). Information from recent outbreak investigations suggests that *L. monocytogenes* may cause a febrile gastroenteritis in normal hosts (41, 85). In 1989, the U.S. Department of Agriculture and the U.S. Food and Drug Administration (FDA) established zero tolerance policies for *L. monocytogenes* in ready-to-eat foods. Between 1989 and 1993, the food industry launched efforts to reduce *Listeria* contamination in processed foods, and dietary recommendations were established and publicized for persons at increased risk of invasive listeriosis. During this 4-year interval there was a 40% decline in the incidence of listeriosis in nine active surveillance areas across the United States (98).

## MICROBIAL ADAPTATION: ENVIRONMENTAL CONDITIONS AND ANTIMICROBIAL RESISTANCE

Natural selection is important in the emergence of pathogens. Some pathogens are able to survive in harsh environmental conditions. *Enterobacter sakazakii*, which causes brain abscesses in children, can survive in dry conditions and has been recovered from powdered infant formula (35). *E. coli* O157:H7 strains have been shown to be acid tolerant (71), and some serotypes of *Salmonella* are known to be thermotolerant (66).

The therapeutic use of an antimicrobial agent, either in human or animal populations, creates a selective pressure that favors survival of bacterial strains with resistance to the agent (99). Antimicrobial-resistant strains of *Salmonella* have become increasingly prominent (47, 62). Studies of patients in the United States with *Salmonella* infections demonstrate an increase in the prevalence of antimicrobial-resistant *Salmonella* infections from 17% of isolates in the late 1970s to 33% in 1996 (47). Compared to patients with susceptible infections, patients with antimicrobial-resistant infections are more likely to require hospitalization and to be hospitalized for longer periods (62).

During the 1990s, *Salmonella* serotype Typhimurium definitive type 104 (DT 104) emerged in the United Kingdom. By 1996 DT 104 was the second most common cause of human salmonellosis in England and Wales; 4,006 isolates were reported from humans in that year alone (108). Over 90% of all DT 104 isolates were resistant to ampicillin, chloramphenicol, streptomycin, sulfonamides, and tetracycline (R-type ACSSuT), and 30% of strains also showed resistance to trimethoprim and ciprofloxacin (108). Surveillance for DT 104 infections in the United Kingdom indicates high hospitalization and fatality rates compared with infections caused by other *Salmonella* serotypes. In one study, 41% of patients with multiresistant DT 104 infection required hospitalization, and 3% died (107). In the

United Kingdom, illness has been associated with contact with farm animals and with consumption of foods such as beef, pork sausages, and chicken. The organism has been isolated primarily from cattle but has also been isolated from poultry, sheep, and pigs (107).

*Salmonella* Typhimurium DT 104 is emerging in the United States. In 1995, a study of a national sample of *Salmonella* Typhimurium isolates submitted to CDC showed that 28% of 976 strains had the ACSSuT resistance pattern, compared with 7% in 1990 (30). In 1995, 83% of a sample of 30 *Salmonella* Typhimurium R-type ACSSuT isolates from 10 states were phage typed as DT 104 (30). Among cattle isolates of *Salmonella* Typhimurium from the Pacific Northwest obtained before 1986, none had this R-type, compared with 13% of isolates obtained between 1986 and 1991 and 64% of isolates obtained between 1992 and 1995 (18).

In the 1980s, European nations began to use fluoroquinolones for the treatment of infectious diseases of livestock. The introduction of fluoroquinolones in poultry production was temporally associated with the emergence of fluoroquinolone-resistant *C. jejuni* in humans (43). In the United States, fluoroquinolones have been approved for limited use in the treatment of a specific disease of poultry (104). In 1996, CDC and FDA began surveillance for the emergence of resistance to fluoroquinolones and other antimicrobial agents in *Salmonella* isolates from human and animal sources (104). Monitoring the prevalence of fluoroquinolone-resistant infections is important to assess the magnitude of the problem and to guide therapeutic recommendations.

## CHANGES IN THE FOOD INDUSTRY

### Globalization of the Food Supply

As the diversity of foods in the marketplace has increased, illnesses have been associated with commercial internationally distributed foods. In 1992, an outbreak of cholera in Maryland was caused by coconut milk imported from southeast Asia (103). In 1994, outbreaks of *Shigella sonnei* infections in the United Kingdom, Norway, and Sweden were associated with lettuce grown in southern Europe (45). An outbreak of *Salmonella* serotype Agona in Europe, North America, and the Middle East was associated with a children's snack food imported from the Middle East (61). In 1989, four outbreaks of staphylococcal food poisoning in the United States were associated with eating mushrooms canned in the People's Republic of China (65).

### Outbreaks Associated with Fruits and Vegetables

Many consumers have increased their intake of fresh fruits and vegetables in response to health promotion efforts (e.g., the National Cancer Institute recommendation to eat five servings of fruits and vegetables a day) (22). Although fresh produce may be nutritious, as consumption has increased, the number of reported outbreaks associated with these types of foods has also increased. In the United States since 1990, food-borne outbreaks have been associated with sliced melons (*Salmonella* spp.) (80), scallions (*Shigella flexneri*) (38), unpasteurized apple cider

(*E. coli* O157:H7) (17) and apple juice (*E. coli* O157:H7) (36), freshly squeezed orange juice (*Salmonella* serotype Hartford) (39), lettuce (*E. coli* O157:H7) (1, 53), raspberries (*C. cayetanensis*) (52), alfalfa sprouts (*Salmonella* spp. and *E. coli* O157:H7) (68, 30a), and sliced tomatoes (*Salmonella* spp.) (109) (Table 2). The fresh produce consumed during these outbreaks was harvested in the United States as well as Mexico and Central America (Table 2). As demand for produce has increased in the United States more produce is being imported from Mexico and Central America (49). Seasonally, >75% of fresh fruits and vegetables are imported and consumed within days of harvest (49) (Fig. 2). During the winter months from 1989 through 1992, 33 to 70% of cantaloupes, 57 to 72% of green onions, 69 to 79% of cucumbers, and 20 to 64% of tomatoes were harvested in Mexico (49) (Fig. 2). There are many points where produce can become contaminated during growth and harvesting, processing and washing, distribution (usually by truck), and final processing (slicing, shredding, and peeling) (102) (Fig. 3). The surface of plants and fruits may be contaminated by soil, manure, or by feces of animals or agricultural workers. It is unknown whether contamination is more likely to occur when produce is grown outside the United States; however, water quality in other countries may be of particular concern. Use of unclean water supplies can lead to the contamination of produce because water is used to irrigate and wash produce and to make ice used to keep produce cool during trucking. The extra handling required to prepare salads and salad bars and the time delay between preparation and consumption associated with salad bars may increase the potential for produce to cause illness (49). Pathogens on the surface of produce such as melons can be

**Table 2.** Selected fruit- and vegetable-associated outbreaks of food-borne disease in the United States and Canada between 1990 and 1997[a]

| Yr | Pathogen | Vehicle | No. of cases | No. of states or provinces affected | Source(s) |
|----|----------|---------|--------------|-------------------------------------|-----------|
| 1990 | *Salmonella* Chester | Cantaloupe | 245 | 30 | Central America |
| 1990 | *Salmonella* Javiana | Tomatoes | 174 | 4 | United States |
| 1990 | Hepatitis A virus | Strawberries | 18 | 2 | United States |
| 1991 | *Salmonella* Poona | Cantaloupe | >400 | 23 | United States, Central America |
| 1993 | *E. coli* O157:H7 | Apple cider | 23 | 1 | United States |
| 1993 | *Salmonella* Montevideo | Tomatoes | 84 | 3 | United States |
| 1994 | *Shigella flexneri* | Scallions | 72 | 2 | Central America |
| 1995 | *Salmonella* Stanley | Alfalfa sprouts | 242 | 17 | Unknown |
| 1995 | *Salmonella* Hartford | Orange juice | 63 | 21 | United States |
| 1995 | *E. coli* O157:H7 | Leaf lettuce | 70 | 1 | United States |
| 1996 | *E. coli* O157:H7 | Leaf lettuce | 49 | 2 | United States |
| 1996 | *Cyclospora cayetanensis* | Raspberries | 978 | 20 | Central America |
| 1996 | *E. coi* O157:H7 | Apple juice | 70 | 4 | United States |
| 1997 | *S.* Infantis / Anatum | Alfalfa sprouts | 109 | 4 | United States |
| 1997 | *E. coli* O157:H7 | Alfalfa sprouts | 64 | 2 | United States |

[a]Adapted from reference 102 and data from the Division of Bacterial and Mycotic Diseases, National Center for Infectious Diseases, CDC.

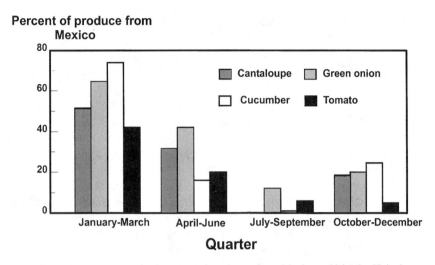

**Figure 2.** Percentage of selected produce items from Mexico sold in the United States, by quarter, 1989 to 1992. Source: reference 49.

transferred to the inner surface of produce during cutting and can then multiply if held at room temperature (80).

### Centralization of the Food Supply

The consolidation of food industries has implications for the epidemiology of food-borne disease. The trend toward increased market size and wider geographic

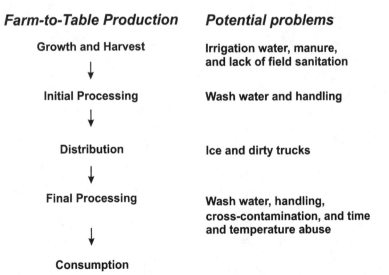

**Figure 3.** Potential sites of contamination during farm-to-table production of produce. Adapted from reference 49.

distribution of products from large centralized food processors carries a risk for larger outbreaks of food-borne disease (21). In 1985, an outbreak of salmonellosis associated with contaminated milk from a large Midwestern dairy resulted in approximately 250,000 illnesses (84). In 1994, a nationwide outbreak of *Salmonella* serotype Enteritidis occurred when ice cream premix was hauled in tanker trucks that had not been thoroughly sanitized after transporting raw liquid egg (50). An estimated 224,000 cases of salmonellosis occurred following consumption of contaminated ice cream. Contamination of mass-produced foods may also cause dispersed outbreaks that are difficult to detect, particularly when the level of contamination of the food item is low. In an outbreak of *E. coli* O27:H20 infections associated with a French soft cheese, illnesses were reported in four nations. In the United States, illnesses were reported in only 5 of 16 (31%) states where the product was distributed (67). The pathogen could not be cultured from most cheese specimens; however, one cheese specimen yielded *E. coli* O27 organisms at a concentration of 10,000 organisms per gram (67).

## CHANGES IN THE POPULATION

### Human Demographics

Demographic changes occurring in industrialized nations have resulted in an increase in the proportion of the population with heightened susceptibility to severe food-borne infections. In the United States, a growing segment of the population has immune impairment as a consequence of infection with human immunodeficiency virus (HIV), age, or underlying chronic disease (37). An estimated 650,000 to 900,000 people in the United States are infected with HIV (59). People with compromised immunity caused by infection with HIV have higher reported rates of salmonellosis, campylobacteriosis, and listeriosis than people not infected with HIV (3, 5). *Salmonella* (and possibly *Campylobacter*) infections are more likely to be severe, recurrent, or persistent (3, 5). Furthermore, extraintestinal disease caused by *Salmonella* and *L. monocytogenes* infection is more likely to be reported among HIV-infected persons than among the general population (3, 5).

The proportion of persons in the United States with age-related susceptibility to food-borne disease has steadily increased as the median age of the population has risen. In 1900 less than 5% of the United States population was older than 65 years of age (24); by 2040, 20% of the population will be older than 65 (25) (Fig. 4). The prevalence of persons with increased susceptibility to food-borne disease because of chronic diseases, such as non-insulin-dependent diabetes, also has increased. The prevalence of diagnosed non-insulin-dependent diabetes in the United States tripled between 1960 and 1993 and has increased eightfold between 1935 and 1993 (60). For every diagnosed case of non-insulin-dependant diabetes, it is estimated that there is one undiagnosed case (60).

Medical technologies including organ transplantation and other tertiary treatments have also extended the life expectancy of persons with chronic diseases. In the 1970s, for example, the 5-year survival rate for Hodgkin's lymphoma was

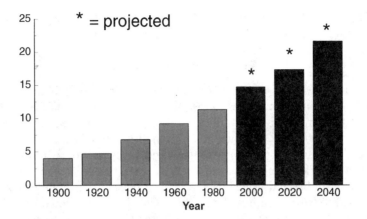

**Figure 4.** Percentage of U.S. population over 65 years of age, from 1900 to 2040. Source: U.S. Bureau of the Census.

approximately 50%; by 1985 the 5-year survival rate approached 80%. The survival rate for all cancers combined also has increased (71a).

### Changes in Behavior

Changes in consumer food-related behaviors can reveal previously unrecognized microbial food-borne hazards. As noted previously, as consumers have increased their consumption of fresh produce the number of recognized outbreaks caused by these products has also increased. Preferences for any raw or lightly cooked food can also place people at increased risk for food-borne illness. Consumption of raw foods of animal origin, including raw oysters (105), unpasteurized milk (110), and ground beef, is particularly hazardous (28). Anecdotes about the health properties of raw foods may interfere with health messages about the risks associated with eating raw foods.

Another change in consumer behavior is shown by the increase in the percentage of spending on food eaten away from home in the United States during recent decades. Fast-food restaurants and salad bars were rare 50 years ago but are primary sites for food in today's society. By the 1990s, outbreaks that occurred outside the household accounted for almost 80% of reported outbreaks in the United States (12). While this may reflect outbreak settings that are most likely to be recognized and thus reported to health officials, other factors common to such food venues may also contribute, such as the pooling of eggs, holding of hazardous foods at temperatures that permit amplification of pathogens, quick and incomplete cooking of foods such as hamburgers, and cross-contamination of cooked foods.

The trend toward eating away from the home may also decrease the opportunity for in-home food safety instruction. These developments have occurred as health educators in secondary schools have emphasized other important health concerns such as substance abuse, HIV infection, and obesity over consumer safety issues including food safety education (88). In a survey of 1,415 United States adults who prepared meals in the home, one third reported that they did not routinely wash hands or cutting boards after handling raw meat or poultry (4).

## Travel and Immigration

International travel has increased dramatically during the 20th century. In 1950, there were 5 million international tourist arrivals worldwide; by 2010, this number is projected to increase to 937 million (75). Travelers can become infected with food-borne pathogens that are uncommon in their nation of residence, and this can complicate diagnosis and treatment when illness occurs after they return home. Occasionally the pathogen is carried home to infect people who did not travel. Cases of cholera (44) and brucellosis (42) have occurred in nontravelers who ate contaminated foods brought into the United States by international travelers. Cholera has also occurred among nontravelers infected by an asymptomatic foodhandler who had recently returned from Central America (2). International travelers visiting developing countries are at particular risk for travelers' diarrhea, which is a catchall term for illnesses associated with a variety of bacterial, viral, and parasitic agents. The primary risk factor is exposure to fecally contaminated food or water. In these countries, both cooked and uncooked foods can be hazardous if handled improperly. Especially risky are tap water, iced beverages, street-vended foods, foods that are not well cooked, or foods held at room temperature for 4 hours or more after cooking (26).

In the mid-1990s, between 500,000 and 1,500,000 legal aliens were admitted to the United States each year (56). This immigration has also contributed to the epidemiology of food-borne disease because some reports of food-borne illnesses involve transmission through foods consumed primarily by immigrant groups (69). Infections caused by *Clonorchis sinensis*, a parasitic flatworm with two intermediate hosts, freshwater snails not indigenous to North America and freshwater fish, are reported almost exclusively in southeast Asian immigrant communities with imported illnesses (96). Outbreaks of trichinosis have become relatively rare in the United States as cooking pork thoroughly has become a widespread cultural practice. An exception occurred in 1990 when Laotian immigrants in Iowa prepared and ate undercooked pork, a traditional food, in celebration of a wedding (94). In some parts of Asia, raw gallbladders of certain animals are consumed in the belief that doing so will improve eyesight and general health; eating raw carp gallbladders has caused acute hepatitis and renal failure in Asian immigrants living in the United States (27). The epidemiology of human brucellosis in California has shifted from an occupational disease of animal husbandry to a food-borne disease most frequently affecting Hispanics who consume raw dairy products, often while abroad (34).

## APPROACHES TO IMPROVED PREVENTION AND CONTROL

### Emerging Pathogens: Surveillance and Public Health Response

The public health infrastructure consists of the personnel (epidemiologists, laboratorians, support staff) and the tools (computers and diagnostic laboratory equipment) necessary to conduct surveillance, investigation, and prevention activities to protect the public's health. Deterioration of the public health infrastructure increases the potential for under-reporting of food-borne infections (16). In the mid-1990s, for example, 12 states had no personnel dedicated to food-borne disease surveillance, largely because of budget restrictions at the state and local levels (16). Surveillance for infectious diseases in this environment may be inadequate. Public health surveillance for food-borne infections in the United States and in other countries is critical to improve prevention. Cooperation between private laboratories, clinicians, and public health agencies is important to diagnose and report infections, characterize isolates, and investigate the source of infections.

Most food-borne disease surveillance is passive. In the United States, CDC maintains national laboratory-based surveillance for *Salmonella*, *Shigella*, *Campylobacter*, and *E. coli* O157:H7, among other pathogens. State and territorial health departments report information on isolates to CDC through an electronic system, the Public Health Laboratory Information System (11). Rapid statistical analysis of this surveillance information can detect unusual clustering of infections by time or geographic area compared with an historical baseline and can lead to early recognition of outbreaks (68). Information from physician-based reporting is also transmitted electronically to CDC and, like laboratory-based surveillance, is used to monitor secular trends in infections due to food-borne pathogens. However, these passive surveillance systems are prone to considerable under-reporting because only a small fraction of ill patients seek medical care, many clinicians do not routinely obtain stool cultures from patients with diarrhea, not all laboratories culture for certain food-borne pathogens, and not all laboratories report isolates to health officials. It has been estimated that for every case of salmonellosis reported to CDC, approximately 20 to 100 cases go unreported (31).

Active surveillance can help to more accurately determine the burden of illness caused by specific food-borne pathogens, increase the timeliness of information, and provide a baseline against which to monitor the effectiveness of control measures. The Foodborne Diseases Active Surveillance Network (FoodNet) was designed to determine more precisely the burden of food-borne illness in the United States through active surveillance and related studies. As the principal food-borne disease component of CDC's Emerging Infections Program (EIP), FoodNet is a collaborative project among CDC, participating EIP sites, the U.S. Department of Agriculture (USDA), and FDA. FoodNet was established in 1995 in five locations: Minnesota, Oregon, and selected counties in Georgia, California, and Connecticut; in 1997, it was expanded to include selected counties in Maryland and New York (6). The total population of these sites, or catchment areas, in January 1998 was 20.3 million people, or 7.7% of the population of the United States.

In addition to more precisely determining the frequency and severity of food-borne diseases that occur in the United States, the objectives of FoodNet are to provide a network for responding to new and emerging bacterial, parasitic, and viral food-borne diseases of national importance, and to identify the source of specific food-borne diseases. By monitoring the burden of food-borne illness over time, FoodNet will help to determine if new food safety initiatives, such as the USDA Pathogen Reduction and Hazard Analysis Critical Control Point (HACCP)

Rule, are effective in decreasing the number of cases of food-borne disease in the United States each year. Information gained through this network will also lead to new interventions and prevention strategies for addressing the public health problem of food-borne diseases (6).

Since January 1996, information has been collected on culture-confirmed cases of *Salmonella, Shigella, Campylobacter, E. coli* O157:H7, *Listeria, Yersinia,* and *Vibrio* infections among residents of the catchment areas; this information is transmitted electronically to CDC. The result is a comprehensive and timely database of food-borne illness in a well-defined population. Data from 1996 surveillance have shown dramatic regional variation in the rates of illnesses caused by various pathogens (Fig. 5). For example, among FoodNet sites there is an increased rate of *Campylobacter* infections in California, an increased rate of *E. coli* O157:H7 infection in Minnesota, and increased rates of *Shigella* infections in California and Georgia (6).

## Improvements in Laboratory Techniques

Molecular typing and subtyping methods are important tools to help detect outbreaks. *Salmonella* serotyping has helped to elucidate the associations between specific serotypes and certain food vehicles, such as serotype Enteritidis and eggs, or serotype Heidelberg and chickens (100). A newer subtyping technique, pulsed-field gel electrophoresis (PFGE), has also been invaluable in food-borne disease surveillance and response (10). PFGE has enhanced surveillance for *E. coli* O157: H7 infections by helping to distinguish sporadic background infections from those that are outbreak related (9, 70) and has helped to link geographically dispersed cases (36) or outbreaks (53). Recently, CDC and selected state public health laboratories have established a computer network to rapidly analyze and compare PFGE patterns of *E. coli* O157:H7 isolates. This network will aid in swift recognition of cases caused by strains with virtually identical DNA fingerprints, sug-

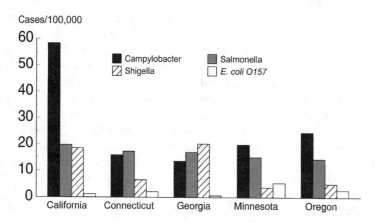

**Figure 5.** Annual incidence (per 100,000 population) of laboratory-confirmed cases of *Campylobacter, Salmonella, Shigella,* and *E. coli* O157:H7 infections, by selected sites, 1996. Source: reference 6.

gesting exposure to a common source and helping to rapidly recognize potential connections among geographically dispersed cases (95).

## Food Production and Handling

The prevention of food-borne disease depends on careful handling of raw products and finished foods. Hazards can be introduced at any point from farm to table. Fortunately, technologies are available to prevent some food-borne diseases. The 20th century's revolution in food sanitation and hygiene was made possible through the application of environmental health technologies. These included refrigeration, chlorination of water, sewage treatment, pasteurization of milk (23), and shellfish monitoring (37a). Once implemented, these technologies successfully reduced sporadic illnesses and outbreaks associated with many food commodities.

New technologies and industrial engineering hold the prospect of improving food safety. Among the most promising technologies are heat treatment of raw and finished ingredients, antibacterial rinses, and pasteurization (33). When technologies are systematically applied to food production to prevent food-borne illnesses, the process is called an HACCP program (33). HACCP programs, originally developed to assure the safety of foods used in the space program, require food industries to identify points in food production where contamination may occur and processes that may pose hazards for the safety of foods. Industry has the lead responsibility for eliminating these potential food-borne hazards, while regulatory agencies monitor each industry's success in eliminating the sources of contamination. Technologies being explored include chlorination of drinking and rinse waters used by food industries, provision of microbiologically safe food and water to food animals, sanitary food animal production, hygienic slaughter, and food irradiation (93). HACCP programs, which focus on preventing food contamination versus conducting endpoint tests to detect contamination after it has occurred, are being implemented by the red meat, poultry, and seafood industries. A risk-based HACCP inspection system allows resources to be targeted toward hazards, emphasizing industry responsibility and governmental oversight for food-borne disease control strategies.

## Food Safety Standards for International Trade

Recent initiatives to reduce international barriers to trade are likely to increase the quantity and diversity of agricultural products crossing national borders. The two major free trade agreements of importance to the United States include the General Agreement on Tariffs and Trade (GATT) and the North American Free Trade Agreement (NAFTA). GATT constitutes a collection of agreements designed to reduce international barriers to trade. Member countries are required to be nondiscriminatory to imports from different foreign countries and to apply the same criteria for imported products as they do for domestic products. Further trade liberalization under GATT has been negotiated in a series of eight "rounds" since 1948. The most recent, in 1994, resulted in the formation of the World Trade Organization (WTO). The WTO agreements supersede but incorporate agreements of GATT and are expected to result in a significant increase in imports worldwide.

Similarly, NAFTA, signed by the United States, Canada, and Mexico, will eventually remove all barriers to trade and could also increase imports to the United States.

The WTO recognizes the sanitary standards and guidelines for food safety developed by the Codex Alimentarius Commission of the Food and Agriculture Organization/World Health Organization as the accepted international standard. The Commission is an intergovernmental body with a membership of 159 governments as of 1 November 1997 (78). It has no authority over member governments to oblige them to accept Codex standards since the standards are only recommendations for use as national food regulations. The Codex Alimentarius (Latin for Food Law or Food Code) currently comprises over 300 standards, guidelines, and other recommendations relating to food quality, composition, and safety (78). The Codex includes standards for most of the principal foods, whether processed, semiprocessed, or raw (78). Associated with these standards are documents such as codes of hygiene and good manufacturing practices (GMPs) and recognized methods of analysis and sampling. The "Principles of food import and export inspection and certification" set out the rules for government-to-government assurances that basic quality requirements, including food safety, are met (78). Governments which accept Codex standards allow free distribution of a product provided that the product meets all relevant requirements of the standard (78).

## Changing Populations

Preparers of meals are the last critical control point before foods reach the table. Interventions to promote safe food preparation practices are needed (58). Food preparers can reduce the risk of food-borne diseases with a few practical food-handling precautions. Thorough heating of potentially hazardous foods will kill pathogens, and refrigeration will prevent their multiplication. Cross-contamination of foods can be avoided by separating cooked and raw foods and preventing contamination of cooked foods by drippings from raw foods. Foodworkers should wash hands, cutting boards, and contaminated surfaces as warranted to prevent cross-contamination. Consumers can reduce the risk of food-borne infections by avoiding high-risk foods, such as runny eggs, hamburgers that are pink at the center, and raw shellfish (106). Education efforts through government, academic, industry, and consumer partnerships should include general food safety information as well as education that is food specific (high-risk foods), site specific (nursing homes and restaurants), and population specific (persons with immune impairment, travelers, etc.).

## CONCLUSIONS

Each link in the production, preparation, and delivery of food can serve as a hazard or an opportunity to prevent that hazard. Food-borne disease surveillance provides a basis for detecting disease and identifying points at which new strategies are needed to protect the food supply. Existing technologies (e.g., pasteurization, chlorination, and refrigeration) and new technologies (e.g., HACCP and food irradiation) are promising methods of food protection. Health education focused on those most at risk for food-borne illnesses may reduce the risk of some food-borne diseases by encouraging consumers to avoid high-risk foods. However, as we approach the 21st century, new and emerging pathogens, changes in food production, and changing populations will continue to affect the safety of our food supply.

## REFERENCES

1. **Ackers, M., B. Mahon, E. Leahy, T. Damrow, L. Hutwagner, T. Barrett, W. Bibb, P. Hayes, P. Griffin, and L. Slutsker.** 1996. An outbreak of *Escherichia coli* O157:H7 infections associated with leaf lettuce consumption, Western Montana, abstr. K43, p. 257. *In Abstracts of the 36th Interscience Conference on Antimicrobial Agents and Chemotherapy.* American Society for Microbiology, Washington, D.C.

2. **Ackers, M., R. Pagaduan, G. Hart, K. D. Greene, S. Abbot, E. D. Mintz, and R. V. Tauxe.** 1997. Cholera and sliced fruit: probable secondary transmission from an asymptomatic carrier in the United States. *Int. J. Infect. Dis.* **1:**212–214.

3. **Altekruse, S. F., F. H. Hyman, K. C. Klontz, B. T. Timbo, and L. K. Tollefson.** 1994. Foodborne bacterial infections in individuals with the human immunodeficiency virus. *South. Med. J.* **87:**169–173.

4. **Altekruse, S. F., D. A. Street, S. B. Fein, and A. S. Levy.** 1996. Consumer knowledge of food-borne microbial hazards and food-handling practices. *J. Food Prot.* **59:**287–294.

5. **Angulo, F. J., and D. L. Swerdlow.** 1995. Bacterial enteric infections in persons infected with human immunodeficiency virus. *Clin. Infect. Dis.* **21**(Suppl. 1):S84–S93.

6. **Angulo, F. J., A. C. Voetsch, D. Vugia, J. L. Hadler, M. Farley, C. Hedberg, P. Cieslak, D. Morse, D. Dwyer, D. L. Swerdlow, and the FoodNet Working Group.** 1998. Determining the burden of human illness from foodborne diseases: CDC's Emerging Infections Program Foodborne Diseases Active Surveillance Network (FoodNet). *Vet. Clin. N. Am.* **14:**165–172.

7. **Archer, D. L., and J. E. Kvenberg.** 1985. Incidence and cost of foodborne diarrheal disease in the United States. *J. Food Prot.* **48:**887–894.

8. **Ashford, R. W.** 1979. Occurrence of an undescribed coccidian in man in Papua New Guinea. *Ann. Trop. Med. Parasitol.* **73:**497–500.

9. **Banatvala, N., A. R. Magnano, M. L. Cartter, T. J. Barrett, W. F. Bibb, L. L. Vasile, P. Mshar, M. A. Lambert-Fair, J. Green, N. H. Bean, and R. V. Tauxe.** 1996. Meat grinders and molecular epidemiology: two supermarket outbreaks of *Escherichia coli* O157:H7 infection. *J. Infect. Dis.* **173:**480–483.

10. **Barrett, T. J., H. Lior, J. H. Green, R. Khakhria, J. G. Wells, B. P. Bell, K. D. Greene, J. Lewis, and P. M. Griffin.** 1994. Laboratory investigation of a multistate food-borne outbreak of *Escherichia coli* O157:H7 by using pulsed-field gel electrophoresis and phage typing. *J. Clin. Microbiol.* **32:**3013–3017.

11. **Bean, N. H., S. M. Martin, and H. Bradford.** 1992. PHLIS: an electronic system for reporting public health data from remote sites. *Am. J. Public Health* **82:**1273–1276.

12. **Bean, N. H., J. S. Goulding, C. Lao, and F. J. Angulo.** 1996. Surveillance for Foodborne Disease Outbreaks—United States, 1988–1992. *In:* CDC Surveillance summaries, October 25, 1996. *Morbid. Mortal. Weekly Rep.* **45**(No. SS-5):1–66.

13. **Bell, B. P., M. Goldoft, P. M. Griffin, M. A. Davis, D. C. Gordon, P. I. Tarr, C. A. Bartelson, J. H. Lewis, T. J. Barrett, J. G. Wells, R. Baron, and J. Kobayashi.** 1994. A multistate outbreak of *Escherichia coli* O157:H7-associated bloody diarrhea and hemolytic uremic syndrome from hamburgers. *JAMA* **272:**1349–1353.

14. **Bell, D.** 1995. Forces that have helped shape the U.S. egg industry: the last 100 years. *Poultry Tribune,* p. 30–43.

15. **Bennett, J. V., S. D. Holmberg, M. F. Rogers, and S. L. Solomon.** 1987. Infectious and parasitic diseases, p. 102–114. *In* R. W. Amler and H. B. Dull (ed.), *Closing the Gap: the Burden of Unnecessary Illness.* Oxford University Press, New York, N.Y.

16. **Berkelman, R. L., R. T. Bryan, M. T. Osterholm, J. W. LeDuc, and J. M. Hughes.** 1994. Infectious disease surveillance: A crumbling foundation. *Science* **264:**368–370.

17. **Besser, R. E., S. M. Lett, T. Weber, M. P. Doyle, T. J. Barrett, J. G. Wells, and P. M. Griffin.** 1993. An outbreak of diarrhea and hemolytic uremic syndrome from *Escherichia coli* O157:H7 in fresh pressed apple cider. *JAMA* **269:**2217–2220.

18. **Besser, T. E., M. Goldoft, and C. C. Gay.** 1996. Emergence of *Salmonella typhimurium* DT 104 in humans and animals in the Pacific Northwest. *In 51st Annual International Conference on Diseases in Nature Communicable to Man Annual.* Washington State Health Department, Seattle.

19. **Black, R. E., and S. Slome.** 1988. *Yersinia enterocolitica. Infect. Dis. Clin. North Amer.* **2:**625–641.

20. **Blake, P. A., M. H. Merson, R. E. Weaver, D. G. Hollis, and P. C. Heublin.** 1979. Disease caused by a marine *Vibrio.* Clinical characteristics and epidemiology. *N. Engl. J. Med.* **300:**1–5.

21. **Blaser, M. J.** 1996. How safe is our food? Lessons from an outbreak of salmonellosis. *N. Engl. J. Med.* **334:**1324–1325.

22. **Bowersox, J.** 1992. Top July stories are "5 a day," new cancer risks. *J. Natl. Cancer Inst.* **84:** 1149–1150.

23. **Bryan, F. L.** 1983. Epidemiology of milk-borne diseases. *J. Food Prot.* **46:**637–649.

24. **Bureau of the Census.** 1993. *Population Projections of the United States, by Age, Sex, Race, and Hispanic origin: 1993–2050.* U.S. Government Printing Office, Washington, DC.

25. **Bureau of the Census.** 1990. *1990 Census of Population. General Population Characteristics.* U.S. Government Printing Office, Washington, DC.

26. **Centers for Disease Control and Prevention.** 1994. *Health Information for International Travel.* U.S. Department of Health and Human Services, Atlanta, Ga.

27. **Centers for Disease Control and Prevention.** 1995. Acute hepatitis and renal failure following ingestion of raw carp gallbladders—Maryland and Pennsylvania, 1991 and 1994. *Morbid. Mortal. Weekly Rep.* **44:**555–556.

28. **Centers for Disease Control and Prevention.** 1995. Outbreak of *Salmonella* serotype Typhimurium infection associated with eating raw ground beef—Wisconsin, 1994. *Morbid. Mortal. Weekly Rep.* **44:**905–909.

29. **Centers for Disease Control and Prevention.** 1996. *Vibrio vulnificus* infections associated with eating raw oysters—Los Angeles. *Morbid. Mortal. Weekly Rep.* **45:**621–624.

30. **Centers for Disease Control and Prevention.** 1997. Multidrug resistant *Salmonella* serotype Typhimurium—United States, 1996. *Morbid. Mortal. Weekly Rep.* 46:308–310.

30a.**Centers for Disease Control and Prevention.** Unpublished data.

31. **Chalker, R. B., and M. J. Blaser.** 1988. A review of human salmonellosis: III. Magnitude of *Salmonella* infection in the United States. *Rev. Infect. Dis.* **10:**111–124.

32. **Chew, K. K.** 1993. Ecologic changes related to declines of oyster stocks in Chesapeake Bay. *Aquac. Mag.* March/April:73–76.

33. **Childers, A. B., and S. L. Rohrer.** 1992. A new food safety strategy for tropical America. *Ann. N.Y. Acad. Sci.* **653:**376–379.

34. **Chomel, B. B., E. E. DeBess, D. M. Mangiamele, K. F. Reilly, T. B. Farver, R. K. Sun, and L. R. Barret.** 1994. Changing trends in the epidemiology of human brucellosis in California from 1973 to 1992: a shift toward foodborne transmission. *J. Infect. Dis.* 170:1216–1223.

35. **Clark, N. C., B. C. Hill, C. M. O'Hara, O. Steingrimsson, and R. C. Cooksey.** 1990. Epidemiologic typing of *Enterobacter sakazakii* in two neonatal nosocomial outbreaks. *Diagn. Microbiol. Infect. Dis.* **13:**467–472.

36. **Cody, S. H., K. Glynn, J. Farrar, L. Cairns, R. Alexander, M. Samadpour, J. Lewis, S. Abbot, R. Bryant, B. Swaminathan, M. Fyfe, R. Hoffman, J. Mohle-Boetani, J. Kobayashi, P. Griffin, and D. Vugia.** 1997. International outbreak of *Escherichia coli* O157:H7 infection associated with unpasteurized commercial apple juice, p. 10. *In Proceedings of the 46th Annual Conference of the Epidemic Intelligence Service.* Centers for Disease Control and Prevention, Atlanta, Ga.

37. **Collins, J. G.** 1993. *Prevalence of Selected Chronic Conditions: United States, 1986–88. Vital Health Stat. Ser. 10* **182:**1–87.

37a. **Committee on Sanitary Control of the Shellfish Industry in the United States.** 1925. Report of the Committee on Sanitary Control of the Shellfish Industry in the United States. *Public Health Reports*, suppl. 53. U.S. Public Health Service, Washington, D.C.

38. **Cook, K. A., T. Boyce, C. Langkop, K. Kuo, M. Swartz, D. Ewert, E. Sowers, J. Wells, and R. Tauxe.** 1995. Scallions and shigellosis: a multistate outbreak traced to imported green onions, p. 36. *In Proceedings of the 44th Annual Conference of the Epidemic Intelligence Service.*

39. **Cook, K. A., D. Swerdlow, T. Dobbs, J. Wells, N. Puhr, G. Hlady, C. Genese, L. Finelli, B. Toth, D. Bodager, and P. Griffin.** 1996. Fresh-squeezed *Salmonella*: An outbreak of *Salmonella hartford* associated with unpasteurized orange juice—Florida, p. 38. *In Proceedings of the 44th Annual Conference of the Epidemic Intelligence Service.* Centers for Disease Control and Prevention, Atlanta, Ga.

40. **Council for Agricultural Science and Technology.** 1994. *Foodborne Pathogens: Risks and Consequences.* Task Force report 122. Council for Agricultural Science and Technology, Ames, Iowa.

41. **Dalton, C. B., C. C. Austin, J. Sobel, P. S. Hayes, W. F. Bibb, L. M. Graves, B. Swaminathan, M. E. Proctor, and P. M. Griffin.** 1997. An outbreak of gastroenteritis and fever due to *Listeria monocytogenes* in milk. *N. Engl. J. Med.* **336:**100–105.

42. **Eckman, M. R.** 1975. Brucellosis linked to Mexican cheese. *JAMA* **232:**636–637.

43. **Endtz, H. P., G. J. Ruijs, B. van Klingeren, W. H. Jansen, T. van der Reyden, and R. P. Mouton.** 1991. Quinolone resistance in *Campylobacter* isolated from man and poultry following the introduction of fluoroquinolones in veterinary medicine. *J. Antimicrob. Chemother.* **27:**199–208.

44. **Finelli, L., D. Swerdlow, K. Mertz, H. Ragazzoni, and K. Spitalny.** 1992. Outbreak of cholera associated with crab brought from an area with epidemic disease. *J. Infect. Dis.* **166:**1433–1436.

45. **Frost, J. A., M. B. McEvoy, C. A. Bentley, Y. Andersson, and B. Rowe.** 1995. An outbreak of *Shigella sonnei* infection associated with consumption of iceberg lettuce. *Emerg. Infect. Dis.* **1:**6–9.

46. **Gellin, B. G., and C. V. Broome.** 1989. Listeriosis. *JAMA* **261:**1313–1320.

47. **Glynn, M. K., P. Dabney, C. Bopp, and F. Angulo.** 1997. Emergence of multiresistant *Salmonella* serotype Typhimurium DT 104 R-type ACSSuT in the United States, p. 14. *In Proceedings of the 44th Annual Conference of the Epidemic Intelligence Service.* Centers for Disease Control and Prevention, Atlanta, Ga.

48. **Griffin, P.M.** 1995. *Escherichia coli* O157:H7 and other enterohemorrhagic *Escherichia coli*, p. 739–761. *In* M. J. Blaser, P. D. Smith, J. I. Ravdin, et al. (ed.), *Infections of the Gastrointestinal Tract.* Raven Press, Ltd., New York, N.Y.

49. **Hedberg, C. W., K. L. MacDonald, and M. T. Osterholm.** 1994. Changing epidemiology of food-borne disease: a Minnesota perspective. *Clin. Infect. Dis.* **18:**671–682.

50. **Hennessy, T. W., C. W. Hedberg, L. Slutsker, K. E. White, J. M. Besser-Wiek, M. E. Moen, J. Feldman, W. W. Coleman, L. M. Edmonson, K. L. MacDonald, and M. T. Osterholm.** 1996. A national outbreak of *Salmonella enteritidis* infections from ice cream. *N. Engl. J. Med.* **334:**1281–1286.

51. **Henzler, D. J., and H. M. Opitz.** 1992. The role of mice in the epizootiology of *Salmonella enteritidis* infection on chicken layer farms. *Avian Dis.* **36:**625–631.

52. **Herwaldt, B. L., M. L. Ackers, and the *Cyclospora* Working Group.** 1997. An outbreak in 1996 of cyclosporiasis associated with imported raspberries. *N. Engl. J. Med.* **336:**1548–1556.

53. **Hilborn, E. D., J. Mermin, P. Mshar, L. Slutsker, R. Mshar, J. Farrar, M. Vance, M. Lambert-Fair, T. Furgalack, D. Vugia, and J. Hadler.** 1997. A multistate outbreak of *Escherichia coli* O157:H7 infections associated with mesclun mix lettuce, p. 33. *In Proceedings of the 46th Annual Conference of the Epidemic Intelligence Service.* Centers for Disease Control and Prevention, Atlanta, Ga.

54. **Hlady, W. G., and K. C. Klontz.** 1996. The epidemiology of *Vibrio* infections in Florida, 1981–1993. *J. Infect. Dis.* **173:**1176–1183.

55. **Huang, P., J. T. Weber, D. M. Sosin, P. M. Griffin, E. G. Long, J. J. Murphy, F. Kocka, C. Peters, and C. Kallick.** 1995. The first reported outbreak of diarrheal illness associated with *Cyclospora* in the United States. *Ann. Intern. Med.* **123:**409–414.

56. **Immigration and Naturalization Service.** 1995. *Legal Immigrations, 1990–1995.* Department of Justice, Washington, D.C.

57. **Kapperud, G., E. Skjerve, K. Hauge, A. Lysaker, I. Aalmen, S. M. Ostroff, and M. Potter.** 1993. Epidemiological investigation of risk factors for *Campylobacter* colonization in Norwegian broiler flocks. *Epidemiol. Infect.* **111:**45–55.

58. **Kapperud, G., P. A. Jenum, B. Stray-Pedersen, K. K. Melby, A. Eskild, and J. Eng.** 1996. Risk factors for *Toxoplasma gondii* infection in pregnancy. *Am. J. Epidemiol.* **144:**405–412.

59. **Karon, J. M., P. S. Rosenberg, G. McQuillan, M. Khare, M. Gwinn, and L. R. Petersen.** 1996. Prevalence of HIV infection in the United States, 1984 to 1992. *JAMA* **276:**126–131.

60. **Kenny, S. J., R. E. Aubert, and L. S. Geiss.** 1995. Prevalence and incidence of non-insulin dependant diabetes, p. 47–67. *In* M. I. Harris, P. H. Bennett, E. J. Boyko, et al. (ed.), *Diabetes in America.* 2nd ed. National Institutes of Health, Bethesda, Md.

61. **Killalea, D., L. R. Ward, D. Roberts, J. de Louvois, F. Sufi, J. M. Stuart, P.G. Wall, M. Susman, M. Schweiger, P. J. Sanderson, I. S. T. Fisher, P. S. Mead, O. N. Gill, C. L. R. Bartlett, and B. Rowe.** 1996. An outbreak of *Salmonella agona* infection in England and the United States caused by contamination of a ready-to-eat savoury snack. *Br. Med. J.* **313:**1105–1107.

62. **Lee, L. A., N. D. Puhr, E. K. Maloney, N. H. Bean, and R. V. Tauxe.** 1994. Increase in antimicrobial-resistant *Salmonella* infections in the United States, 1989–1990. *J. Infect. Dis.* **170:**18–34.

63. **Levine, W. C., J. F. Smart, D. L. Archer, N. H. Bean, and R. V. Tauxe.** 1991. Foodborne disease outbreaks in nursing homes, 1975 through 1987. *JAMA* **266:**2106–2109.

64. **Levine, W. C., J. W. Buehler, N. H. Bean, and R. V. Tauxe.** 1991. Epidemiology of nontyphoidal *Salmonella* bacteremia during the human immunodeficiency virus epidemic. *J. Infect. Dis.* **164:**81–87.

65. **Levine, W. C., R. W. Bennet, Y. Choi, K. J. Henning, J. R. Rager, K. A. Hendricks, D. P. Hopkins, R. A. Gunn, and P. M. Griffin.** 1996. Staphylococcal food poisoning caused by imported canned mushrooms. *J. Infect. Dis.* **173:**1263–1267.

66. **Liu, T. S., G. H. Snoeyenbos, and V. L. Carlson.** 1969. Thermal resistance of *Salmonella senftenberg* 775W in dry animal feeds. *Avian Dis.* **13:**611–631.

67. **MacDonald, K. L., M. Eidson, C. Strohmeyer, M. E. Levy, J. G. Wells, N. D. Puhr, K. Wachsmuth, N. T. Hargrett, and M. L. Cohen.** 1985. A multistate outbreak of gastrointestinal illness caused by enterotoxigenic *Escherichia coli* in imported semisoft cheese. *J. Infect. Dis.* **151:**716–720.

68. **Mahon, B. E., A. Pönkä, W. N. Hall, K. Komatsu, S. E. Dietrich, A. Siitonen, G. Cage, M. A. Lambert-Fair, N. H. Bean, P. M. Griffin, and L. Slutsker.** 1995. An international outbreak of Salmonella infections caused by alfalfa sprouts grown from contaminated seeds. *J. Infect. Dis.* **175:**876–882.

69. **Mead, P. S., and E. D. Mintz.** 1995. Ethnic eating: foodborne disease in the global village. *Infect. Dis. Clin. Pract.* **5:**319–323.

70. **Mead, P. S., L. Finelli, M. A. Lambert-Fair, D. Champ, J. Townes, L. Hutwagner, T. J. Barrett, K. Spitalny, and E. D. Mintz.** 1997. Risk factors for sporadic infection with *Escherichia coli* O157:H7. *Arch. Intern. Med.* **157:**204–208.

71. **Miller, L. G., and C. W. Kaspar.** 1994. *Escherichia coli* O157:H7 acid tolerance and survival in apple cider. *J. Food Prot.* **57:**460–464.

71a.**Miller, B. A., L. A. G. Ries, B. F. Hankey, et al. (ed.).** 1993. SEER Cancer Statistics Review 1973–1990. National Cancer Institute, Bethesda, Md.

72. **Mishu, B., A. A. Ilyas, C. L. Koski, F. Vriesendorp, S. D. Cook, F. A. Mithen, and M. J. Blaser.** 1993. Serologic evidence of previous *Campylobacter jejuni* infection in patients with the Guillain-Barré syndrome. *Ann. Intern. Med.* **118:**947–953.

73. **Mishu, B., J. Koehler, L. A. Lee, D. Rodrigue, F. H. Brenner, P. Blake, and R. V. Tauxe.** 1994. Outbreaks of *Salmonella enteritidis* infections in the United States, 1985–1991. *J. Infect. Dis.* **169:**547–552.

74. **National Marine Fisheries Service.** 1995. *Monthly Oyster Landings by Region.* National Oceanic and Atmospheric Administration, Silver Spring, Md.

75. **Paci, E.** 1995. Exploring new tourism marketing opportunities around the world. *In Proceedings of the Eleventh General Assembly of the World Tourism Organization.* Cairo, Egypt.
76. **Passaro, D. J., R. Reporter, L. Mascola, L. Kilman, G. Malcolm, H. Rolka, S. B. Werner, and D. J. Vugia.** 1996. Epidemic illness caused by *Salmonella enteritidis* infection in Los Angeles County: the predominance of phage type 4. *West. J. Med.* **165:**126–130.
77. **Pearson, A. D., M. Greenwood, T. D. Healing, D. Rollins, M. Shahamat, J. Donaldson, D. M. Jones, and R. R. Colwell.** 1993. Colonization of broiler chickens by waterborne *Campylobacter jejuni. Appl. Environ. Microbiol.* **59:**987–996.
78. **Randell, A. W., and A. J. Whitehead.** 1997. Codex Alimentarius: food safety standards for international trade. *Rev. Sci. Tech. Off. Int. Epizoot.* **16:**313–321.
79. **Relman, D. A., T. M. Schmidt, A. Gajadhar, M. Sogin, J. Cross, K. Yoder, O. Sethabutr, and P. Echevarria.** 1996. Molecular phylogenetic analysis of *Cyclospora*, the human intestinal pathogen, suggests that it is closely related to *Eimeria* species. *J. Infect. Dis.* **173:**440–445.
80. **Ries, A. A., S. Zaza, C. Langkop, R. V. Tauxe, and P. A. Blake.** 1990. A multistate outbreak of *Salmonella chester* linked to imported cantaloupe, abstr. 915, p. 238. *In Abstracts of the 30th Interscience Conference on Antimicrobial Agents and Chemotherapy.* American Society for Microbiology. Washington, DC.
81. **Riley, L. W, R. S. Remis, S. D. Helgerson, H. B. McGee, J. B. Wells, B. R. Davis, R. J. Hebert, E. S. Olcott, L. M. Johnson, N. T. Hargrett, P. A. Blake, and M. L. Cohen.** 1983. Hemorrhagic colitis associated with a rare *Escherichia coli* serotype. *N. Engl. J. Med.* **308:**681–685.
82. **Rodrigue, D. C., R. V. Tauxe, and B. Rowe.** 1990. International increase in *Salmonella enteritidis*: a new pandemic? *Epidemiol. Infect.* **105:**1–7.
83. **Rodrigue, D. C., D. N. Cameron, N. D. Puhr, F. W. Brenner, M. St Louis, I. K. Wachsmuth, and R. V. Tauxe.** 1992. Comparison of plasmid profiles, phage types, and antimicrobial resistance patterns of *Salmonella enteritidis. J. Clin. Microbiol.* **30:**854–857.
84. **Ryan, C. A., M. K. Nickels, N. T. Hargrett-Bean, M. E. Potter, T. Endo, L. Mayer, C. W. Langkop, C. Gibson, R. C. McDonald, R. T. Kenny, N. D. Puhr, P. J. McDonnell, R. J. Martin, M. L. Cohen, and P. A. Blake.** 1987. Massive outbreak of antimicrobial-resistant salmonellosis traced to pasteurized milk. *JAMA* **58:**3269–3274.
85. **Schlech, W. F.** 1997. *Listeria* gastroenteritis—old syndrome, new pathogen. *N. Engl. J. Med.* **336:**1302.
86. **Schuchat, A., B. Swaminathan, and C. V. Broome.** 1991. Epidemiology of human listeriosis. *Clin. Microbiol. Rev.* **4:**169–183.
87. **Siegler, R. L., A. T. Pavia, R. D. Christofferson, and M. K. Milligan.** 1994. A 20-year population based study of postdiarrheal hemolytic uremic syndrome in Utah. *Pediatrics* **94:**35–40.
88. **Small, M. L., L. Kann, B. C. Pateman, R. S. Gold, and L. J. Koble.** 1995. School health education. *J. School Health* **65:**30–311.
89. **Snoeyenbos, G. H., C. F. Smyzer, and H. Van Roekel.** 1969. *Salmonella* infections of the ovary and peritoneum of chickens. *Avian Dis.* **13:**668–670.
90. **Soave, R.** 1996. *Cyclospora:* an overview. *Clin. Infect. Dis.* **23:**429–437.
91. **Sobel, J., A. Hirshfeld, K. Mctigue, C. Nichols, C. Burnette, S. Mottice, F. Brenner, G. Malcolm, and D. L. Swerdlow.** 1996. *Salmonella* Enteritidis phage type 4 pandemic reaches Utah, abstr. LB27, p. 12. *In Program Addendum, Abstracts of the 36th Interscience Conference on Antimicrobial Agents and Chemotherapy.* American Society for Microbiology. Washington, DC.
92. **St. Louis, M. E., D. L. Morse, M. E. Potter, T. M. DeMelfi, J. J. Guzewich, R. V. Tauxe, and P. A. Blake.** 1988. The emergence of grade A shell eggs as a major source of *Salmonella enteritidis* infections: new implications for the control of salmonellosis. *JAMA* **259:**2103–2107.
93. **Steele, J. H., and R. E. Engel.** 1992. Radiation processing of foods. *J. Am. Vet. Med. Assoc.* **201:**1522–1529.
94. **Stehr-Green, J. K., and P. M. Schantz.** 1986. Trichinosis in Southeast Asian refugees in the United States. *Am. J. Public Health* **76:**1238–1239.
95. **Stephenson, J.** 1997. New approaches for detecting and curtailing foodborne microbial infections. *JAMA* **277:**1337–1340.
96. **Sun, T.** 1980. Clonorchiasis: a report of four cases and discussion of unusual manifestations. *Am. J. Trop. Med. Hyg.* **29:**1223–1227.

97. **Swerdlow, D. L., L. A. Lee, R. V. Tauxe, N. H. Bean, and J. Q. Jarvis.** 1990. Reactive arthropathy following a multistate outbreak of *Salmonella typhimurium* infections, abstr. 916, p. 239. *In Abstracts of the 30th Interscience Conference on Antimicrobial Agents and Chemotherapy.* American Society for Microbiology. Washington, D.C.

98. **Tappero, J. W., A. Schuchat, K. A. Deaver, L. Mascola, and J. D. Wenger.** 1995. Reduction in the incidence of human listeriosis in the United States. Effectiveness of prevention efforts? *JAMA* **273:**1118–1122.

99. **Tauxe, R. V., S. D. Holmberg, and M. L. Cohen.** 1989. The epidemiology of gene transfer in the environment, p. 377–403. *In* S. B. Levy and R. V. Miller (ed.), *Gene Transfer in the Environment.* McGraw-Hill, New York, N.Y.

100. **Tauxe, R. V.** 1991. *Salmonella:* a postmodern pathogen. *J. Food Prot.* **54:**563–568.

101. **Tauxe, R. V.** 1992. Epidemiology of *Campylobacter jejuni* infections in the United States and other industrialized nations, p. 9–20. *In* I. Nachamkin, S. Tompkins, M. Blaser (ed.) *Campylobacter jejuni: Current Status and Future Trends.* American Society for Microbiology. Washington, D.C.

102. **Tauxe, R. V.** 1997. Emerging foodborne diseases: an evolving public health challenge. *Emerg. Infect. Dis.* **3:**425–434.

103. **Taylor, J. L., J. Tuttle, T. Pramukul, K. O'Brien, T. J. Barrett, B. Jolbitado, Y. L. Lim, D. Vugia, J. G. Morris, Jr., and R. V. Tauxe.** 1993. An outbreak of cholera in Maryland associated with imported commercial coconut milk. *J. Infect. Dis.* **167:**1330–1335.

104. **Tollefson, L.** 1996. FDA reveals plans for antimicrobial susceptibility monitoring. *J. Am. Vet. Med. Assoc.* **208:**459–460.

105. **Tuttle, J., S. Kellerman, and R. V. Tauxe.** 1994. The risks of raw shellfish: what every transplant patient should know. *J. Transplant. Coord.* **4:**60–63.

106. **U.S. Food and Drug Administration.** 1995. *Food Code: Recommendations of the United States Public Health Service.* National Technical Information Service, Springfield, Va.

107. **Wall, P. G., D. Morgan, K. Lamden, M. Ryan, M. Griffin, E. J. Threlfall, L. R. Ward, and B. Rowe.** 1994. A case control study of infection with an epidemic strain of multiresistant *Salmonella typhimurium* DT 104 in England and Wales. *Commun. Dis. Rep.* **4:**R130–135.

108. **Wall, P. G., D. Ross, P. Van Somern, L. R. Ward, J. Threlfall, and B. Rowe.** 1997. Features of the epidemiology of multidrug resistant *Salmonella typhimurium* DT 104 in England and Wales, p. 565–567. *In Proceedings of Salmonella and Salmonellosis '97.*

109. **Wood, R. C., C. Hedberg, K. White, K. MacDonald, and M. Osterholm.** 1991. A multi-state outbreak of *Salmonella javiana* infections associated with raw tomatoes, p. 69. *In Proceedings of the 40th Annual Conference of the Epidemic Intelligence Service.* Centers for Disease Control and Prevention, Atlanta, Ga.

110. **Wood, R. C., K. L. Macdonald, and M. T. Osterholm.** 1992. *Campylobacter* enteritis outbreaks associated with drinking raw milk during youth activities. A 10-year review of outbreaks in the United States. *JAMA* **268:**3228–3230.

111. **World Health Organization.** 1995. *Report of the WHO Surveillance Programme for Control of Foodborne Infections and Intoxications in Europe: Sixth Report, 1990–1992.* Federal Institute for Health Protection of Consumers and Veterinary Medicine, FAO/WHO Collaborating Centre for Research and Training in Food Hygiene and Zoonoses, Berlin, Germany.

*Emerging Infections 2*
Edited by W. M. Scheld, W. A. Craig, and J. M. Hughes
© 1998 ASM Press, Washington, D.C.

*Chapter 16*

# From Prions to Parasites: Issues and Concerns in Blood Safety

*Rima F. Khabbaz and Mary Chamberland*

In the United States each year, approximately 4 million persons receive blood transfusions from about 12 million donations collected from volunteer blood donors. In addition, another 12 million units of plasma are collected by plasmapheresis from paid donors. Some of the plasma recovered from whole blood units is used as fresh frozen plasma and the rest, as is pheresed plasma, is fractionated to manufacture plasma-derived products, such as immunoglobulin (Ig) preparations, clotting factors concentrates, and albumin.

Over the last decade, numerous efforts have been directed at decreasing the risk of transmission of infectious agents through transfusion. Multiple approaches have been successfully combined to achieve a safe blood supply. The current risk of the major transfusion-transmitted viral infections is very low: the observed incidence of human immunodeficiency virus (HIV), hepatitis B virus (HBV), and hepatitis C virus (HCV) infections from transfusion is so low that mathematical modeling has been used to estimate the risk of acquiring these infections by transfusion. In general, the residual risk for viral transmission can be due to preseroconversion "window period" donations, immunologically variant viruses, nonseroconverting chronic carriers, or screening test errors. The residual risk of transmission of HIV and HBV by screened blood is almost exclusively due to "window period" donations (i.e., donations from recently infected donors who have not developed detectable markers of infection) (Table 1) (11, 46, and 66). The larger residual risk of HCV transmission is due to a longer window period, relatively less sensitive screening tests, and the existence of nonserocoverting immunosilent chronic carriers (Table 1) (4, 66). Third-version anti-HCV tests will likely lower the risk of HCV transmission by transfusion (33).

Since blood is a biologic product, it is a natural vehicle for transmission of infectious agents, and until an artificial blood substitute is developed, the risk of transfusion-transmitted infections will probably never be zero. However, progress

*Rima F. Khabbaz and Mary Chamberland* • Division of Viral and Rickettsial Diseases, National Center for Infectious Diseases, Centers for Disease Control and Prevention, Atlanta, Georgia 30333.

**Table 1.** Estimated risk and window period of infectivity for transmission of HIV, HBV, and HCV through transfusion

| Virus | Risk per unit donated | Window period (days) |
|-------|----------------------|---------------------|
| HIV-1 | 1:450,000 (66) to 1:660,000 (46) | 16[a] |
| HBV | 1:63,000 (66) to 1:500,000 (4) | 59 |
| HCV | 1:10,000 (4) to 1:103,000 (66) | 82 |

[a]Median time to presence of detectable p24 antigen.

in donor selection, donor screening by serologic testing and other markers of infection, the development and use of viral inactivation procedures for plasma-derived products, and changes in transfusion practices have brought us ever closer to this goal. Blood donors today are routinely interviewed to exclude persons with a history of exposures or behaviors that increase their risk of harboring transmissible agents. Improved ascertainment of risk behaviors is being sought through more extensive questioning of donors (19, 82). All blood donations are routinely screened for syphilis, HBV, HCV, human T-cell lymphotropic virus type 1 (HTLV-I), HIV type 1 (HIV-1), and HIV-2, and selected donations are additionally screened for cytomegalovirus.

In recent years, blood safety has been the focus of increased attention (41, 80). Blood safety issues have been numerous and varied and have encompassed a wide range of microorganisms and concerns. This chapter will review select topics to illustrate recent challenges in this area, including those posed by emerging infections that may be transmissible by blood.

## REDUCING THE RISK OF HIV, HBV, AND HCV TRANSMISSION

Since 1992, the use of recombinant protein-based enzyme immunosorbent assays (EIAs) for HIV-1 and HIV-2 to screen donated blood has reduced the infectious window period (i.e., the time from infection to development of detectable HIV antibodies) to 25 days (12), resulting in an estimated risk of one transmission per 450,000 to 660,000 screened units of blood (46, 66). To further reduce this risk, HIV-1 p24 antigen screening of all blood and plasma donations was instituted in March 1996. HIV-1 p24 antigen detects infection about 6 days before antibodies develop (12). It was therefore estimated that four to six infectious donations, not captured by the serologic screening, might be detected annually. In the first year of p24 antigen screening, one antigen positive/antibody negative donation was detected, and a second one was identified shortly thereafter (70).

Recent advances in nucleic acid amplification technologies, including PCR, offer superior approaches (e.g., nucleic acid screening of donors) for further decreasing the residual risks of virus transmission. PCR testing can further reduce the window period of HIV-1 to an estimated 11 days (12), the HBV window period to 25 days (42), and the HCV window period to 59 days (3). Another advantage of nucleic acid testing is the detection of seronegative, immunosilent, infected persons. Both HBV and HCV seronegative, PCR-positive carriers have been found in studies of blood donors in Germany (79). The application of highly sensitive nucleic acid amplification to screen large numbers of single donor units in the high volume blood bank setting will be challenging and require complete automation as well as improvements in sample processing and validation of methodologies to retain high sensitivity and avoid potential contamination and error problems. Several manufacturers are addressing this challenge and developing combination (multiplex) viral RNA/DNA detection systems. It is expected that licensure and implementation of these assays might take at least 3 to 5 years (11).

Nucleic acid screening assays are unlikely to replace serologic screening assays, as the serologic assays have an excellent overall track record and because of the desire to retain multiple layers of safety. In Europe, PCR testing of pools of plasma used in manufacturing plasma-derived products has been adopted as an additional measure to reduce the viral load in the starting material, before it is subjected to viral inactivation steps. Because of the complexities of current nucleic acid amplification technology for single unit testing, strategies involving testing of pooled samples have been proposed as an initial step. Testing of PCR pools will require the selection and validation of the optimal pool size to be used. The U.S. Food and Drug Administration (FDA) has indicated that the testing of pools of a manageable number of donors will be viewed as donor screening and that identification and notification of donors with positive results will be required. Using seroconverting plasma donor panels, the American Red Cross and the National Genetics Institute have recently evaluated the sensitivity of PCR testing of pools of 500 donor samples. A median window period reduction of 1.6 to 2.8 days over the window period achieved by serologic screening and HIV p24 antigen testing was noted for HIV-1, and a median window period reduction of 20 days was seen for HCV (71). Testing of pools of a variable number of donor samples is also being undertaken to assess and validate workable algorithms and matrices and to address technical questions of stability, sensitivity, and specificity (25).

## THE CHALLENGE OF VARIANT STRAINS OF HIV

HIV strains are classified into different groups based on nucleic acid sequence analysis. HIV-1 and HIV-2 are at the extreme of this diversity (40). Most circulating HIV strains around the world belong to "major" (group M) HIV-1 subtypes. Group M is composed of 10 distinct subtypes, designated A through J. HIV-1 subtype B is the predominant subtype in the United States (Figure 1). Screening EIAs for HIV-1 use immunodominant regions of the B subtype. These assays are also highly sensitive for HIV-1 subtypes A to H (40). HIV-2, which is endemic in many countries in West Africa, has been transmitted by transfusion of blood and blood products in Europe (59). Epidemiologic and donor testing data indicate that the prevalence of HIV-2 among blood donors in the United States is very low. Nevertheless, because of the potential for transmission by blood and blood products and the availability of licensed combination HIV-1/HIV-2 EIAs, the FDA recommended in June 1992 that blood and plasma donors be screened for antibodies to HIV-2. No cases of transfusion-acquired HIV-2 infection have been reported in the United States, and only three HIV-2 seropositive units have been found among whole-blood and plasma donors (72).

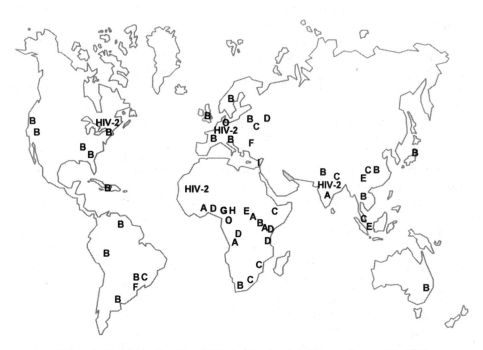

**Figure 1.** Worldwide diversity of HIV isolates (reprinted from reference 40). HIV-1 group M subtypes A through I are represented on the map by letters A through I, and group O is represented by the letter O. The map is not an exhaustive list of all reported subtypes, nor does it include isolated reports or recently imported cases.

An "outlier" group of HIV-1 strains, known as group O HIV-1 strains, has been identified and characterized. The number of group O infections reported worldwide is small, and most have occurred among persons in West and Central African countries (40). HIV-1 group O infections are inconsistently detected by current EIAs for antibodies to HIV-1 (62). To date, studies of blood donors in the United States have not found any evidence of infection with HIV-1 group O (17). Recently, the first two HIV-1 group O infections among persons in the United States were reported; both persons were originally from Africa and neither was a blood donor (17, 74). Efforts are under way to modify existing HIV EIAs to improve detection of group O strains without compromising sensitivity for the group M viruses. As an interim measure, in December 1996 the FDA recommended that donors at increased risk for HIV-1 group O infection (e.g., residence in areas where group O strains are endemic) be deferred from donating blood or plasma.

## TRANSMISSION OF HCV FROM AN IVIg PREPARATION

Intravenous Ig (IVIg) preparations made by cold ethanol fractionation of large plasma pools have been safely used in the United States since the early 1980s to provide antibody replacement for persons with immunodeficiency disorders and for the treatment of persons with immune-mediated diseases. The first and only outbreak of HCV infection associated with contaminated IVIg was reported in the United States in 1994 (16). Infection was associated with lots of Gammagard (Baxter Healthcare Corporation, Deerfield, Ill.), produced from plasma screened by second-version anti-HCV assays. The implicated lots of IVIg were positive for HCV RNA. The most likely explanation for this outbreak was that the second-version tests may have removed most of the complexing antibodies from plasma used to make IVIg, resulting in more HCV in the Ig fraction than in the non-Ig fraction. In addition, manufacture of this particular product did not include a viral inactivation step as a further measure for product safety. As a result of this investigation, the FDA has been working with manufacturers to add one or more viral inactivation/removal procedures in the production of all Ig products. Although this step has been accomplished for IV-administered products, similar procedures are still being finalized for incorporation into the manufacture of intramuscularly administered Ig products. As an interim measure, the FDA has required all nonvirally inactivated Ig products to be screened with PCR tests for HCV RNA; only those products that test negative are released for distribution. Of note, intramuscular Ig has never been associated with the transmission of any infectious disease in the United States. The transmission of HCV from an IVIg product emphasizes the need for vigilance and demonstrates how changes in manufacturing processes, including those in which new steps are introduced specifically to reduce the potential of viral transmission, may inadvertently result in increased transmission.

## THE CHALLENGE OF NONENVELOPED VIRUSES

Plasma-derived products, such as Ig preparations, clotting factor concentrates, and albumin, are made from large pools of plasma. In addition to donor screening and testing, the safety of these products also derives from viral inactivation procedures, such as heat or solvent-detergent treatment (54). Currently used viral inactivation procedures have virtually eliminated transmission of HIV, HBV, and HCV. However, these procedures do not effectively inactivate nonenveloped viruses, such as parvovirus B19 (B19) and hepatitis A virus (HAV) that lack a lipid envelope and are consequently relatively heat stable.

B19 was discovered in the mid-1970s in the sera of healthy blood donors being screened for HBV surface antigen (20). B19 infection is fairly ubiquitous among humans, with reported seroprevalence rates of 29 to 79% among adult blood donors. The virus is primarily transmitted from person to person, presumably through direct contact with respiratory secretions. In the normal host, B19 causes a self-limited infection, often asymptomatic or associated with a mild rash illness in children (i.e., erythema infectiosum) or a self-limited arthropathy, most commonly in women. More severe and chronic clinical manifestations have been described in immunocompromised patients, such as patients with HIV disease or leukemia, and self-limited but potentially severe aplastic crises occur in patients with sickle cell disease and other preexisting anemias (51, 78). Fetal infections can result in nonimmune fetal hydrops and fetal death (49). Estimates of B19 viremia in blood donors have ranged from 0 to 2.6 per 10,000 (78). Transmission from single-donor blood is believed to be rare and nonconsequential for most recipients. However, a high percentage of pooled plasma products contains B19 DNA and poses a risk of transmitting the virus. The seroprevalence of B19 is higher among hemophilia patients than among age-matched controls (83). The clinical significance of B19 among hemophilia patients has not been determined (61).

Cases of posttransfusion HAV infection have been reported but are infrequent (32). HAV infection is characteristically acute and self-limited, and blood donor selection procedures exclude persons with prodromal symptoms. However, as for many other viral infections, viral particles may be present in the blood before symptoms develop and result in the occasional transmission of HAV by blood transfusion. The deferral of donors who report a history of close contact with a patient with viral hepatitis likely limits this occurrence. Clusters of HAV infections transmitted from factor concentrates have occurred among patients with hemophilia in Europe in the early 1990s (55) and in South Africa (43), and more recently in the United States (69). Vaccination of chronic recipients of products made from pooled plasma with the recently licensed hepatitis A vaccine has been recommended (16).

The transmission of B19 and HAV by virally inactivated products raises a concern about unknown and emerging infections that may have properties similar to these viruses and be able to survive in these products. Novel improved viral inactivation procedures are needed to prevent transfusion-associated transmission of these nonenveloped viruses.

## THE CHALLENGE OF NEWLY DISCOVERED VIRUSES

Hepatitis G virus (HGV) and human herpesvirus 8 (HHV-8) are two newly discovered viruses that pose very different challenges to blood safety. HGV, a flavivirus, is fairly prevalent among blood donors; 1 to 2% of healthy blood donors have evidence of infection (1). Despite its name, HGV has not been shown to cause either acute or chronic liver disease (5). However, multiple lines of evidence suggest that HGV is a blood-borne viral infection. First, elevated prevalence rates of HGV RNA have been reported in populations with increased exposure to blood and blood products, including IV drug users, patients who require hemodialysis, and persons with hemophilia (2). Second, acute HGV infection has been temporally associated with transfusion receipt among persons known to be HGV RNA negative before transfusion (1). Third, in the small number of instances in which all donors of blood products provided to transfusion recipients with acute HGV infection could be evaluated, at least one HGV-infected donor was identified (1). These same studies, however, were unable to document convincingly that HGV was associated with the development of disease (i.e., frank hepatitis). Until more information is learned about the pathogenicity of HGV and a serologic assay is developed, the need and ability to screen blood and plasma donors remain unresolved (2).

HHV-8, also known as Kaposi's sarcoma-associated virus, is a newly discovered herpesvirus that has been associated with both HIV- and non-HIV-related Kaposi's sarcoma. Until very recently, the lack of standardized testing procedures of proven sensitivity to detect antibodies to the virus has limited study of this new virus.

Nonetheless, because HHV-8 is found in peripheral blood mononuclear cells (PBMCs), there has been speculation and concern that transfusion of blood, particularly cellular components, might result in transmission of this virus. However, seroprevalence surveys among various population groups suggest that HHV-8 is more likely sexually transmitted, rather than blood-borne. In general, seroprevalence rates for HHV-8 among persons (both HIV-seropositive and HIV-seronegative) with exposure to blood and blood products have been comparable to those for healthy, HIV-seronegative individuals (30, 44, 48).

More direct evidence regarding the transmissibility of HHV-8 through blood and blood products will require follow-up of recipients from known infected donors. Operskalski et al. evaluated the HIV- and HHV-8-infected donors of blood products given to 14 transfusion recipients (13 of whom received cellular components and one who received fresh frozen plasma); 10 of the 14 recipients became infected with HIV, but none tested positive for HHV-8 (60). Blackbourn et al. recently reported finding infectious (demonstrated by reverse-transcription-PCR) HHV-8 from the blood of a healthy U.S. blood donor; follow-up evaluation of this donor's previous recipients has been initiated (8). Although initial seroprevalence and donor-recipient pairs studies are reassuring, further evaluation is needed.

## THE CHALLENGE OF PRIONS: CJD

Creutzfeldt-Jakob disease (CJD) is a rare, invariably fatal degenerative disease believed to be caused by an unconventional, disinfection-resistant infectious agent (22). The likely causative agent is a prion, which is a conformationally altered form of a normal plasma membrane protein. Iatrogenic CJD has occurred after corneal transplantation, through contaminated electroencephalograph (EEG) electrodes and neurosurgical instruments, and in recipients of human pituitary-derived growth hormone and dura mater grafts. The CJD agent has been reported occasionally in the blood of CJD patients at low titers, and inoculation of PBMCs and some derivatives of plasma from CJD patients into rodent brains has resulted in CJD-like lesions (26, 56, 75, 76). These studies have raised concerns regarding the transmissibility of the agent of CJD by blood. However, to date there have been no confirmed reports of CJD resulting from receipt of blood or blood products. Epidemiologic case-control studies have shown no increase in the frequency of transfusions among CJD patients compared with controls (21, 28, 45, 50). National mortality data for CJD in the United States show a relatively stable annual rate of about 1 case per million (38). Thus, despite regular blood donation by persons who subsequently develop CJD, blood transfusions do not appear to be amplifying CJD in this population. National mortality data also show no reports of CJD in patients with hematologic conditions, such as sickle cell disease and thalassemia, that require frequent transfusion (Table 2). The epidemiologic data therefore suggest that the risk of CJD, if any, from transfusion must be very small. An ongoing search for CJD in hemophilia patients who have received products from a large number of donors over their lifetimes has failed, to date, to find any CJD case in this population (29). Studies of recipients of blood from donors who subsequently developed CJD have similarly not detected CJD (35, 73).

**Table 2.** CJD deaths and death rates by age group in the United States, 1979 to 1994[a]

| Age group (yr) | No. of deaths | Death rate per million persons | No. with hemophilia A, hemophilia B, thalassemia, or sickle-cell disease |
|---|---|---|---|
| 0–44 | 80 | 0.03 | 0 |
| 45–59 | 652 | 1.15 | 0 |
| ≥60 | 2,910 | 4.58 | 0 |

[a]Modified from reference 38.

Nevertheless, concerns for this theoretical risk have led to policies in the United States to defer donors at increased risk of CJD, such as donors with a family history of CJD, recipients of human pituitary-derived growth hormone, and recipients of dura mater grafts. Concomitant with deferral of these donors, remaining products from their previous donations as well as previous donations from CJD-diagnosed donors are recalled, and recipients of these products are notified of the recall. These policies pose difficulties and threaten the availability of life-saving products; other suggested approaches to decrease the theoretical risk of CJD, such as deferring older donors, may also possibly negatively impact blood safety (13).

## BACTERIAL CONTAMINATION

The incidence and range of adverse clinical outcomes from bacterial contamination of blood have been poorly characterized (68, 81). From 1986 through 1991, the FDA received reports of 182 transfusion-associated fatalities, of which 29 (16%) were caused by bacterial contamination of blood products (18, 39). However, the incidence of both fatal and nonfatal bacterium-associated transfusion-related complications is likely underestimated (18, 81). Recently, the U.S. General Accounting Office estimated that the rate of bacterium-associated adverse reactions from random donor platelet pools was 0.6 per 1000 pooled units (80).

Platelets are stored in agitated oxygen-permeable containers at room temperature for a maximum of 5 days before infusion (81). These conditions will sustain rapid growth of a variety of aerobic organisms, including *Staphylococcus* spp. and (less commonly) gram-negative rods. In one study, Morrow et al. prospectively recorded adverse clinical events during a 42-month period among oncology patients who received platelet transfusions (58). They found that transfusion-associated bacterial sepsis occurred overall in 1 of 4,200 platelet transfusions; however, the incidence of transfusion-associated sepsis was higher for transfusions of multidonor, pooled platelet transfusions compared with transfusions of single-donor, apheresis platelets. In this same study, Morrow also observed that sepsis rates increased with length of storage. Febrile reactions temporally associated with platelet transfusion in this study were not uncommon, ranging from 5% of recipients of multidonor transfusions to nearly 2% of recipients of single-donor transfusions. Although fevers are often ascribed to an immune response to transfused white blood cells, it is likely that some proportion represents undetected bacteremia.

Transfusion of red blood cells has been associated with bacterial sepsis, most often due to *Yersinia enterocolitica*, which grows readily in refrigerated blood. From November 1985 through November 1996, the Centers for Disease Control and Prevention (CDC) received 21 reports of sepsis, including 12 deaths, associated with transfusion of red blood cells contaminated with *Y. enterocolitica* (18). Similar to that reported for platelet-related bacteremia, the risk for sepsis increases with duration of storage of red blood cells, and most episodes are associated with erythrocytes stored for ≥25 days (68, 81). The risk for red blood cell-associated sepsis has been estimated to be one per 500,000 units transfused (23); similarly, Au-Buchon has estimated that 1 of every 1,000,000 units may be associated with endotoxin-induced septic shock caused by gram-negative bacteria (6).

Bacterial contamination can occur at one or more points in the collection, processing, pooling, and transfusion of blood. Various approaches have been suggested to reduce the possibility of contamination, including screening prospective donors for recent gastrointestinal illness that may be indicative of infection with *Y. enterocolitica* (77) and reducing the time that blood components can be stored before transfusion (68); however, such proposals have been countered with concerns that their implementation would eliminate significant numbers of healthy donors or uncontaminated units (69). Bacteriologic monitoring of units by Gram staining or culturing techniques has been reported to lack adequate sensitivity, specificity, feasibility, timeliness, and predictive value for clinically significant complications (7, 58, 81). More promising approaches under development include chemiluminescence-linked nucleic acid probes, PCR, and radiometric techniques (81).

Because rates of bacteria-associated transfusion reactions in the United States are unknown, CDC, in collaboration with national blood collection organizations, has initiated a prospective study to determine the rates of bacteria-associated transfusion reactions from whole blood, red blood cells, and platelets (18). This study will establish standardized definitions and systematic procedures for the recognition, reporting, and clinical, epidemiologic, and laboratory evaluation of adverse transfusion reactions in recipients of contaminated blood or blood components.

## TRANSFUSION-RELATED PARASITIC DISEASE CONCERNS

Several parasitic agents have recently caused concern for blood safety. Hundreds of cases of babesiosis have been reported in the United States, mostly from the Northeast. Of these, fewer than 25 cases of transfusion-associated babesiosis, mostly caused by *Babesia microti* but also by the more recently recognized WA1-type *Babesia* parasite, have been reported (31, 36, 57). The parasite survives blood banking conditions and is transmissible by transfusion of red blood cells and platelet concentrates (27). With the expansion of deer populations in the northeastern United States, concerns exist that the incidence of transfusion-transmitted babesiosis may increase (63). The tick vector and animal reservoir of the *Babesia* more recently found in the northwestern United States remain to be identified. Current strategies for prevention of transfusion-transmitted *Babesia* rely on questioning donors for history of babesiosis and on performing a hematocrit determination at

the time of donation. Babesiosis classically manifests as a febrile illness with hemolytic anemia, but infection can also cause chronic asymptomatic or mildly symptomatic parasitemia. The risk for severe disease is higher in the elderly, asplenic,
and immunocompromised patient.

Chagas' disease, a vector-borne disease caused by the parasite *Trypanosoma
cruzi*, is endemic in parts of Central and South America and Mexico. The most
common mode of acquisition is by contact with the feces of reduvid bugs. If
untreated, Chagas' disease can result in lifelong, asymptomatic parasitemia; infected individuals can in turn transmit the disease through transfusion. Receipt of
blood transfusions is the most common means of transmission in some areas of
endemicity (65). The immigration of thousands of persons from areas where *T.
cruzi* is endemic and increased international travel have raised concerns about the
increased potential for transfusion-transmitted Chagas' disease in North America
(68). It has been estimated that at least 100,000 persons with chronic *T. cruzi*
infection reside in the United States (65). To date, there have been three reported
cases of Chagas' disease from transfusions in the United States and one in Canada;
all four patients were immunocompromised and developed acute, symptomatic disease that facilitated their recognition (65, 68). The American Red Cross has
conducted limited look-back studies of recipients of blood and blood products that
were seropositive for *T. cruzi* and found no evidence of transmission, suggesting
that the transmission rate in the United States may be no higher than 10% (47, 80).
More recent studies conducted among donor populations that included persons
more likely to have been born in or traveled to countries where the disease is
endemic have found approximately 0.1% of donors to be seropositive for antibodies
to *T. cruzi* (9, 47, 67, 80). Extrapolating from these studies, Dodd has estimated
that the overall risk for *T. cruzi* infection is 1 in 42,000 per unit of donated blood
in the United States (80).

Visceral leishmaniasis, caused by organisms in the *Leishmania donovani* species
complex, can be associated with parasitemia and therefore with the potential for
transmission by blood transfusion. Transmission of leishmaniasis by blood transfusion has been reported only in rare instances (fewer than 15 cases worldwide),
and no case of any type of leishmaniasis acquired by blood transfusion has been
reported in the United States (37). Concern about the potential for transmission of
leishmanias through blood transfusion occurred when a previously undescribed type
of leishmaniasis was found to affect a small number of persons who had been
deployed to the Persian Gulf as part of Operation Desert Storm (52). To date, the
Department of Defense has parasitologically confirmed 12 cases of this unusual
type of visceral leishmaniasis, called viscerotropic leishmaniasis, among the almost
700,000 deployed personnel (52, 53). Viscerotropic leishmaniasis is unusual in that
it is caused by a parasite (*Leishmania tropica*) that typically causes cutaneous
leishmaniasis, but in this instance the parasite invades the internal organs of the
body. Parasitic confirmation is difficult and requires an invasive procedure, such as
bone marrow or lymph node aspiration, and infected persons have generally had
low levels of the parasites. In November 1991, as a precautionary measure, the
U.S. Department of Defense and the American Association of Blood Banks recommended that all persons who had traveled to the Persian Gulf after 1 August

1990, be deferred as blood donors. The ban was lifted in 1993, and no additional cases of viscerotropic leishmaniasis were identified during the nearly 14 months of the ban (34).

## CONCLUSIONS

As this chapter illustrates, a variety of issues and challenges that include a wide range of microorganisms have emerged in the blood safety arena in the 1990s. Despite the variety and complexity of some of these issues, it is fair to say that in the context of other health-related risks, the risks of acquiring infectious diseases from blood transfusion are quite small. In fact, the U.S. blood supply in the 1990s is among the safest in the world and is safer today than at any time in history (8). The same approaches that have contributed to improved blood safety, including donor selection, testing, viral inactivation procedures, improved transfusion practices, and surveillance, are expected to continue to play a major role in dealing with these challenges and other potential threats to blood safety. Further reduction in the risk of transfusion-associated infections through these approaches is possible. However, as new potential threats are considered and as new and improved technologies become available, a balance will need to be reached between concerns for safety and availability of needed life-saving products. While technologic advances offer the possibility of further reduction in the residual risk of many transfusion-associated infections through improved testing or microbial inactivation steps, careful consideration of costs and benefits of additional procedures will be necessary to prevent a negative impact on supply. In addition, changes in procedures and practices, including the introduction of improved tests, might inadvertently result in new unanticipated risks. Careful monitoring of transfusion-associated infections through surveillance is key to protecting the blood supply from known pathogens and to monitoring for the emergence of new infectious agents.

The approaches to dealing with emerging infections include the need to assess the risk of transmission of emerging agents and to develop and evaluate effective prevention strategies when needed, including diagnostic tests for screening, deferral policies, and improved viral inactivation procedures. Education of physicians and transfusion recipients regarding the benefits and risks associated with receipt of blood and blood products is an important adjunct to prevention efforts so that informed decisions can be made.

## REFERENCES

1. **Alter, H. J., Y. Nakatsuji, J. Melpolder, J. Wages, R. Wesley, J. W. Shih, and J. P. Kim.** 1997. The incidence of transfusion-associated hepatitis G virus infection and its relation to liver disease. *N. Engl. J. Med.* **336:**747–754.
2. **Alter, H. J.** 1997. G-pers creepers, where'd you get those papers? A reassessment of the literature on the hepatitis G virus. *Transfusion* **37:**569–572. (Editorial).
3. **Alter, H. J.** 1995. To C or not to C: these are the questions. *Blood* **85:**1681–1695.
4. **Alter, M. J.** 1995. Residual risk of transfusion-associated hepatitis, p. 23. *In Programs and Abstracts of the NIH Consensus Development Conference on Infectious Disease Testing for Blood Transfusions.* National Institutes of Health, Bethesda, Md.

5. **Alter, M. J., M. Gallagher, T. T. Morris, L. A. Moyer, E. L. Meeks, K. Krawczynski, J. P. Kim, and H. S. Margolis.** 1997. Acute non-A-E hepatitis in the United States and the role of hepatitis G virus infection. *N. Engl. J. Med.* **336:**741–746.

6. **AuBuchon, J. P.** 1997. Blood transfusion options: improving outcomes and reducing costs. *Arch. Pathol. Lab. Med.* **121:**40–47.

7. **Barrett, B. B., J. W. Andersen, and K. C. Anderson.** 1993. Strategies for the avoidance of bacterial contamination of blood components. *Transfusion* **33:**228–233.

8. **Blackbourn, D. J., J. Ambroziak, E. Lennette, M. Adams, B. Ramachandran, and J. A. Levy.** 1997. Infectious human herpesvirus 8 in a healthy North American blood donor. *Lancet* **349:**609–611.

9. **Brashear, R. J., M. A. Winkler, J. D. Schur, H. Lee, J. D. Burczak, H. J. Hall, and A. A. Pan.** 1995. Detection of antibodies to *Trypanosoma cruzi* among blood donors in the southwestern and western United States. I. Evaluation of the sensitivity and specificity of an enzyme immunoassay for detecting antibodies to *T. cruzi*. *Transfusion* **35:**213–218.

10. **Bresee, J. S., E. E. Mast, P. J. Coleman, M. J. Baron, L. B. Schonberger, M. J. Alter, M. M Jonas, M. Y. Yu, P. M. Renzi, and L. C. Schneider.** 1996. Hepatitis C virus infection associated with administration of intravenous immune globulin: a cohort study. *JAMA* **276:**1563–1567.

11. **Busch, M. P., S. L. Stramer, and S. H. Kleinman.** 1997. Evolving applications of nucleic acid amplification assays for prevention of virus transmission by blood components and derviaties, p. 123–176. *In* G. Garratty (ed.), *Application of Molecular Biology to Blood Transfusion Medicine.* American Association of Blood Banks, Bethesda, Md.

12. **Busch, M. P., L. L. L. Lee, G. A. Satten, D. R. Henrard, H. Farzadegan, K. E. Nelson, S. Read, R. Y. Dodd, and L. R. Petersen.** 1995. Time course of detection of viral and serologic markers preceding human immunodeficiency virus type 1 seroconversion: implications for screening of blood and tissue donors. *Transfusion* **35:**91–97.

13. **Busch, M. P., S. A. Glynn, and G. B. Schreiber.** 1997. Potential increased risk of virus transmission due to exclusion of older donors because of concern over Creutzfeldt-Jakob disease. *Transfusion* **37:**996–1002.

14. **Centers for Disease Control.** 1990. Human T-lymphotropic virus type I screening in volunteer blood donors—United States, 1989. *Morb. Mortal. Weekly Rep.* **39:**915.

15. **Centers for Disease Control.** 1991. Public Health Service inter-agency guidelines for screening donors of blood, plasma, organs, tissues, and semen for evidence of hepatitis B and hepatitis C. *Morbid. Mortal. Weekly Rep.* **40(RR-4):**1–17.

16. **Centers for Disease Control and Prevention.** 1996. Prevention of hepatitis A through active or passive immunization: Recommendations of the Advisory Committee on Immunization Practices. *Morbid. Mortal. Weekly Rep.* **45(RR-15):**1–30.

17. **Centers for Disease Control and Prevention.** 1996. Identification of HIV-1 group O infection—Los Angeles County, California. *Morbid. Mortal. Weekly Rep.* **45:**561–565.

18. **Centers for Disease Control and Prevention.** 1997. Red blood cell transfusions contaminated with *Yersinia enterocolitica*—United States, 1991–1996, and initiation of a national study to detect bacteria-associated transfusion reactions. *Morbid. Mortal. Weekly Rep.* **46:**553–555.

19. **Conry-Cantelina, C., J. C. Melpolder, and H. J. Alter.** 1997. Intranasal drug use among volunteer whole blood donors: results of a survey. *Transfusion* **37(9S):**99S. (Abstract.)

20. **Cossart, Y. E., A. M. Field, B. Cant, and D. Widdows.** 1975. Parvovirus-like particles in human sera. *Lancet* **i:**72–73.

21. **Davanipour, Z., M. Alter, E. Sobel, D. M. Asher, and D. C. Gajdusek.** 1985. A case-control study of Creutzfeldt-Jakob disease. Dietary risk factors. *Am. J. Epidemiol.* **122:**443–451.

22. **DeArmond, S. J., and S. P. Prusiner.** 1995. Etiology and pathogenesis of prion diseases. *Am. J. Pathol.* **146:**785–811.

23. **Dodd, R. Y.** 1994. Adverse consequences of blood transfusion: quantitative risk estimates. p. 1. *In* S. T. Nance (ed.), *Blood Supply Risks, Perceptions and Prospects for the Future.* American Association of Blood Banks, Bethesda, Md.

24. **Dodd, R. Y.** 1995. Scaling the heights. *Transfusion* **35:**186–188. (Editorial.)

25. **Dodd, R. H., G. D. Griffin, A. Conrad, R. I. F. Smith, P. L. Page, and S. L. Stramer.** 1997. Pilot study to determine the feasibility of PCR testing of pooled donor samples for HBV, HCV, HAV and parvovirus B19. *Transfusion* **37**(9S):1S. (Abstract).

26. **Dreslys, J. P., C. Lasmezas, and D. Dormont.** 1994. Selection of specific strains in iatrogenic Creutzfeldt-Jakob disease. *Lancet* **343**:848–849.

27. **Eberhard, M. L., E. M. Walker, and F. J. Steurer.** 1995. Survival and infectivity of *Babesia* in blood maintained at 25°C and 2-4°C. *J. Parasitol.* **81**:790–792.

28. **Esmonde, T. F., R. G. Will, J. M. Slattery, R. Knight, R. Harries-Jones, R. de Silva, and W. B. Matthews.** 1993. Creutzfeldt-Jakob disease and blood transfusion. *Lancet* **341**:205–207.

29. **Evatt, B.** Unpublished data.

30. **Gao, S. J., L. Kingsley, M. Li, W. Zheng, C. Parravicini, J. Ziegler, R. Newton, C. R. Rinaldo, A. Saah, J. Phair, R. Detels, Y. Chang, and P. S. Moore.** 1996. KSHV antibodies among Americans, Italians and Ugandans with and without Kaposi's sarcoma. *Nat. Med.* **2**:925–928.

31. **Gerber, M. A., E. D. Shapiro, P. J. Krause, R. G. Cable, S. J. Badon, and R. W. Ryan.** 1994. The risk of acquiring Lyme disease or babesiosis from a blood transfusion. *J. Infect. Dis.* **170**:231–234.

32. **Giacoia, G. P., and D. O. Kasprisin.** 1989. Transfusion-acquired hepatitis A. *South. Med. J.* **82**:1357–1360.

33. **Gretch, D.** 1997. Diagnostic tests for hepatitis C, p. 45. *In Program and Abstracts of NIH Consensus Development Conference on Management of Hepatitis C.* National Institutes of Health, Bethesda, Md.

34. **Gunby, P.** 1993. Desert Storm veterans now may donate blood; others call for discussion of donor tests. *JAMA* **269**:451–452.

35. **Heye, N., S. Hensen, and N. Muller.** 1994. Creutzfeldt-Jakob disease and blood transfusion. *Lancet* **343**:298–299.

36. **Herwaldt, B. L., A. M. Kjemtrup, P. A. Conrad, R. C. Barnes, M. Wilson, M. G. McCarthy, M. H. Sayers, and M. L. Eberhard.** 1997. Transfusion-transmitted babesiosis in Washington State: first reported case caused by a WA1-type parasite. *J. Infect. Dis.* **175**:1259–1262.

37. **Herwaldt, B. L.** Unpublished data.

38. **Holman, R. C., A. S. Khan, E. D. Belay, and L. B. Schonberger.** 1996. Creutzfeldt-Jakob disease in the United States, 1979–1994: using national mortality data to assess the possible occurrence of variant cases. *Emerg. Infect. Dis.* **2**:333–337.

39. **Hoppe, P. A.** 1992. Interim measures for detection of bacterially contaminated red cell components. *Transfusion* **32**:199–201. (Editorial).

40. **Hu, D. J., T. O. Dondero, M. A. Rayfield, J. R. George, G. Schocketman, H. W. Jaffe, E. C. Luo, M. L. Kalish, B. G. Weniger, C. P. Pau, C. A. Schable, and J. W. Curran.** 1996. The emerging genetic diversity of HIV: the importance of global surveillance for diagnostics, research, and prevention. *JAMA* **275**:210–216.

41. **Institute of Medicine.** 1995. HIV and the blood supply: an analysis of crisis decision making. National Academy Press, Washington, D.C.

42. **Jagodzinski, L., F. Kraus, and P. Garrett.** 1994. Detection of hepatitis B viral sequences in early HBV infection. *Transfusion* **34**(S):37S.

43. **Kedda, M. A., M. C. Kew, R. J. Cohn, S. P. Field, R. Schwyzer, E. Song, and F. Fernandes-Costa.** 1995. An outbreak of hepatitis A among South African patients with hemophilia: evidence implicating contaminated factor VIII concentrate as the source. *Hepatology* **22**:1363–1367.

44. **Kedes, D. H., E. Operskalski, M. Busch, R. Kohn, J. Flood, and D. Ganem.** 1996. The seroepidemiology of human herpesvirus 8 (Kaposi's sarcoma-associated herpesvirus): distribution of infection in KS risk groups and evidence for sexual transmission. *Nature Med* **2**:918–924.

45. **Kondo, K., and Y. Kuroiwa.** 1982. A case control study of Creutzfeldt-Jakob disease: association with physical injuries. *Ann. Neurol.* **11**:377–381.

46. **Lackritz, E. M., G. A. Satten, J. Aberle-Grasse, R. Y. Dodd, V. P. Raimondi, R. S. Janssen, W. F. Lewis, E. P. Notari IV, and L. R. Petersen.** 1995. Estimated risk of transmission of the human immunodeficiency virus by screened blood in the United States. *N. Engl. J. Med.* **333**:1721–1725.

308     Khabbaz and Chamberland

47. **Leiby, D. A., E. J. Read, B. A. Lenes, A. J. Yund, R. J. Stumpf, L. V. Kirchhoff, and R. Y. Dodd.** 1997. Seroepidemiology of *Trypanosoma cruzi*, etiologic agent of Chagas' disease, in U.S. blood donors. *J. Infect. Dis.* **176:**1047–1052.
48. **Lennette, E., D. J. Blackbourn, and J. A. Levy.** 1996. Antibodies to human herpesvirus type 8 in the general population and in Kaposi's sarcoma patients. *Lancet* **348:**858–861.
49. **Levy, R., A. Weissman, G. Blomberg, and Z. J. Hagay.** 1997. Infection by parvovirus B19 during pregnancy: a review. *Obstet. Gynecol. Surv.* **52:**254–259.
50. **Little, B. W., J. Mastrianni, A. L. DeHaven, et al.** 1993. The epidemiology of Creutzfeldt-Jakob disease in eastern Pennsylvania. *Neurology* **43:**A316. (Abstract).
51. **Luban, N. L. C.** 1994. Human parvoviruses: implications for transfusion medicine. *Transfusion* **34:** 821–827.
52. **Magill, A. J., M. Grogl, R. A. Gasser Jr, W. Sun, and C. N. Oster.** 1993. Visceral infection caused by *Leishmania tropica* in veterans of Operation Desert Storm. *N. Engl. J. Med.* **328:**1383–1387.
53. **Magill, A. J., M. Grogl, S. C. Johnson, and R. A. Grasser.** 1994. Visceral infection due to *Leishmania tropica* in veterans of Operation Desert Storm who presented 2 years after leaving Saudi Arabia. *Clin. Infect. Dis.* **19:**805–806.
54. **Mannucci, P. M.** 1993. Clinical evaluation of viral safety of coagulation factor VIII and IX concentrates. *Vox Sang.* **64:**197–203.
55. **Mannucci, P. M., S. Gdovin, A. Gringeri, M. Colombo, A. Mele, N. Schinaia, N. Ciavarella, S. U. Emerson, and P. H. Purcell.** 1994. Transmission of hepatitis A to patients with hemophilia by factor VIII concentrates treated with organic solvent and detergent to inactivate viruses. *Ann. Intern. Med.* **120:**1–7.
56. **Manuelides, E. E., J. H. Kim, J. R. Mericangas, and L. Manuelides.** 1985. Transmission to animals of Creutzfeldt-Jakob disease from human blood. *Lancet* **ii:**896–897.
57. **Mintz, E. D., J. F. Anderson, R. G. Cable, and J. L. Hadler.** 1991. Transfusion-transmitted babesiosis: a case report from a new endemic area. *Transfusion* **31:**365–368.
58. **Morrow, J. F., H. G. Braine, T. S. Kickler, P. M. Ness, J. D. Dick, and A. K. Fuller.** 1991. Septic reactions to platelet transfusions: a persistent problem. *JAMA* **266:**555–558.
59. **O'Brien, T. R., J. R. George, and S. D. Holmberg.** 1992. Human immunodeficiency virus type 2 infection in the United States: epidemiology, diagnosis, and public health importance. *JAMA* **267:** 2775–2779.
60. **Operskalski, E. A., M. P. Busch, J. W. Mosley, and D. Kedes.** 1997. Blood donations and viruses. *Lancet* **349:**1327.
61. **Ragni, M. V., W. C. Koch, and J. A. Jordan.** 1996. Parvovirus B19 infection in patients with hemophilia. *Transfusion* **36:**238–241.
62. **Pau, C. P., J. Hud, C. Spruill, C. Schable, E. Lackritz, M. Kai, J. R. George, M. A. Rayfield, T. J. Dondero, A. E. Williams, M. P. Busch, A. E. Brown, F. E. McCutchan and G. Schochetman.** 1996. Surveillance for human immunodeficiency virus type 1 group O infections in the United States. *Transfusion* **36:**398–400.
63. **Popovsky, M. A.** 1991. Transfusion-transmitted babesiosis. *Transfusion* **31:**296–298.
64. **Schable, S., L. Zekeng, P. Chou-Pong, D. Hu, L. Kaptue, L. Gurtler, T. Dondero, J. M. Tsague, G. Schochetman, and H. Jaffe.** 1994. Sensitivity of United States HIV antibody tests for detection of HIV-1 group O infections. *Lancet* **344:**1333–1334.
65. **Schmunis, G. A.** 1991. *Trypanosoma cruzi*, the etiologic agent of Chagas' disease: status in the blood supply in endemic and nonendemic countries. *Transfusion* **31:**547–557.
66. **Schreiber, G. B., M. P. Busch, S. H. Kleinman, and J. J. Korelitz.** 1996. The risk of transfusion-transmitted viral infections. *N. Engl. J. Med.* **334:**1685–1690.
67. **Schulman, I. A., M. D. Appleman, S. Saxena, A. L. Hiti, and L. V. Kirchoff.** 1997. Specific antibodies to *Trypanosoma cruzi* among blood donors in Los Angeles, California. *Transfusion* **37:** 727–731.
68. **Sloand, E. M., E. Pitt, and H. G. Klein.** 1995. Safety of the blood supply. *JAMA* **274:**1368–1373.
69. **Soucie, J. M., B. H. Robertson, and B. P. Bell.** Hepatitis A virus infections associated with clotting factor concentrate in the United States. Submitted for publication.

70. **Stramer, S. L., J. Haberle-Grasse, J. P. Brodsky, M. P. Busch, and E. M. Lackritz.** 1997. US blood donor screening with p24 antigen (Ag); one year experience. *Transfusion* **37**(9S):1S. (Abstract.)

71. **Stramer, S. L., R. A. Porter, J. P. Brodsky, A. Conrad, G. F. Smith, and R. Y. Dodd.** 1997. Sensitivity of HIV and HCV detection by pooled PCR testing. *Transfusion* **37**(9S):98S. (Abstract.)

72. **Sullivan, M., A. Williams, E. Guido, R. Melter, C. Schable, and S. Stramer.** 1997. Detection and characterization of an HIV type 2 antibody positive blood donor in the U.S. *Transfusion* **37**(9S):58S. (Abstract.)

73. **Sullivan, M. T., L. B. Schonberger, D. Kessler, A. E. Williams, and R. Y. Dodd.** 1997. Creutzfeldt-Jakob Disease (CJD) investigational lookback study. *Transfusion* **37**(9S):2S. (Abstract.)

74. **Sullivan, P. S., A. N. Do, K. Robbins, M. Kalish, S. Subbarao, D. Pieniazek, C. Schable, G. Afaq, J. Markowitz, R. Myers, J. M. Joseph, and G. Benjamin.** 1997. Surveillance for variant strains of HIV: Subtype G and group O HIV-1. *JAMA* **278**:292. (Letter.)

75. **Tamai, Y., H. Kojuma, R. Kitajima, M. Kalish, S. Subbarao, D. Pieniazek, C. Schable, G. Afaq, J. Markowitz, R. Myers, J. M. Joseph, and G. Benjamin.** 1992. Demonstration of the transmissible agent in tissue from a pregnant woman with Creutzfeldt-Jakob disease. *N. Engl. J. Med.* **327**:649.

76. **Tateishi, J.** 1985. Transmission of Creutzfeldt-Jakob disease from human blood and urine into mice. *Lancet* **ii**:1074.

77. **Tipple, M. A., L. A. Bland, J. J. Murphy, M. J. Arduino, A. L. Panlilio, J. J. Farmer III, M. A. Tourault, C. R. Macpherson, J. E. Menitove, and A. J. Grindon.** 1990. Sepsis associated with transfusion of red cells contaminated with *Yersinia enterocolitica*. *Transfusion* **30**:207.

78. **Torok, T. J.** 1995. Human parvovirus B19, p. 668–702. *In* J. S. Remington and J. O. Klein (ed.), *Infectious Diseases of the Fetus and Newborn Infant.* W. B. Saunders, Philadelphia, Pa.

79. **Tuma, W., V. Schottstedt, and G. Bunger.** 1997. PCR mini-pool testing of all donations from a large blood bank. *In Program of Cambridge Healthtech Institutes Conference on Blood Safety Screening.* Cambridge Healthtech Institute, Newton Upper Falls, Mass.

80. **U.S. General Accounting Office.** 1997. *Blood Supply: Transfusion-Associated Risks.* Government Printing Office, Washington, D.C.

81. **Wagner, S. J., L. I. Friedman, and R. Y. Dodd.** 1994. Transfusion-associated bacterial sepsis. *Clin. Micro. Rev.* **7**:290–302.

82. **Williams, A. E., R. A. Thomson, G. B. Schreiber, M. J. Arduino, A. L. Panlilio, J. J. Farmer III, M. A. Tourault, C. R. Macpherson, J. E. Menitove, and A. J. Grindon.** 1997. Estimates of infectious disease risk factors in US blood donors. *JAMA* **277**:967–972.

83. **Williams, M. D., B. J. Cohen, A. C. Beddall, K. J. Pasi, P. P. Mortimer, and F. G. Hill.** 1990. Transmission of human parvovirus B19 by coagulation factor concentrates. *Vox Sang.* **58**:177–181.

*Emerging Infections 2*
Edited by W. M. Scheld, W. A. Craig, and J. M. Hughes
© 1998 ASM Press, Washington, D.C.

*Chapter 17*

# CDC's Global Efforts To Address Emerging Diseases

*James W. LeDuc and James M. Hughes*

The 1992 Institute of Medicine (IOM) report *Emerging Infections: Microbial Threats to Health in the United States* was the first comprehensive attempt to crystallize the rising concern among the scientific and public health communities that much of the world, including the United States, had become complacent in the fight against infectious diseases (7). This concern was stimulated in part by the ongoing pandemic of human immunodeficiency virus (HIV) and AIDS but certainly was not limited to this devastating disease. The IOM report posed several challenges to the Centers for Disease Control and Prevention (CDC) as the nation's prevention agency, and CDC responded by developing a strategic plan, released in 1994, entitled *Addressing Emerging Infectious Disease Threats: a Prevention Strategy for the United States* (2). The plan contained four primary goals: (i) to improve surveillance efforts to better detect, promptly investigate, and monitor emerging pathogens, the diseases they cause, and the factors influencing their emergence; (ii) to foster applied research to integrate laboratory science and epidemiology to optimize public health practice; (iii) to strengthen prevention and control through enhanced communication of public health information about emerging diseases and prompt implementation of prevention strategies; (iv) to improve the national infrastructure needed to fulfill these goals by increasing local, state, and federal public health capacity to support surveillance and implement prevention and control programs. These four goals became the pillars of the CDC program in emerging infectious diseases.

## FOUNDATIONS FOR GLOBAL ACTIVITIES

These same four goals were later used as the basis for the United States government interagency plan, *Infectious Disease—a Global Health Threat*, issued in 1995 by the National Science and Technology Council Committee on International

*James W. LeDuc and James M. Hughes* • National Center for Infectious Diseases, Centers for Disease Control and Prevention, Atlanta, GA 30333.

Science, Engineering, and Technology (CISET) Working Group on Emerging and Re-emerging Infectious Diseases (11). The CISET report expands on these fundamental goals and broadens the perspective from national to global. The report calls for all U.S. government agencies involved in health to collaborate in implementing the comprehensive interagency plan. As a result, approximately 30 government agencies, from the Departments of Agriculture, Commerce, Defense, Health and Human Services, State, and others, are working together to implement specific objectives drawn from these four primary goals. Formal endorsement through a Presidential Decision Directive (NSTC-7) has emphasized the critical importance of implementing this strategy (4). The CISET report has become a central document in development of the U.S. global strategy to address emerging infectious diseases.

As the CISET report was being finalized, the World Health Organization crafted these same basic goals into a formal resolution, *Communicable diseases prevention and control: new, emerging and re-emerging infectious diseases* (WHA48.13), which was considered during the 1995 World Health Assembly (21). This and a companion resolution calling for revision and updating of the *International Health Regulation* were well received and fully endorsed by the Assembly, thereby becoming part of the global agenda for health (20). Similar plans containing the same basic goals and objectives have now been endorsed by most of the World Health Organization (WHO) regional offices and many of the member nations (12).

Most recently, during the Denver summit of eight leaders from the highly industrialized nations, discussions included specific mention of the growing threat of emerging infectious diseases and led to endorsement of the same four fundamental goals defined in the CDC, CISET, and WHO plans, with special emphasis on enhancing the global capacity for disease surveillance and response and for coordination of outbreak investigations.

The net result of all these activities is that a solid foundation has been laid on a global level that is consistent and clearly focused on CDC's four basic goals (Table 1). This remarkable consensus among global leaders on the need to systematically address the growing threat of infectious diseases provides the basis for a truly coordinated global approach in response to this challenge.

## COLLABORATIONS WITH THE WORLD HEALTH ORGANIZATION

The transition from plan development to implementation has already begun through several specific initiatives. Within CDC, review of the existing capacity of the 31 WHO Collaborating Centers designated within the National Center for In-

**Table 1.** Essential goals common to all plans to address emerging infectious diseases

Improve surveillance to better detect and respond to emerging infectious diseases
Foster applied research activities
Improve prevention and control programs
Build national and international capacity to achieve these goals

fectious Diseases (NCID) is under way to ensure that these centers are adequately prepared to fulfill their terms of reference and provide the services each has agreed upon (Table 2). Over $2 million has been invested to upgrade these centers and to offer them an opportunity to collaborate in addressing common problems with other WHO Collaborating Centers elsewhere in the United States and abroad. An example of such a collaboration is the current work under way by the center for plague, located in the Division of Vector-Borne Infectious Diseases at Fort Collins, Colo., which recently hosted a meeting of the directors of virtually every plague laboratory in the world. These experts discussed recent advances in laboratory techniques and exchanged information on the epidemiological characteristics of plague in their respective countries. The result has been the formation of an important global resource comprised of scientists who are well acquainted, have a greater level of confidence and respect for their colleagues, and are much better prepared to share information, strains, and techniques in the future.

CDC is also assisting WHO by providing seconded staff and some financial support to both the new Division of Emerging and Other Communicable Diseases

**Table 2.** WHO Collaborating Centers located in the NCID

Antimicrobial Resistance
Arthropod-Borne Viruses, Western Hemisphere
*Clostridium botulinum*
Cysticercosis
Dengue and Dengue Hemorrhagic Fever
Research, Training, and Eradication of Dracunculiasis
Foodborne Disease Surveillance
Viral Hemorrhagic Fevers
Reference and Research on Viral Hepatitis
Reference and Research on Human Immunoglobulins Subclasses
HIV/AIDS
Surveillance, Epidemiology and Control of Influenza
Evaluating and Testing New Insecticides
Leptospirosis
Lyme Borreliosis
Control and Elimination of Lymphatic Filariasis
Malaria Control in Africa
Measles Virus Diagnostics
Prevention and Control of Epidemic Meningitis
Mycoses in North America
Reference and Research on Plague Control
Poliovirus and Enterovirus Surveillance
Reference and Research on Rabies
Respiratory Viruses Other than Influenza
Rickettsial Diseases
Rotavirus and the Agents of Viral Gastroenteritis
*Shigella*
Smallpox and Other Poxvirus Infections
Staphylococcal Phage Typing
Reference and Research on Syphilis Serology
*Vibrio cholerae* O1 and O139

Surveillance and Control, which is leading the WHO emerging disease efforts, and to the efforts toward global eradication of polio, among other projects at WHO Headquarters.

## COLLABORATIONS WITH THE PAN AMERICAN HEALTH ORGANIZATION

The CDC is working closely with the Pan American Health Organization (PAHO), the WHO regional office for the Americas, to implement a regional plan to address emerging infectious diseases. CDC has provided support for staff directing this program and has participated in several regional meetings. These included a meeting of the task force on surveillance for emerging and re-emerging infectious diseases held in Toronto, Canada, in November 1996; a workshop to define priorities for institutional strengthening for the diagnosis and epidemiological surveillance of emerging diseases in Goiania, Brazil, in March 1996; and subsequent meetings in Rio de Janeiro and Manaus, Brazil, to further develop regional surveillance strategies (14, 15).

CDC, PAHO, and representatives of several Latin American countries met recently in Manaus, Brazil, to establish an Amazon regional network for surveillance of emerging viral diseases (Fig. 1). Laboratory directors of research and public health facilities from Colombia, Venezuela, Peru, Bolivia, and Brazil agreed to share common laboratory diagnostic reagents and procedures to systematically examine specimens from patients suffering from febrile (dengue-like) illnesses, noncardiogenic adult respiratory distress syndrome, febrile icteric syndrome, and hemorrhagic fevers. If possible, each collaborating laboratory will test 2,000 sera from patients seen in its country over the next 12 months for evidence of infection with specific pathogens (Table 3). Results of this ongoing testing will be informally shared among the participating laboratories; if these preliminary collaborations are successful, the network participants may expand their collaborations to monitoring antibiotic resistance for community-acquired bacterial infections, assessing the resistance patterns of malaria, and exchanging information on other diseases endemic in the region. Network participants may also expand their collaborations to more formally address unexplained deaths and very serious illnesses following a study design similar to one now used in the United States (16).

Plans are likewise under development to establish a second Latin American collaborative network, this one involving the Southern Cone nations of South America. Collaborators will be drawn from Argentina, Chile, Uruguay, Paraguay, Brazil, and Bolivia and will consider regionally important diseases such as hantavirus pulmonary syndrome and influenza. An organizational meeting was held in April 1998 in Buenos Aires, Argentina.

## BILATERAL AND MULTILATERAL AGREEMENTS

Several bilateral and multilateral agreements are now in place that offer excellent opportunities for CDC and other U.S. government agencies dealing in health to collaborate internationally in addressing emerging infectious diseases and to im-

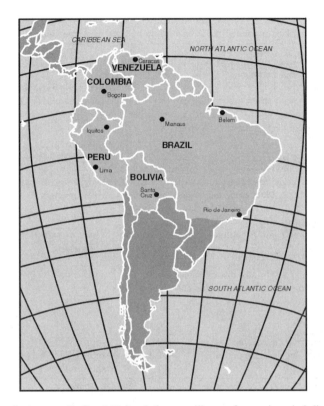

**Figure 1.** Amazon Regional Network for surveillance of emerging viral diseases, showing locations of key collaborating laboratories.

plement the recommendations outlined in the CISET report (Table 4). The United States and European Union (E.U.) are collaborating under the New Trans Atlantic Agenda Task Force on Communicable Diseases. Three working groups have been established: surveillance and response; research and training; and capacity evaluation and building. Each working group is cochaired by representatives from the U.S. and E.U. sides, with the surveillance group led on the U.S. side by CDC, the research group by the National Institutes of Health (NIH), and the capacity strengthening group by the United States Agency for International Development (USAID).

Specific work plans have been developed and are being implemented; for example, under the surveillance and response working group, significant progress is being made in exchanging information on food-borne illnesses using information from the European Enter-net surveillance system and the U.S. FoodNet program (19). Enter-net is a collaborative effort among public health laboratories within the E.U. that provides member countries with information regarding food-borne infections such as those from salmonella or *Escherichia coli*, then shares that information to determine if similar strains have been involved in outbreaks elsewhere. The network was, for example, quite valuable in recognizing a recent international

**Table 3.** Summary of syndromes to be examined and initial and secondary pathogens to be screened by collaborating laboratories of the Amazon Region Emerging Infectious Disease Network

| Initial screen | Secondary screen |
|---|---|
| **Undifferentiated febrile syndrome** | |
| Malaria, dengue (types 1, 2, 3, and 4), Oropouche fever, Mayaro fever, group C arbovirus infections, yellow fever, Venezuelan equine encephalitis, leptospirosis, influenza, Q fever | Ehrlichioses, rickettsioses, parvovirus B-19 infection, measles, rubella, hepatitis A, hepatitis B, hepatitis C |
| **Hemorrhagic fever syndrome** | |
| Dengue, yellow fever, leptospirosis, arenavirus infections (Machupo, Guanarito, and others) | Ehrlichiosis, rickettsioses, hepatitis B, hepatitis C, hantavirus infection |
| **Febrile icteric syndrome** | |
| Leptospirosis, yellow fever, hepatitis A, hepatitis B, hepatitis C | Hepatitis D (only if patient is hepatitis B virus positive), hepatitis E |
| **Adult (noncardiogenic) respiratory distress syndrome** | |
| Influenza, hantavirus infection (hantavirus pulmonary syndrome), legionellosis, Q fever, psittacosis | |
| **Sudden unexpected death syndrome**[a] | |
| Culture, histopathology | Immunohistopathology, nucleic acid probes with PCR, electron microscopy |

[a]Initial screen conducted locally, secondary screen conducted at a reference laboratory.

outbreak of salmonellosis associated with a commercial snack food widely distributed in both Europe and the United States (8, 18).

Representatives from the E.U. and U.S. involved in monitoring food-borne diseases recently met to discuss expanding the network of Enter-net collaborators. Laboratory directors from Latvia, Poland, Hungary, Israel, Japan, Canada, South Africa, Australia, and the Czech Republic were invited to consider participating in an expanded Enter-net. Efforts are also progressing on greater exchange of information on antimicrobial resistance using the same network of collaborators.

The U.S.-Japan Common Agenda has also offered an excellent opportunity to implement emerging infectious diseases activities. NIH has taken the lead for the United States in coordinating the technical aspects of these collaborations, and four specific targets for activity have been defined: dengue and dengue hemorrhagic fever, acute respiratory infections, enterohemorrhagic *E. coli*, and antimicrobial

**Table 4.** Bilateral and multilateral initiatives on emerging infectious diseases involving CDC and international partners, 1998

United States-European Union New Trans-Atlantic Agenda Task Force on Communicable Diseases
United States-Japan Common Agenda
United States-South Africa Binational Commission (Gore-Mbeki Commission)
United States-Russia Binational Commission (Gore-Chernomyrdin Commission)

resistance. Activities are not limited to exchanges between the United States and Japan; they include interactions with public health officials and scientists in many Pacific Rim nations. This was the case in a recent meeting held in Bangkok, Thailand, when public health officials and scientists gathered to discuss each of these four targets for activity. Again, the fundamental approach in addressing these issues has focused on the four basic goals of improving surveillance, conducting applied research, strengthening adequate infrastructure, and improving prevention and control strategies.

Two important bilateral initiatives are under way through the auspices of the office of the Vice President: the Gore-Mbeki Binational Commission with South Africa and the Gore-Chernomyrdin Commission with Russia. Both programs include active efforts to address emerging infectious diseases. In South Africa, special efforts are being made to enhance national surveillance to specifically address the challenges of sexually transmitted diseases, tuberculosis, and viral hemorrhagic fevers.

In Russia, collaborations are under way to address nosocomial infections, sexually transmitted diseases, and viral hemorrhagic fevers; various training activities are included. In addition, the Gore-Chernomyrdin Commission offered an excellent opportunity for CDC collaborations with Russian scientists and health officials to address the recent epidemic of diphtheria. Work with Russian counterparts in the field of tuberculosis was dramatically increased by the significant funding recently announced by the Soros Foundation. CDC is now working with the Russian Ministry of Health, the Public Health Research Institute (selected by the Soros Foundation to implement the tuberculosis (TB) efforts with Russian partners), and USAID to develop demonstration projects in Russia. These projects will include both investment in diagnostic and research laboratories in Moscow and demonstration projects applying the WHO-recommended directly observed therapy, short course, for treatment of patients. Site selection for these demonstration projects is still under way and has included consideration of several oblasts and discussions of addressing the problem of TB within the Russian prison system.

In addition to the collaborations on TB, major efforts are under way within the framework of the Gore-Chernomyrdin Commission by the American International Health Alliance (AIHA), CDC, and the Russian Ministry of Health to address hospital-acquired infections in Russia. AIHA published a basic infection control manual for Russia and the Newly Independent States (NIS) in 1997 and distributed copies to hospital epidemiologists and other health care professionals at a recent workshop in Atlanta. This manual will be used as a teaching tool and as a major everyday resource document by infection control experts in Russia and the NIS. It will be an essential element of existing training plans to help build Russian capacity in hospital infection control. One component of the overall hospital infection control effort is to include specific activities to build individual hospital capacity for routine bacterial culture and susceptibility testing for common nosocomial pathogens. Plans call for this effort to eventually expand to systematic regional and national surveillance for antimicrobial resistance.

CDC is collaborating with the U.S. National Academy of Sciences in a major new effort to assist Russian scientists from the former biological warfare facilities to redirect their resources and skills to peaceful uses. Under this initiative, pilot collaborative projects have been established between scientists from CDC, the United States Army Medical Research Institute of Infectious Diseases, U.S. universities, and scientists from Russian laboratories to work on various emerging diseases and significant health problems in Russia. Current projects include development of an improved diagnostic test for a regionally important liver fluke, genetic analysis of hepatitis C viruses, collaborations on studies of the epidemiology of hemorrhagic fever with renal syndrome in Far Eastern Russia, strain analysis of tuberculosis isolates, and genetic analysis of monkeypox viruses, including isolates from the recent episode of human transmission in central Africa. Each of these projects is well under way, and collectively they demonstrate the potential for meaningful and productive collaborations with Russia to reduce the global threat of biological weapons, including their potential use by terrorists (10).

## OVERSEAS FIELD STATIONS

Permanent field stations are maintained by NCID in Kenya and Guatemala. The Kenyan laboratory is operated as a joint program with the Kenya Medical Research Institute (KEMRI) and the Kenyan Ministry of Health. The laboratory has facilities both in Kisumu in western Kenya and at the KEMRI headquarters in Nairobi. It receives funding from CDC, USAID, and others. The Kisumu field station has been in existence for approximately 25 years and has a long tradition of excellence in research on malaria and other endemic diseases. It has also served as an important training base for Kenyan and foreign scientists. Current activities focus on: (i) an evaluation of permethrin-impregnated bednet efficacy to prevent malaria deaths in children less than 5 years of age; (ii) studies on placental plasmodial infection and its risk of mother-to-infant transmission of HIV type 1; (iii) epidemiologic and immunologic longitudinal study of a cohort of newborn children (the Asembo Bay Cohort Project) to determine acquisition of antibodies to malaria antigens in relation to infection and clinical illness; and (iv) work with the Kenyan Ministry of Health on malaria control activities. Recently, these activities have been expanded to include culture, identification, and determination of antibiotic susceptibility patterns of bacterial pathogens associated with diarrheal illness in western Kenya. The Kisumu malaria field station is also an important collaborating facility in the recently announced Multinational Initiative on Malaria (9). As part of the initiative, the staff of the field station hosted investigators from Africa to discuss malaria during pregnancy, laying the foundation for another specialized collaborative network of investigators addressing a common problem from geographically diverse perspectives.

The Virus Research Center at KEMRI in Nairobi has been a WHO collaborating center for arboviruses and hemorrhagic fever reference and research for many years; however, the past decade has witnessed a decline in the capacity of this important East African resource. In 1995, in response to recognition of yellow fever transmission in Kenya, CDC began a collaboration with KEMRI and WHO to help rebuild the technical capacity of the center by hosting a workshop on yellow fever virus laboratory diagnosis and isolation. Subsequently, CDC provided funding for a virologist to assist the center in building surveillance capacity for yellow fever, as well as other important virus diseases (17). This investment has proven especially valuable, since the laboratory recently played a key central role in addressing the current outbreak of Rift Valley fever which has swept southern Somalia and much of Kenya, killing thousands of domestic livestock and hundreds of humans (22).

The field station in Guatemala is called the Medical Entomology Research and Training Unit. Like the Kenya field station, it is a research unit of the Division of Parasitic Diseases of the National Center for Infectious Diseases. The unit was established in 1978 under a tripartite agreement between the Guatemala Ministry of Health and Social Assistance, the Universidad del Valle de Guatemala, and CDC. Its objectives are to conduct field and laboratory research on important human parasitic diseases prevalent in Central America and to train students and public health professionals in basic and applied public health research. Current activities focus on Chagas' disease, cyclosporiasis, malaria, onchocerciasis, geohelminth infections, and leishmaniasis. The laboratory also serves as the base for a variety of regional public health activities such as epidemiologic surveillance networks regarding emerging infectious diseases. An example of this is the current collaboration on cyclosporiasis involving the Guatemala Ministry of Health and Social Assistance, Ministry of Agriculture, the U.S. Food and Drug Administration, and CDC (6). Because of its geographic information systems capabilities, the laboratory is also designated the regional mapping center for the Onchocerciasis Elimination Program of the Americas, working in conjunction with PAHO and WHO.

CDC maintains a branch of its division of vector-borne infectious diseases in San Juan, Puerto Rico, to specifically address the resurgent problem of dengue and dengue hemorrhagic fever in the Americas and globally (5). Staff collaborates with public health officials throughout the Americas in addressing outbreaks of dengue, monitoring the spread of the four dengue serotypes, recommending strategies for vector control and management of patients, and facilitating in conjunction with PAHO an extensive network of collaborating dengue diagnostic laboratories. The laboratory actively assists in the conduct of periodic proficiency testing for the laboratory network and is a source of reference reagents and technical training. Staff also assists local municipalities in outbreak response and in design and management of active surveillance systems to monitor dengue transmission.

CDC is also increasing collaborations with a number of other countries worldwide. In Vietnam, serious discussions are under way to identify opportunities to enhance existing collaborations. At present, several Vietnamese scientists have visited CDC for extensive training in bacteriology and virology and have now returned to their own laboratories to put into place the technical skills acquired. A WHO-organized collaborative efficacy study of locally produced oral inactivated cholera vaccine is now under way in Viet Nam involving collaborations between the Vietnamese Ministry of Health, CDC, and NIH. In addition, investigators are beginning to work together to study the incidence of both dengue and leptospirosis in Vietnam. Finally, penicilliosis has become an extremely important regional cause of death among immunocompromised HIV-infected individuals. CDC and other groups are working with Vietnamese collaborators to better understand the epidemiology and treatment options of this disease. CDC also maintains field stations in Thailand and Côte d'Ivoire, where investigations focus primarily on HIV, and in Botswana, where investigations are centered on tuberculosis.

During a recent visit to India, Secretary of Health and Human Services Donna Shalala signed an agreement to work collaboratively with Indian public health officials to address emerging infectious disease. The lead agency for the United States is CDC; for India it is the National Institute for Communicable Diseases. Discussions are now under way to explore areas of potential collaborations. These talks focus on dengue and dengue hemorrhagic fever, Japanese encephalitis, HIV and AIDS prevention, tuberculosis prevention and control, and control of sexually transmitted diseases. Training and personnel exchanges are likely to be discussed. Extensive work is now in progress to evaluate a newly developed vaccine for rotaviruses discovered through collaborative studies involving scientists from the All India Institute of Medical Sciences and CDC. The vaccine has been tested for safety and immunogenicity in adult volunteers in the United States and will be analyzed in India. Depending upon the outcome of these trials, the vaccine will be evaluated in infants for its suitability to protect against rotavirus diarrhea (1).

The United States Department of Defense (DOD) maintains a network of overseas medical research facilities where military and civilian experts investigate endemic diseases. In 1997 CDC embarked upon a new collaboration with Naval Medical Research Unit 3 in Cairo, Egypt, by assigning a medical epidemiologist to the laboratory. This scientist is working closely with the staff of the Navy laboratory, the Egyptian Ministry of Health, the Eastern Mediterranean Regional Office of WHO, and the Egyptian Field Epidemiology Training Program to systematically investigate new, emerging, and re-emerging infectious diseases. Initial reports are quite promising, and it is possible that similar secondments may be considered to other DOD laboratories.

## SPECIFIC CHALLENGES

The growing threat of antimicrobial resistance is of major concern and is included in nearly all international activities. As mentioned, this topic is a key component of ongoing work with the E.U., Russia, Kenya, South Africa, and others. One noteworthy effort involves the work of CDC in providing quality control and proficiency testing services to the network of WHO collaborating laboratories being developed to monitor antibiotic resistance patterns globally. At present, CDC scientists coordinate proficiency testing for laboratories that contribute results to WHO to monitor patterns of resistance. This information helps to ensure the quality of the data obtained and to identify collaborating facilities in need of technical assistance. This effort will grow in importance as WHO expands its program in monitoring antimicrobial resistance.

Influenza is one of the most important emerging infectious diseases. The virus is transmitted globally among humans and has reservoir hosts in avian populations, pigs, and other animals. Each year new strains or variants emerge, necessitating modification of the vaccines used to protect human health. In order to determine the most important influenza viruses in circulation, WHO has developed a network of over 100 collaborating laboratories that systematically isolate locally circulating influenza viruses, make preliminary characterization of these isolates, and send representative samples to one of four WHO reference centers for influenza located in Australia, Japan, England, or CDC. These isolates are then further characterized antigenically and genetically, and this information is shared during an annual meeting in Geneva. The meeting objectives are to review global surveillance data, determine the optimum composition for the following year's vaccine, and provide official WHO recommendations for influenza vaccine composition to vaccine manufacturers worldwide.

In addition to serving as one of the primary reference centers for characterization of circulating influenza viruses, CDC in recent years has assisted WHO in expanding the network of collaborating laboratories by providing funding and training opportunities, especially in southern China, where many new influenza viruses may originate. CDC also works collaboratively with WHO in addressing outbreaks of influenza virus, as occurred during the recent outbreak of H5N1 influenza A virus in Hong Kong (3).

One of the largest challenges facing CDC and its global partners in addressing emerging diseases is the lack of well-trained personnel needed to conduct the surveillance, response, and laboratory investigations. In order to begin to build the necessary international capacity, CDC and the Association of State and Territorial Public Health Laboratory Directors have developed a new program dedicated to training scientists through 1- or 2-year fellowships in laboratory sciences. Similar to the established Epidemic Intelligence Service program, Emerging Infectious Diseases Laboratory Fellows are encouraged to work on the front lines of emerging diseases, becoming involved in outbreak investigations and formally setting forth their results through presentations and publications. The 1997–1998 class has 20 fellows; for the first time, the entering 1998–1999 class will include three non-U.S. citizens.

## CONCLUSIONS

The four basic goals originally defined in the CDC plan to address emerging infectious diseases have been embraced both nationally and globally. This convergence of thinking by world leaders in health offers a tremendous opportunity for meaningful international collaboration in addressing the global challenges of emerging infectious diseases. The transition from plan development to implementation has begun, with many focused activities and the promise for additional future collaborations.

### REFERENCES

1. **Bhan, M. K., J. F. Lew, S. Sazawal, et al.** 1993. Protection conferred by neonatal rotavirus infection against subsequent diarrhea. *J. Infect. Dis.* **163:**282–287.
2. **Centers for Disease Control and Prevention.** 1994. *Addressing Emerging Infectious Disease Threats: A Prevention Strategy for the United States.* U.S. Department of Health and Human Services, Public Health Service, Atlanta, Ga.
3. **Fukuda, K.** 1998. Summary of epidemiological studies on influenza A(H5N1) cases in Hong Kong, p. 5. *In International Conference on Emerging Infectious Diseases, Program Addendum.*

4. **Gore, A.** 1996. Emerging infections threaten national and global security. *ASM News* **62:**448–449.
5. **Gubler, D., and G. G. Clark.** 1995. Dengue/dengue hemorrhagic fever: the emergence of a global health problem. *Emerg. Infect. Dis.* **1:**55–57.
6. **Herwaldt, B. L., M. L. Ackers, and the Cyclospora Working Group.** 1997. An outbreak in 1996 of cyclosporiasis associated with imported raspberries. *N. Engl. J. Med.* **336:**1548–1556.
7. **Institute of Medicine.** 1992. *Emerging Infections: Microbial Threats to Health in the United States.* Institute of Medicine, Washington, D.C.
8. **Killalea, D., L. R. Ward, and D. Roberts, et al.** 1996. International epidemiological and microbiological study of outbreak of *Salmonella agona* infection from a ready to eat savoury snack—I: England and Wales and the United States. *Br. Med. J.* **313:**1105–1107.
9. **Mons, B., E. Klasen, R. van Kessel, and T. Nchinda.** 1998. Partnership between South and North crystallizes around malaria. *Science* **279:**498–499.
10. **National Academy of Sciences.** 1997. *Controlling Dangerous Pathogens. A Blueprint for U.S.-Russian Cooperation.* National Academy of Sciences, Washington, D.C.
11. **National Science and Technology Council.** 1995. *Report of the NSTC Committee on International Science, Engineering, and Technology (CISET) Working Group on Emerging and Re-emerging Infectious Diseases.* Executive Office of the President of the United States, Washington, D.C.
12. **Pan American Health Organization.** 1995. *Regional Plan of Action for Combatting New, Emerging, and Re-emerging Infectious Diseases in the Americas. PAHO/HCP/HCT/95.060.* Pan American Health Organization, Washington, D.C.
13. **Pan American Health Organization.** 1996. *Final Report: Workshop To Define Priorities of Institutional Strengthening for the Diagnosis and Epidemiological Surveillance of Emerging Diseases. PAHO/HCT/96.078.* Pan American Health Organization, Washington, D.C.
14. **Pan American Health Organization.** 1997. *Meeting of the Task Force on Surveillance for Emerging and Reemerging Infectious Diseases. PAHO/HCT/97.01.* Pan American Health Organization, Washington, D.C.
15. **Pan American Health Organization.** 1998. *Meeting to Establish a Network of Laboratories for the Surveillance of Emerging Infectious Diseases (EID) in the Amazon Region. PAHO/HCP/HCT/106/98.* Pan American Health Organization, Washington, D.C.
16. **Perkins, B. A., J. M. Flood, R. Danila, et al.** 1996. Unexplained deaths due to possibly infectious causes in the United States: Defining the problem and designing surveillance and laboratory approaches. *Emerg. Infect. Dis.* **2:**47–53.
17. **Sanders, E. S., P. Borus, G. Ademba, G. Kuria, P. M. Tukei, and J. W. LeDuc.** 1996. Sentinel surveillance for yellow fever in Kenya, 1993 to 1995. *Emerg. Infect. Dis.* **2:**236–238.
18. **Shohat, T., M. S. Green, D. Merom, et al.** 1996. International epidemiological and microbiological study of outbreak of *Salmonella agona* infection from a ready to eat savoury snack—II: Israel. *Br. Med. J.* **313:**1107–1109.
19. **U.S. Environmental Protection Agency, U.S. Department of Health and Human Services, and U.S. Department of Agriculture.** 1997. *Food Safety, from Farm to Table. A National Food-Safety Initiative. A Report to the President.* U.S. Environmental Protection Agency, U.S. Department of Health and Human Services, and U.S. Department of Agriculture, Washington, D.C.
20. **World Health Organization.** 1995. *World Health Assembly Resolution, WHA48.7. Revision and Updating of the International Health Regulation.* World Health Organization, Geneva, Switzerland.
21. **World Health Organization.** 1995. *World Health Assembly Resolution, WHA48.13. Communicable Diseases Prevention and Control: New, Emerging and Re-emerging Infectious Diseases.* World Health Organization, Geneva, Switzerland.
22. **World Health Organization, Hemorrhagic Fever Commission.** 1998. Rift Valley fever: East Africa 1997-8, p. 6. *International Conference on Emerging Infectious Diseases, Program Addendum.*

# INDEX